From Bioimaging to Biosensors

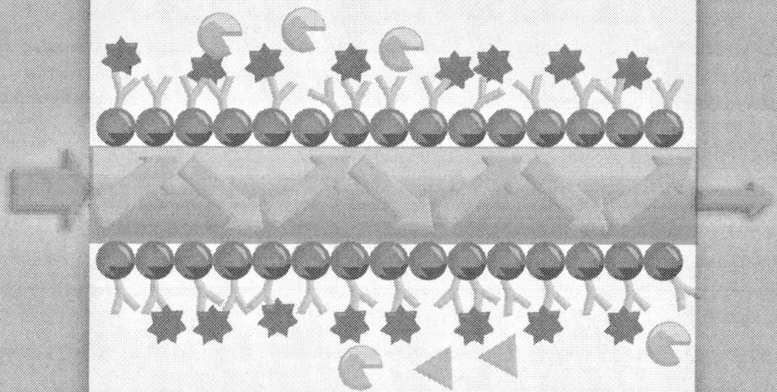

From Bioimaging to Biosensors

Noble Metal Nanoparticles in Biodetection

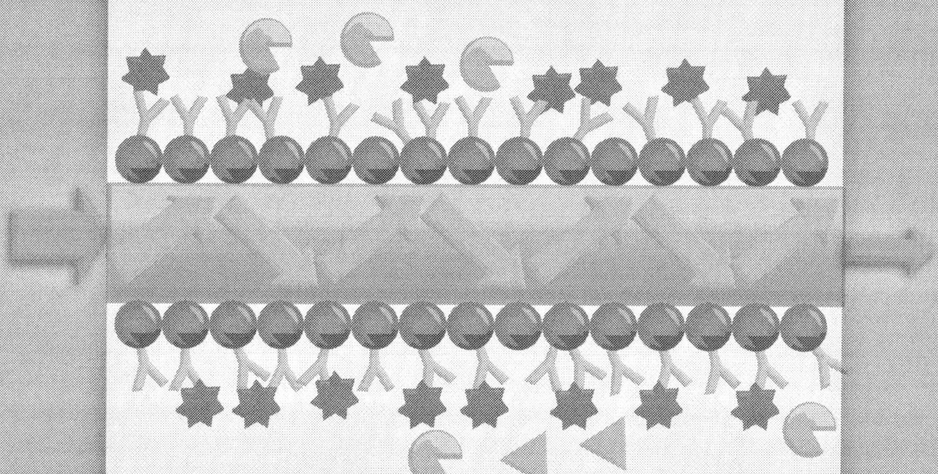

Edited by
Lai-Kwan Chau
Huan-Tsung Chang

Pan Stanford Publishing

Published by

Pan Stanford Publishing Pte. Ltd.
Penthouse Level, Suntec Tower 3
8 Temasek Boulevard
Singapore 038988

Email: editorial@panstanford.com
Web: www.panstanford.com

British Library Cataloguing-in-Publication Data
A catalogue record for this book is available from the British Library.

From Bioimaging to Biosensors: Noble Metal Nanoparticles in Biodetection

ISBN 978-981-4267-24-3 (Hardcover)
ISBN 978-981-4303-10-1 (eBook)

Printed in the USA

Contents

Preface xi

1. Synthesis and Optical Properties of Noble Metal Nanoparticles for Biodetection **1**

Hsing-Ying Lin, Ping-Ji Huang, Chen-Han Huang, Yen-Chieh Wang, and Churng-Ren Chris Wang

1.1 Gold Nanoparticles and Their Biomedical Applications 2

1.2 Synthesis of Gold Nanoparticles 3

1.3 Optical Properties of Noble Metal Nanoparticles 4

1.3.1 Fluorescing Noble Metal Clusters 4

1.3.2 Absorption Spectral Characteristics of Noble Metal Nanorods 5

1.3.3 Scattering Spectra of Noble Metal Nanorods 7

2. Bioconjugation of Noble Metal Nanoparticles and Their Applications to Biolabeling and Bioimaging **11**

Chen-Sheng Yeh, Fong-Yu Cheng, and Chih-Chia Huang

2.1 Introduction 11

2.2 Bioconjugation of Noble Metal Nanoparticles 14

2.2.1 DNA Conjugation 15

2.2.2 Protein, Peptide, and Antibody Conjugation 16

2.2.3 Other Biomolecule Conjugation Methods 18

2.3 Applications of Noble Metal Nanoparticles to Biolabeling and Bioimaging 19

2.3.1 X-Ray Computed Tomography 19

2.3.2 Magnetic Resonance Imaging 19

2.3.3 Optical Imaging 23

2.4 Conclusion and Outlook 24

3. Colorimetric Bioassay Using Noble Metal Nanoparticles **29**

Ming-Feng Huang, Yang-Wei Lin, and Huan-Tsung Chang

3.1 Introduction 30
3.2 Synthesis of Au and Ag NPs 31
3.2.1 Wet Chemical Approaches 32
3.2.2 Stabilization 33
3.2.3 Functionalization 35
3.3 Localized Surface Plasmon Resonance of Au and Ag NPs 37
3.4 Applications 39
3.4.1 Crosslinking Aggregation-Based Assays 39
3.4.1.1 Protein assays 40
3.4.1.2 DNA and RNA assays 43
3.4.1.3 Small analyte assays 45
3.4.2 Non-Crosslinking Aggregation-Based Assays 46
3.4.2.1 DNA assays 47
3.4.2.2 Protein and small analyte assays 48
3.5 Summary 51

4. Slide- and Micoarray-Based Biosensors Using Noble Metal Nanoparticles **57**

Ping-Ji Huang and Lai-Kwan Chau

4.1 Introduction 58
4.2 Localized Surface Plasmon Resonance 60
4.3 Slide-Based LSPR Biosensors 61
4.4 Microarray-Based LSPR Biosensors 70
4.5 Conclusions and Outlook 72

5. Optical Waveguide-Based Biosensors Using Noble Metal Nanoparticles **77**

Lai-Kwan Chau, Chang-Yue Chiang, Wei-Ting Hsu, Shin-Huei Chen, and Shu-Fang Cheng

5.1 Introduction 77
5.2 Principle of the Biosensors 80
5.3 Optical Fiber-Based PPR Biosensor 86

5.4 Planar Waveguide-Based PPR Biosensor 93
5.5 Tubular Waveguide-Based PPR Biosensor 96
5.6 Conclusions and Outlook 98

6. Fabrication of Biosensor Chips 103

Wei Te Wu, Guo-Hua Feng, and Wen Hsin Hsieh

6.1 Photolithography Process 103
6.1.1 Substrate Cleaning 105
6.1.2 Photoresist Selection and Application 107
6.1.3 Photomask Design/Fabrication and Alignment 108
6.1.4 Photoresist Exposure and Development 110
6.2 Soft Lithography 111
6.2.1 Lithography: Deep UV Lithography 112
6.2.2 Electrodeposition: Electroplating 114
6.2.3 Micro Molding: Hot-Embossing and Micro-Injection 116
6.2.4 Bonding 118
6.3 Fabrication of Diffraction Gratings 119
6.3.1 Diamond Ruling 120
6.3.2 Gray-Scale Lithography 120
6.3.3 Holographic Exposure 122
6.3.4 Electron-Beam Direct Writing 123
6.3.5 Nanoimprint Lithography 124
6.4 Manufacture of Optical Fiber Windows 124
6.4.1 Etching Method 127
6.4.2 Polishing Method 128
6.4.3 Ultrashort High-Energy Pulse Laser Processing Method 129
6.5 Conclusions and Outlook 131

7. Microfluidics for Biosensor Chips 135

Shau-Chun Wang

7.1 Introduction 136
7.2 Fabrication of Microfluidic Devices 137
7.3 Particle Plasmon Resonance Detection in Microfluidic Devices Using Noble Metal Nanoparticles 139

7.3.1 Microfluidic Devices to Facilitate PPR Detection 140

7.3.2 Microfluidic Mixer to Improve PPR Detection 142

7.4 Integration of Biosensing Systems Using Noble Metal Nanoparticles with Mass Spectrometer 143

7.5 Fluorescence Spectroscopic Detectionin Microfluidic Devices Using Noble Metal Nanoparticles 146

7.5.1 Applying Gold Nanoparticles as Quenching Acceptors to Förster Resonance Energy Transfer (FRET) Detections 146

7.5.2 Using Silver Nanoparticles in Surface Plasmon Coupled Fluorescence Detection 148

7.5.3 Immobilizing a Catalytic DNA Molecular Beacon on Au Nanoparticle to Detect Pb(II) Species 150

7.6 Other Detection Techniques in Microfluidic Devices Using Noble Metal Nanoparticles 150

7.6.1 Microfluidic Devices to Facilitate Surface-Enhanced Raman Scattering Detections 150

7.6.2 Microfluidic Devices to Facilitate Thermal Lens Detections 151

7.7 Conclusion 152

8. Biodetection Based on Resonance Light Scattering of Noble Metal Nanoparticles 157

Tai-Chia Chiu and Cho-Chun Hu

8.1 Introduction 158

8.2 Basic Theory of RLS 159

8.2.1 RLS of Plasmonic NPs 160

8.3 Applications of NP-Based RLS Techniques 161

8.3.1 Au NPs as RLS Probes 162

8.3.1.1 Small analytes 162

8.3.1.2 Proteins 168

8.3.1.3 DNA 171

8.3.2 Ag NPs as RLS Probes 174

8.3.2.1 Small analytes 174
8.3.2.2 Biopolymers 175
8.4 Conclusions and Outlook 176

9. Photoluminescence of Gold Nanoparticles and Their Applications to Sensing and Cell Imaging 181

Chih-Ching Huang and Yu-Shen Lin

9.1 Introduction 182
9.2 Preparation and Optical Properties of Polymer-Stabilized Au NCs 184
9.3 Preparation and Optical Properties of Thiol-Stabilized Au NCs 188
9.4 Preparation and Optical Properties of Luminescent Au NPs 194
9.5 Applications 199
9.6 Conclusion 205

10. Biodetection Based on Fluorescence Quenching and Surface-Enhanced Fluorescence Using Noble Metal Nanoparticles 211

Yang-Wei Lin, Chi-Wei Liu, and Huan-Tsung Chang

10.1 Introduction 212
10.2 Theory 214
10.2.1 Fluorescence Quenching 218
10.2.2 SEF 221
10.2.2.1 Surface plasmons 221
10.2.2.2 Localized enhancements 226
10.3 Analytical Applications 230
10.3.1 Protein Immunoassays 230
10.3.2 DNA Analysis 235
10.3.3 Other Applications 239
10.4 Conclusions and Outlook 242

11. Surface-Enhanced Raman Scattering Based on Noble Metal Nanoparticles 249

Li-Lin Tay and John E. Hulse

11.1 Introduction 250
11.1.1 Electromagnetic Enhancement Mechanism 251
11.1.2 Consequences of Electromagnetic Enhancement 253

11.1.3 Chemical Enhancement 256
11.1.4 SERS Bioanalytical Applications 257
11.2 NAEB: A Novel SERS-Active Nanoparticle Assemblies 259
11.3 SERS-Based Bioimaging with Multifunctional Nanoparticles 262
11.4 Summary and Outlook 265

12. Mass Spectrometric Bioanalysis Assisted by Noble Metal Nanoparticles **271**

Yen-Hsiu Lin and Wei-Lung Tseng

12.1 Introduction 272
12.2 Nanomaterials in LDI-MS 272
12.2.1 Gold 275
12.2.2 Silver and Platinum 279
12.3 Nanomaterials in TOF-SIMS 281
12.4 Nanomaterials in ICP-MS 284
12.5 Conclusions 286

Index 291

Preface

Over the past two decades, there has been intense research on the development of biodetection techniques for the diagnosis of diseases and environmental analysis of biological agents. Thanks to the recent development in nanotechnology, research has begun to explore new bioimaging and biosensing strategies based on these nanomaterials. One promising approach is to utilize the extraordinary optical properties of noble metal nanoparticles. The absorption and scattering cross sections of noble metal nanoparticles are orders of magnitude stronger than that of organic dyes. Thus, these nanoparticles act as excellent sensors and novel contrast agents for optical detection due to their enhanced absorption and scattering, respectively. Moreover, the localized surface plasmon resonance property of these nanoparticles makes label-free and real-time biodetection possible. This book discusses the fundamental principles of bioimaging and biosensing based on noble metal nanoparticles, reviews auxiliary technologies such as bioconjugation, microfabrication, and microfluidics, provides an account of recent development, and illustrates, with examples, their applications. These reviews include perspectives from analytical chemistry, physical chemistry, materials science, biochemistry, microfluidics, and engineering.

The book starts with a review on the synthesis, characterization, optical properties, and bioconjugation of noble metal nanoparticles, followed by the introduction of various biodetection techniques based on noble metal nanoparticles. In between these topics, microfabrication of biosensing chips and the use of microfluidics to enhance biosensing performance are discussed. The text is intended to provide valuable background for researchers in nanotechnology, chemistry, biology, biomedical engineering, and medicine, especially those with an interest in bioimaging, biosensor, or mass spectrometric bioanalysis.

Lai-Kwan Chau
Huan-Tsung Chang

Chapter 1

Synthesis and Optical Properties of Noble Metal Nanoparticles for Biodetection

Hsing-Ying Lin,[b] Ping-Ji Huang,[a] Chen-Han Huang,[b] Yen-Chieh Wang,[a] and Churng-Ren Chris Wang[a,b,*]

[a]Department of Chemistry and Biochemistry and [b]Center for Nano Bio-Detection, National Chung Cheng University, 168 University Road, Min-Hsiung, Chia-Yi 621, Taiwan

[*]checrw@ccu.edu.tw

The noble metal nanoparticles, mainly in gold related nanostructures, have been recognized widely in various biodetections. We briefly review the synthesis for such nanoparticle systems and provide several model predictions for their optical properties. The surface plasmon associated spectral behaviors for several chosen elements were simulated via classical electrostatic model. The surface plasmon-related absorption and scattering spectra are well known to be strongly dependent on the size, shape, composition, and surrounding medium of nanoparticles. We focus on providing such spectral information for rod-like metal nanoparticles. In addition, absorption spectra are presented in both overall and deconvoluted forms. The later consists of spectra of both longitudinal and transverse surface plasmon modes.

From Bioimaging to Biosensors: Noble Metal Nanoparticles in Biodetection
Edited by Lai-Kwan Chau and Huan-Tsung Chang

ISBN 978-981-4267-24-3 (Hardcover), 978-981-4303-10-1 (eBook)
www.panstanford.com

1.1 Gold Nanoparticles and Their Biomedical Applications

Noble metal, especially gold, nanoparticles have been used for various biomedical applications,[1–8] including as contrast agents for photoacoustic imaging.[9–11] One intriguing property of gold nanoparticles is that their absorption spectra are geometry dependent. The size effect on the surface plasmon absorption of spherical gold nanoparticles was reported to result in the red-shift of the spectral peak red shifting with increasing particle size, with gold nanospheres with diameters of tens of nanometers exhibiting an absorption peak at around 550 nm.[12] However, this misleading report was later realized that the size effects on such nanoparticles reflect in the absorption cross-sections only. The spectral shift in the experimental observation was mis-interpreted with the existence of the shape effect. In contrast, the resonance of peak absorption of gold nanorods depends only weakly on their diameter and overall dimension, with it instead shifting strongly to the longer wavelength with the aspect ratio (defined as the ratio of the length of the major axis to that of the minor axis).[13,14] Laser irradiation at the wavelength corresponding to the peak absorption results in the maximal absorption as well as the maximal photoacoustic signal.

Targeting gold nanoparticles to cancer cells helps in the early detection using photoacoustic imaging due to the large difference in the optical absorption between gold nanoparticles and the tissue.[5] In addition, targeting different cancer cells with bioconjugated gold nanorods having different aspect ratios can also be achieved.[11] The bioconjugated gold nanorods interact with cells that have antigens specific to the conjugated antibody, and hence the cells that bind the bioconjugated gold nanorods can be detected using photoacoustic techniques. Multiple targeting using gold nanorods with different aspect ratios was tested experimentally to demonstrate the feasibility of measuring the expression levels of different oncogenes of cancer cells simultaneously.

In this chapter, we discuss the synthetic schemes developed for various types of dispersed gold nanostructures in aqueous solutions and three different optical properties of noble metal nanoparticles, which are widely adopted in the area of biodetection. In the content for such optical behaviors, we emphasize on the simulated absorption and scattering spectra based on the classical Mie/Drude formalism for 16 chosen metal nanorods. The predictions are expected not only to clearly portrait the material-dependent spectral behaviors, but also to facilitate the material design for future applications of the noble metal nanoparticles.

1.2 Synthesis of Gold Nanoparticles

The development in nanosynthesis of nearly monodispersed gold nanocrystals with controlled sizes and shapes is vital for both fundamental science and their applications. The preparation of dispersed gold nanoparticles in aqueous solution described by Faraday[15] is so far the first well-documented method. Since then, synthesis of other types of noble metal nanocrystals[16–21] and, lately, growth of size- and shape-controlled gold nanocrystals through electrochemical method[13,14,22] and seeded growth[23–25] have also been developed in aqueous solution.

We then focus on the preparation methodologies of gold nanoparticles for the use of biomedical applications, ranging from immunoassay rapid test technology, biomolecular sensing to recent simultaneous cancer diagnosis and therapy. The gold nanostructures aiming for the above applications cover from spherical particles to nanoshells and nanorods.

Synthesis of nearly monodispersed gold nanoparticles in aqueous by the use of standard citrate reduction (SCR) method is probably the most well-known bottom-up wet chemical approach. Its historical development first by Turkevich *et al.*[26] in 1951, and later by Frens[27] in 1973, has been widely recognized. The ingredients and their functions associated with this method have been clearly described and re-investigated recently.[28]

The synthesis of gold nanorods was first demonstrated by using the co-surfactant system under an electrochemical method.[13,14] Thus, the prepared nanorods suspended in an aqueous solution were synthesized inside an electrochemical cell and were stabilized by the cationic co-surfactant capping molecules. Such co-surfactant system is composed of tetradodecylammonium bromide and hexadecyltrimethylammonium bromide. The aspect ratios of gold nanorods can be finely controlled; subsequently the resulting peak absorption of their surface plasmon resonance can be precisely tuned.

A seed-mediated growth method was later developed for several types of gold nanostructures, such as nanorods[23,25] and nanoshells. Gold nanoshells, consisting of a dielectric core with a gold shell of nanometer thickness, were reported by a preparation scheme applying the similar seed-mediated growth method to the coating on a relatively large silica particle.[29] Later, the preparation of hollow gold nanoshells was demonstrated to be achieved through reacting aqueous $HAuCl_4$ solutions with solid templates such as silver nanoparticles.[30]

More recently, gold nanocages were first synthesized by the use of a polymer-assisted followed by a galvanic replacement reaction between solutions containing gold precursor salts and silver nanostructures prepared through polyol reduction.[31]

1.3 Optical Properties of Noble Metal Nanoparticles

The interaction of light with small metal nanoparticles has been of great interest for many years. The visible colors of a few kinds of noble metal nanoparticles are due to the resonant excitation of a collective oscillation of the conduction electrons in the particles termed surface plasmons. The plasmon-related optical properties of metal nanoparticles strongly depend on the size,[32] shape,[33] composition, and surrounding medium of nanoparticles.[34] In this section, typical optical characteristics of noble metal nanoparticles, such as fluorescing, absorption, and scattering are summarized, respectively. The main focus is to present the absorption and scattering spectra for rod-like metal nanoparticles dispersed in water. To further illustrate the transverse and longitudinal components in the associated spectra, the overall absorption spectra were deconvoluted to further reflect the material-dependent trend.

1.3.1 Fluorescing Noble Metal Clusters

The fluorescence of metal clusters and thin films is well established based on the observation of photoluminescence from bulk copper and gold,[35] and on the photoinduced luminescence from noble metals.[36] For example, the photoinduced fluorescence from Ag_3 clusters was observed to center around 500 nm.[37] Silver nanoparticles in water were found to have a fluorescence peak at 465 nm.[38] Embedded silver nanodots were also observed to fluoresce.[39,40] Most of the observed fluorescence was attributed to the radiative recombination of an electron–hole pair between *d* band and *sp*-conduction band above the Fermi level. Due to the plasmon resonance excitation, the local field created around the nanoparticles is found to modify the observed fluorescence.[41]

When the size regime falls into less than ca. 2 nm, gold nanoparticles exhibit the fluorescence property. This unique behavior is believed to be attributed to their sizes becoming comparable to the Fermi wavelength of the electron (ca. 0.7 nm). The quantum size effect occurs and results in molecule-like properties of discrete electronic states and size-dependent fluorescence.[42,43] The photoluminescent properties are attributed to the recombination involving *d*-band excitation.[44] While gold nanoparticles having larger sizes show a size-dependent plasmon absorption band with their free electrons in both the ground and excited states confined to dimensions smaller than their mean free path, ca. 20 nm.

1.3.2 Absorption Spectral Characteristics of Noble Metal Nanorods

Under the limit of classical electrostatic model, the absorption spectra of spherical metal nanoparticles for several tens metal elements have been described previously.[45] The material-dependent optical properties in the range of 200–900 nm can be clearly described. Based on the same classical formalism, we present, in the following two sections, both the absorption and scattering spectra for 16 chosen metal nanorods dispersed in the surround medium of water by the use of classical electrostatic simulation model described previously.[13,22,46–48] Elements of Na, Ti, Mn, Re, Ni, Pd, Pt, Fe, Cu, Ag, Au, Os, Al, Ga, Co, and Rh were selected to portrait the relative individual and group spectral behaviors. The spectra are presented in the wavelength range of 150–1200 nm. Metal nanorods exhibit two surface plasmon components in their absorption and scattering spectra: longitudinal and transverse modes. Depending on the type of material, their relative intensities vary. But, quite similarly, the peak positions of surface plasmon transverse band shift to shorter wavelength, while those of the longitudinal band red-shift as the particle aspect ratios increase.[13,14,49]

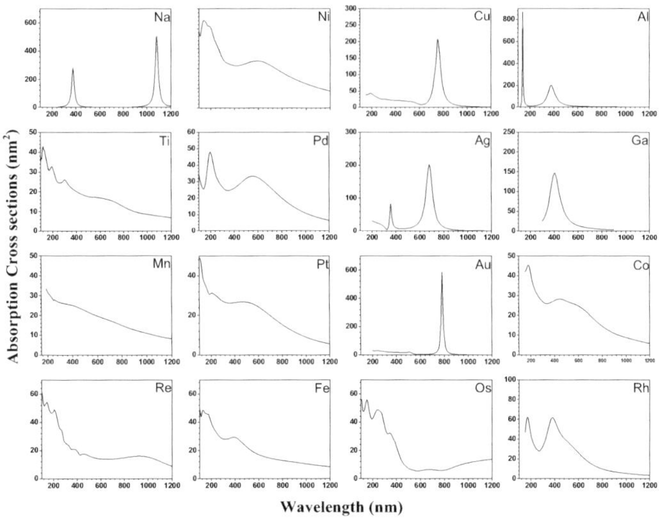

Figure 1.1 Simulated absorption spectra of metallic nanorods. The calculation was based on the classical electrostatic model for prolate nanoparticles with 50 nm in length and 20 nm in diameter.

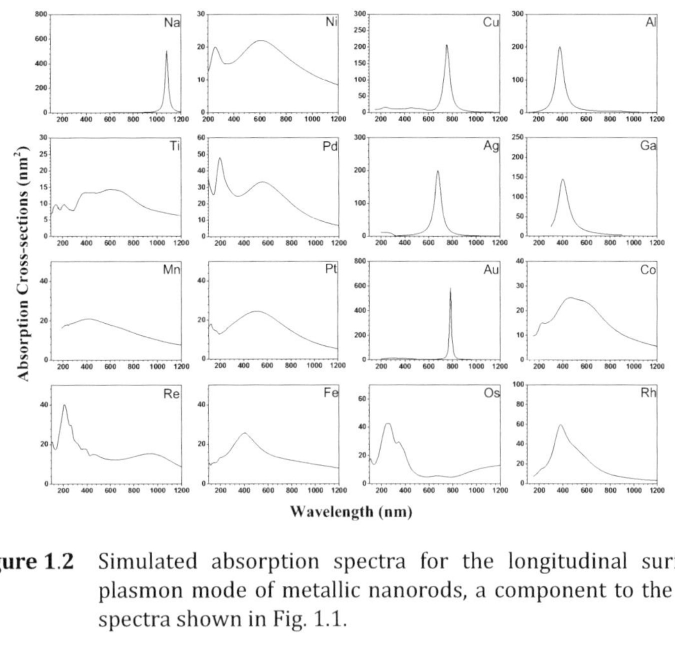

Figure 1.2 Simulated absorption spectra for the longitudinal surface plasmon mode of metallic nanorods, a component to the full spectra shown in Fig. 1.1.

In this section, we present the model predictions for the overall absorption spectra of different metal nanorods with 50 nm in length and 20 nm in diameter (see Fig. 1.1). The calculations were conducted including size correction for the effective mean free path of free electrons. It gives better descriptions to the experimental observations. In terms of the clearly resolved characteristic surface plasmon bands for longitudinal and transverse modes, we found no particular trend by considering the free electron density. Well-resolved surface plasmon bands were observed in the cases of Na, Cu, Ag, Au, Al, and Ga. In addition, absorption spectra for either longitudinal or transverse mode are given in Fig. 1.2 and Fig. 1.3, respectively.

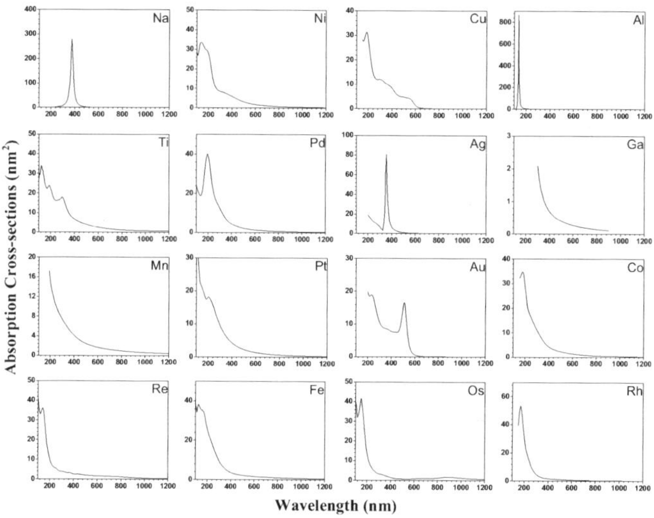

Figure 1.3 Simulated absorption spectra for the transverse surface plasmon mode of metallic nanorods, a component to the full spectra shown in Fig. 1.1.

1.3.3 Scattering Spectra of Noble Metal Nanorods

In the model descriptions, the definitions and originalities for the surface plasmon associated absorption and scattering are different. Basically, the imaginary part of the mean polarizability contributes to the dipole absorption while square of the mean polarizability is responsible for the scattering.[13,46] The results mainly confirm the dominating role of the surface plasmon to both spectra. Peak positions in both absorption and scattering spectra are identical, at least within the resolution limit of simulation, for both longitudinal and transverse bands. By comparing Fig. 1.4 with Fig. 1.1, one can easily notice that the overall spectral appearances in scattering spectra are somewhat different from those obtained in the absorption spectra. The scattering shows relatively much higher intensities in shorter wavelength region due to its characteristic frequency dependence.

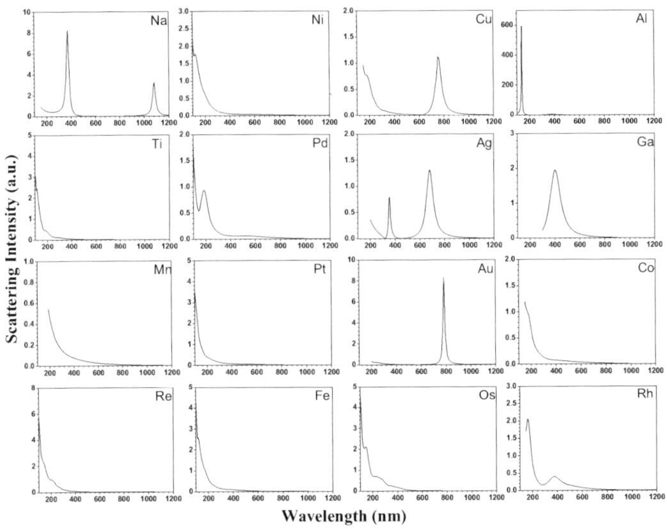

Figure 1.4 Simulated scattering spectra of metallic nanorods. The calculation was based on the classical electrostatic model for prolate nanoparticles with 50 nm in length and 20 nm in diameter.

Acknowledgment

The authors gratefully acknowledge the financial support from the National Science Council of Taiwan in the past years.

References

1. C. M. Niemeyer, *Angew. Chem. Int. Ed.*, **40**, 4128 (2001).
2. A. P. Alivisatos, K. P. Johnsson, X. Peng, T. E. Wilson, C. J. Loweth, M. P. B. Jr., and P. G. Schultz, *Nature*, **382**, 609 (1996).
3. A. K. Boal, F. Ilhan, J. E. DeRouchey, T. Thurn-Albrecht, T. P. Russell, and V. M. Rotello, *Nature*, **404**, 746 (2000).

4. M. A. Hayat, *Colloid Gold: Principles, Methods and Applications* (Academic Press, New York, (1989).
5. J. Kreuter, *Microcapsules and Nanoparticles in Medicine and Pharmacy* (CRC, Boca Raton, (1992).
6. C. C. Lin, Y. C. Yeh, C. Y. Yang, C. L. Chen, G. F. Chen, C. C. Chen, and Y. C. Wu, *J. Am. Chem. Soc.*, **124**, 3508 (2002).
7. C. A. Mirkin, R. L. Letsinger, R. C. Mucic, and J. J. Storhoff, *Nature*, **382**, 607 (1996).
8. T. A. Taton, C. A. Mirkin, and R. L. Letsinger, *Science*, **289**, 1757 (2000).
9. M. A. Eghtedari, J. A. Copland, V. L. Popov, N. A. Kotov, M. Motamedi, and A. A. Oraevsky, *Proc. of SPIE*, **4960**, 76 (2003).
10. P. C. Li, C. R. C. Wang, D. B. Shieh, C. W. Wei, C. K. Liao, C. Poe, S. J. Jhan, A. A. Ding, and Y. N. Wu, *Opt. Express*, **16**, 18605 (2008).
11. P. C. Li, C. W. Wei, C. K. Liao, C. D. Chen, K. C. Pao, C. R. C. Wang, Y. N. Wu, and D. B. Shieh, *IEEE Transactions on Ultrasonics Ferroelectrics and Frequency Control*, **54**, 1642 (2007).
12. S. Link and M. A. El-Sayed, *J. Phys. Chem. B*, **103**, 8410 (1999).
13. S. S. Chang, C. W. Shih, C. D. Chen, W. C. Lai, and C. R. C. Wang, *Langmuir*, **15**, 701 (1999).
14. Y. Y. Yu, S. S. Chang, C. L. Lee, and C. R. C. Wang, *J. Phys. Chem. B*, **101**, 6661 (1997).
15. M. Faraday, *Philos. Trans. R. Soc. London*, **147**, 145 (1857).
16. A. Henglein, *J. Phys. Chem. B*, **104**, 1206 (2000).
17. A. Henglein and M. Giersig, *J. Phys. Chem. B*, **103**, 9533 (1999).
18. A. Henglein and M. Giersig, *J. Phys. Chem. B*, **104**, 6767 (2000).
19. Z. S. Pillai and P. V. Kamat, *J. Phys. Chem. B*, **108**, 945 (2004).
20. T. H. M. Teranishi, T. Tanaka, and M. Miyake, *J. Phys. Chem. B*, **103**, 3818 (1999).
21. Y. C. H. Xiong, B. J. Wiley, J. Wang, M. J. Kim, and Y. Xia, *J. Am. Chem. Soc.*, **129**, 3665 (2007).
22. C.-W. Shih, W.-C. Lai, C.-C. Hwang, S.-S. Chang, and C. R. C. Wang, in *Metal Nanoparticles: Synthesis, Characterization, and Applications*, Eds. D. L. Feldheim and C. A. Foss (Marcel Dekker, Inc., New York, Basel, 2001), p. 163.
23. N. R. Jana, L. Gearheart, and C. J. Murphy, *J. Phys. Chem. B*, **105**, 4065 (2001).
24. C. J. Murphy and N. R. Jana, *Adv. Mater.*, **14**, 80 (2002).
25. B. Nikoobakht and E.-S. M. A., *Chem. Mater.*, **15**, 1957 (2003).

26. J. Turkevich, J. Hillier, and P. C. Stevenson, *Discuss. Faraday Soc.*, **11**, 55 (1951).
27. G. Frens, *Nature Phys. Sci.*, **241**, 20 (1973).
28. X. Xiaohui Ji, X. Song, J. Li, Y. Bai, W. Yang, and X. Peng, *J. Am. Chem. Soc.*, **129**, 13939 (2007).
29. S. J. Oldenburg, R. D. Averitt, S. L. Westcott, and N. J. Halas, *Chem. Phys., Lett.* **288**, 243 (1998).
30. Y. Sun and X. Y., *Anal. Chem.*, **74**, 5297 (2002).
31. J. Y. Chen, F. Saeki, B. J. Wiley, H. Cang, M. J. Cobb, Z.-Y. Li, L. Au, H. Zhang, M. B. Kimmey, X. D. Li, and Y. N. Xia, *Nano Lett.*, **5**, 473 (2005).
32. K. L. Kelly, E. Coronado, L. L. Zhao, and G. C. Schatz, *J. Phys. Chem. B*, **107**, 668 (2002).
33. I. O. Sosa, C. Noguez, and R. G. Barrera, *J. Phys. Chem. B*, **107**, 6269 (2003).
34. T. K. Sau, A. L. Rogach, F. Jackel, T. A. Klar, and J. Feldmann, *Adv. Mater.*, **22**, 1805 (2010).
35. A. Mooradian, *Phys. Rev. Lett.*, **22**, 185 (1969).
36. G. T. Boyd, Z. H. Yu, and Y. R. Shen, *Phys. Rev., B* **33**, 7923 (1986).
37. D. Ievlev, I. Rabin, W. Schulze, and G. Ertl, *Chem. Phys. Lett.*, **328**, 142 (2000).
38. Z. Jiang, W. Yuan, and H. Pan, *Spectrochim. Acta Part A: Mol. Biomol., Spectrosc.* **61**, 2488 (2005).
39. J. Zheng and R. M. Dickson, *J. Am. Chem. Soc.*, **124**, 13982 (2002).
40. Y. Dai, X. Hu, C. Wang, D. P. Chen, X. W. Jiang, C. S. Zhu, B. K. Yu, and J. R. Qiu, *Chem. Phys. Lett.*, **439**, 81 (2007).
41. S. Link and M. A. Ei-Sayed, *Annu. Rev. Phys. Chem.*, **54**, 331 (2003).
42. J. Zheng, P. R. Nicovich, and R. M. Dickson, *Annu. Rev. Phys. Chem.*, **58**, 409 (2007).
43. J. Zheng, C. Zhang, and R. M. Dickson, *Phys. Rev. Lett.*, **93**, 077402 (2004).
44. P. Apell, R. Monreal, and S. Lundqvist, *Phys. Scr.*, **38**, 174 (1988).
45. J. A. Creighton and D. G. Eadon, *J. Chem. Soc., Faraday Trans.*, **87**, 3881 (1991).
46. M. Kerker, *The Scattering of Light and Other Electromagnetic Radiation* (Academic Press, New York, 1969).
47. C. W. Kuo and C. R. C. Wang, *Curr. Nanosci.*, **6**, 619 (2010).
48. D.-S. Wang and M. Kerker, *Phys. Rev. B*, **24**, 1777 (1981).
49. B. M. I. vanderZande, M. R. Bohmer, L. G. J. Fokkink, and C. Schonenberger, *J. Phys. Chem. B*, **101**, 852 (1997).

Chapter 2

Bioconjugation of Noble Metal Nanoparticles and Their Applications to Biolabeling and Bioimaging

Chen-Sheng Yeh*, **Fong-Yu Cheng, and Chih-Chia Huang**

Department of Chemistry, National Cheng Kung University, Tainan, Taiwan
*csyeh@mail.ncku.edu.tw

Noble metal nanoparticles are attractive biolabeling and bioimaging materials in biomedicine because of their unique optical properties. The most important purpose of *in vitro* biolabeling and bioimaging is the selective and specific observation of interesting molecules, substrates, or regions. To reach these goals, bioconjugation of noble metal nanoparticles are used to create novel complexes with unique characteristics for targeting specific molecules. The applications of the bioconjugation of these nanoparticles depend on what substrates are conjugated on the particle surfaces and which functions are provided. This chapter describes the bioconjugation of noble metal nanoparticles and their biolabeling and bioimaging applications.

2.1 Introduction

Noble metal nanoparticles have gained interest in recent years because of their unique chemical and physical properties, and their

From Bioimaging to Biosensors: Noble Metal Nanoparticles in Biodetection
Edited by Lai-Kwan Chau and Huan-Tsung Chang

ISBN 978-981-4267-24-3 (Hardcover), 978-981-4303-10-1 (eBook)
www.panstanford.com

wide range of potential applications including surface plasmon resonance (SPR),[1] surface-enhanced Raman scattering (SERS),[2] biosensing,[3] and use in optoelectronic devices.[4] Noble metal nanoparticles exhibit a strong optical extinction wavelength due to localized surface plasmon resonance (LSPR) of their free electrons upon excitation by an electromagnetic field. Therefore, these nanoparticles are usually used as label markers and optical probes for molecular imaging.

Through appropriate surface modification, most noble nanoparticles exhibit high transportation property and prevent rapid blood clearance rendering tumor-specific targeting ability.[5,6] Noble metal nanoparticles undergo surface modification to exhibit better stability, good biocompatibility, lower cytotoxicity, better water solubility, and specific targeting. Cytotoxicity and biocompatibility are two important factors when using biolabeling and bioimaging probes of noble metal nanoparticles in live cells, organs, and bodies. They affect the retention time of the nanoparticles in live cells, organs, and bodies, and the sufficient tracking time for the detection of bioimages. For example, PEG-modified Au nanoparticles can increase the circulation time in blood compared to Au nanoparticles without any surface modification.[7] PEG provides the biocompatible property to reduce the uptake of live cells during blood circulation. The importance of specific targeting of nanoparticles is that biomolecule-conjugated noble metal nanoparticles can target the diseased region, e.g., tumors, and provide signals that are detected by optical instruments when applied to detect cancer cells. The accurate labels and images help us clearly diagnose pathological changes. To only observe a specific substrate in a complex system, biomolecule-conjugated nanoparticles with specific targeting ability can be used to target the goal substrate, and the nanoparticles can then be tracked using an optical system. All applications emphasize the importance of surface functionality of the nanomaterials, which if used to their advantage can successfully exploit the properties of the nanoparticles. As a result, the design of attaching molecules to nanoparticles is an important area of research. To enable promising biomedical applications of nanoparticles, the chemistry involved should be environmentally benign, specific, compatible in aqueous solution, lead to minimum side products, and be highly reproducible.

Bioconjugation of noble metal nanoparticles mainly takes place through covalent bonds and electrostatic interactions.[8–11] Common covalent bond-conjugation methods use metal-thiol bonds directly between noble metal nanomaterials and biomolecules or cross-link agents such as (1-ethyl-3-(3-dimethylaminopropyl) carbodiimide) (EDC), which links amine and carboxylic acid groups; 4-(*N*-Maleimidomethyl)cyclohexane-1-carboxylic acid 3-sulfo-*N*-hydroxysuccinimide ester (sulfo-SMCC), which links amine and thiol groups; and the azide-acetylene system.[12] For electrostatic interactions, the nanoparticles and biomolecules should be oppositely charged. The formation of covalent bonds is stronger compared to electrostatic interactions, and hence, the biomolecules are difficult to detach from the nanoparticle surface. In addition, electrostatic adsorption offers very little control over the orientation of bound molecules. Orientation and conformational changes in biomolecules during adsorption on nanoparticles can reduce their binding affinities and activities.[13] Non-specific conjugation sites (random conjugations) of biomolecules result in some problems, for example, the active sites of biomolecules may be blocked and the activities disappear. Generally, the activities of biomolecules are affected (increase or decrease) when their conformation produces some changes. Hence, it is important that the activities of biomolecules are kept after conjugation with noble metal nanoparticles and still show functional performance.

To achieve the *Great Aspiration* for reduction of death for cancer patients, a new approach in detecting cancer in the early stage is highly desired. Biomedical imaging provides contrast information to interest tissues and organs for analytic and diagnostic purpose. Therefore, it is requisite to develop helpful imaging methods to improve sensitivity and resolution of biological imaging. The time of data acquisition and financial cost are also required to consider for further biomedical development. Furthermore, different imaging techniques may provide complementary information in biological interpretation.

Since the 1950s, Au nanoparticles have been used as radioactive agents.[14] Additionally, Au nanoparticles conjugated to antibodies have been used for biological staining in electron microscopy since the 1980s.[15,16] Nanoparticles provide an opportunity to develop non-invasive methodologies as multifunctional diagnostic and therapeutic agents ranging from clinical diagnosis to cellular biology and drug discovery. It is well known that Au nanoparticles possess unique size- and shape-dependent physical and chemical properties.[16–18] Very recently, gold quantum dots (QDs) were found to exhibit molecule-like properties and were used as a fluorescent probe.[19,20] Research on nonlinear optical imaging in live cells and implanted tumors has been carried out using metal nanomaterials (nanoparticles, nanorods, and nanoshells) as a contrast tools. Metallic nanoparticles also exhibit unique surface plasmon behavior[16] and are used as unique optical probes for colorimetric sensing[21] and reflection imaging[18] as well as used in ultrasensitive SERS detection in bioimaging.[22,23] Chapters 3, 9, and 11 discuss biodetection based on colorimetry, photoluminescence, and SERS of noble metal nanoparticles, respectively.

Considerable effort has been devoted to fabricating noble nanoparticle-based contrast agents to improve local contrast enhancement.[4] Medical imaging diagnostics include magnetic resonance imaging (MRI), positron emission tomography (PET), CT, ultrasound, and optical imaging. Optical imaging methods (absorption, scattering, and fluorescence), however, display better sensitivity but suffer from low tissue penetration depths. Metal nanoagents with light absorption, scattering, and emission in the near-infrared window of 700–900 nm are particularly powerful at large penetration depths of light irradiation in most biological media and living tissues. Moreover, noble metal nanomaterials with various shapes, such as gold nanorods, nanoshells, and nanocages, provide a variety of bioimaging contrast agents.[16–18,24,25]

2.2 Bioconjugation of Noble Metal Nanoparticles

Recent advances in the biomolecular modification[26] of noble metal nanoparticles have led to widespread interest in their properties and applications.[27] Many biomolecules have been successfully conjugated on the surface of noble metal nanoparticles for biosensors,[28] SERS,[29] X-ray contrast agents,[30] and two-photon luminescence (TPL) imaging.[31] In these cases the bioconjugation of noble metal nanoparticles play an important role for their specific applications.

2.2.1 DNA Conjugation

Noble metal nanoparticle-DNA conjugates, especially Au nanoparticle-DNA conjugates, have been utilized in many applications, including hybridization sensing,[32] self-assembly,[33] and delivery.[34] Covalent attachment of DNA to noble metal nanoparticles is straightforward and generally accomplished by thiol linkers.[35] The DNA are usually modified at the terminal base with thiol groups, and the thiol groups can directly react with the nanoparticles and to form covalent Au-S bonds (Fig. 2.1). The length of DNA can affect the conjugated numbers on the particle surface. The density of the conjugated DNA numbers also affects the stability in solvents. The DNA-conjugated noble metal nanoparticles can be stable in aqueous solution under higher salt concentrations as the conjugated DNA helps them resist salt effects.

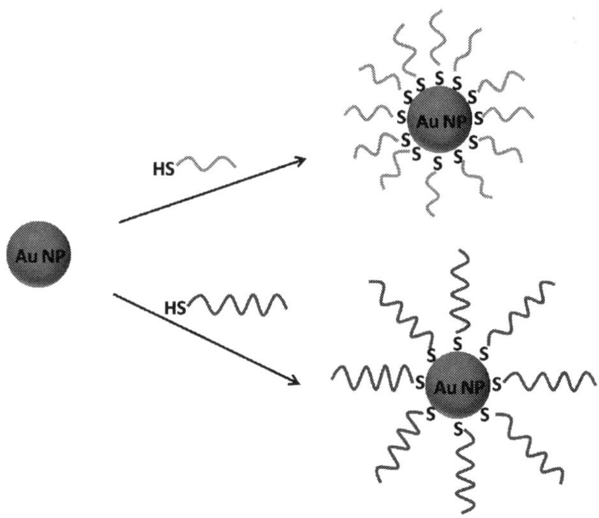

Figure 2.1 Conjugation of Au nanoparticles with thiol-modified DNA. Short DNA and long DNA affect the conjugated numbers on the nanoparticle surface.

Oligonucleotide-conjugated noble metal nanoparticles can hybridize with complementary oligonucleotide. This idea is used to design DNA detection assays. For example, light scattering techniques are employed to demonstrate the specific binding to specific DNA (Fig. 2.2). This scenario is that the DNA-conjugated

Au nanoparticles specifically and selectively recognize DNA targets of interest. Subsequently, the targeted DNAs produce signals (light scattering) detected by optical measurement. The colors observed from the light scattering of noble metal nanoparticles depend on their compositions, shapes, and diameters.[36] If DNAs are conjugated with different noble metal nanomaterials, DNA-conjugated particles can detect many different DNAs of interest at the same time because of the different colors originating from distinct noble nanoparticles. Taton *et al.* had shown a two-color DNA sandwich assay.[37] Different diameter gold nanoparticle probes were used to give specific targeting for detection of interesting subjects on a chip. The signals from different nanoparticles with distinct color provided clear detection for targeted subjects.

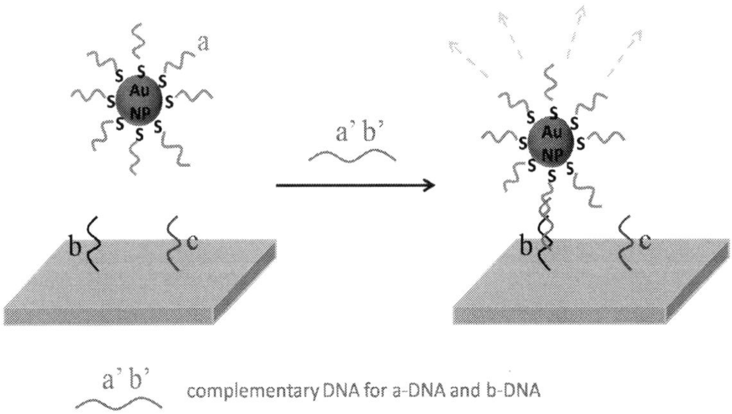

Figure 2.2 DNA detection assay using light scattering. The a-DNA-conjugated Au nanoparticles can specifically and selectively bind to b-DNA after adding complementary a′b′-DNA, but c-DNA is not able to hybridize with a-DNA-conjugated Au nanoparticles. Thus, the site of b-DNA can observe responded color using light scattering, while the site of c-DNA has no signal.

2.2.2 Protein, Peptide, and Antibody Conjugation

Proteins, peptides, and antibodies have been extensively utilized to conjugate with noble metal nanomaterials for biomedical studies.[38–40] To directly conjugate with noble metal nanoparticles, biomolecules may use their residual thiol groups to attach to the nanoparticle surfaces and to form covalent metal-S bonds. Another conjugation method is electrostatic interaction using the surface charge of biomolecules to adsorb on the particle surfaces with opposite charges. It should be noted that these two conjugation methods may cause biological activities or functions to disappear due to the randomly conjugated sites in the biomolecules. When biomolecules are conjugated with nanoparticles through covalent bonds or electrostatic interactions, they may undergo some changes in their conformation. The conformation of biomolecules is an important factor to affect the performance of activities and functions. Sen *et al.* showed that bovine serum albumin (BSA) proteins exhibited conformational changes that affected the efficiency of surface energy transfer (SET) after conjugation with Au nanoparticles.[40] If the reactive sites in the biomolecules are not specific but random, the orientation and conformation is hindered and resulting in changes in efficiency. To decrease this effect, conjugation at specific sites in the biomolecules is required. For example, Liao *et al.* successfully conjugated antibodies on the Au nanorods and kept the orientation of antibodies.[39] They used (n-hydroxysuccinimide-PEG-thiol) to incubate with the Au nanorods, and thiol groups were then attached to the nanorod surfaces to form Au–S bonds. The terminally functional groups, NHS groups, were exposed on the nanorod surfaces, and the antibodies reacted with the NHS groups of NHS-PEG-S-Au nanorods.[41] In this case, antibodies only used their amine groups, not other groups, so their orientation had no change after conjugating with NHS-PEG-S-Au nanorods resulting in the antibodies kept their bio-activity for specific targeting. Figure 2.3 shows the commonly used strategies to conjugate biomolecules on the noble metal nanoparticles. These conjugations are suitable for most biomolecules such as proteins, antibodies, lipases, peptides, DNA, and enzymes, and even chemical compounds. In Fig. 2.3A, the surfaces of noble metal nanoparticles expose the amine group, and the biomolecules contribute the thiol group to form the conjugate using sulfosuccinimidyl-4-(*N*-maleimidomethyl) cycholhexane-1-carboxylate (SMCC).[42] Similar results are seen in EDC conjugation methods (Fig. 2.3B). The EDC serves as bioconjugation linker to form covalent binding between the amine-exposed nanoparticles and the carboxylic group of biomolecules. In addition to EDC and SMCC conjugating methods, there are still many useful chemical-conjugated methods to link nanoparticles and biomolecules. For example, Brennan *et al.* used azide-modified Au nanoparticles to react with acetylene-modified lipases, utilizing the copper (I)-catalyzed 1,2,3-triazole formation between azides and terminal acetylenes.[38]

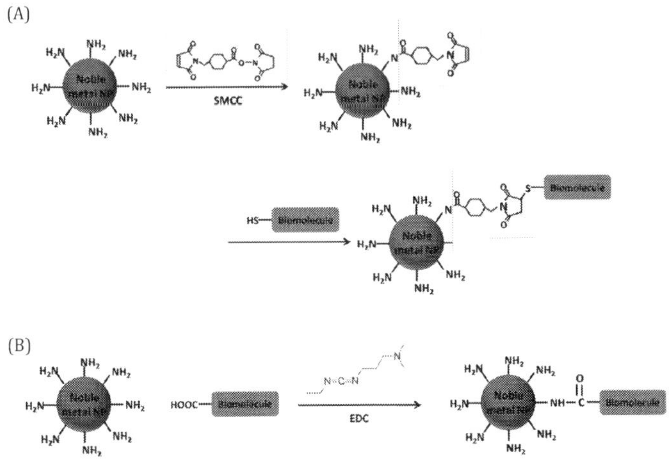

Figure 2.3 Conjugation methods of noble metal nanoparticles with biomolecules using (A) SMCC and (B) EDC. SMCC is a cross-link for combination of amine and thiol groups and EDC is a reagent for combination of amine and carboxylic acid groups to form amide bonds.

2.2.3 Other Biomolecule Conjugation Methods

Conjugation of noble metal nanoparticles with biomolecules proceeds not only through the formation of covalent bonds and electrostatic interactions but also through host–guest systems. The host–guest interactions can be seen in biomolecule systems such as antibody–antigen, protein A (or protein G)-immunoglobulin G (IgG) and biotin-avidin. The advantages of host–guest systems are high selectivity and specification and the strong interaction between the host and guest substrates. In these systems, the orientation and conformation of biomolecules does not undergo any change, and thus, the biomolecules can keep their biological functions and bioactivities. For examples, biotin-modified DNA, peptides, and antibodies can specifically target avidin-coated Au nanoparticles.[43,44] Recently, similar conjugating strategies (inorganic metal ion–biomolecules systems) with specific and strong interactions were used to attach biomolecules on noble metal nanoparticles. A metal chelate, nitrilotriacetic acid (NTA)-nickel (II) with highly selectively conjugated with polyhistidine (His) tags, because His tags can be readily engineered on most proteins for a specific interaction to nickel. NTA-Ni-Au nanoparticles have shown high specific targeting efficiency to histidine-tagged proteins or peptides for specific tumor-targeting.[45,46]

2.3 Applications of Noble Metal Nanoparticles to Biolabeling and Bioimaging

2.3.1 X-Ray Computed Tomography

X-ray computed tomography (CT) is one of common tools used in medical diagnosis. Iodine-based molecules are frequently used contrast agents for CT because of the high X-ray absorption coefficient of iodine. Iodinated compounds, however, make only very short imaging times and can cause toxicity in kidneys. The use of gold nanoparticle as a contrast agent is an attractive alternative. Due to its higher X-ray absorption coefficient than iodine (1.94 cm^2/g at 100 keV), the feasibility of using gold nanomaterials (5.16 cm^2/g at 100 keV) as a potential CT contrast agent *in vivo* is currently under studies. For example, PEG-coated gold nanoparticles[6] and gold nanoparticles within gum arabic matrix[47] are able to generate high efficient *in vivo* CT angiogram images of the heart and vessels. The PEG-hybrid gold nanoparticles had not only clearly enhanced the CT signal for the aorta, but also obtained long circulation times *in vivo* with better biocompatibility than the iodinated imaging agent (Ultravist®).[6] The additional experiments based on the intravenous injection of PEG-hybrid gold nanoparticles into hepatoma-bearing rats also exhibited a clear CT contrast in hepatoma tissue. It is noted that the gold nanoparticles provided additional potential functionality in the therapeutic applications once the gold nanoparticle exposed to high energy irradiation.[47,48]

2.3.2 Magnetic Resonance Imaging

The development of new contrast agents based on Au nanoparticles for MR imaging is progressing now. Significant effort has demonstrated the combinations of MR imaging materials with promising biolabling agents. For example, Au/DOTA-Gd^{3+} hybrids were developed to raise the contrast enhancement sensitivity and to prolong the tracking and imaging time for diagnosis.[49] The Au nanocarriers carried hundreds of DOTA ligands. Accordingly, approximate 150 of DOTA molecules were estimated anchoring onto 2 nm Au nanoparticles. This resulted in a higher relaxivity (r_1 = 585 mM^{-1} s^{-1} in particle concentration) for T_1-contrast enhancement than DOTA-Gd agent alone (3 mM^{-1} s^{-1}). When the Au nanorods joined with Fe_3O_4 nanoparticles, an ehanced r_2 relaxivity (248.1 mM^{-1} s^{-1}) was observed as compared with free Fe_3O_4 nanoparticles (63.5 mM^{-1} s^{-1}), thus increasing the T_2-weighting signal.[50] The composites of Gd-based particles[51] or iron oxide nanoparticles combined with Au nanoshells were also fabricated for MR imaging and NIR-therapeutic applications.[52,53] Kim *et al.* presented a versatile nanostructures composed of a dielectric silica core deposited by superparamagnetic iron oxide (SPIO) nanoparticles, and a thin layer of gold coverings on the surface.[52] The magnetic gold nanoshell can act as a negative MR contrast agent and a NIR radiation absorber for destruction of cancer cells when exposed to a femtosecond NIR laser. In another study, a gold layer was formed onto the surface of γ-Fe_2O_3 nanoparticles through a hydroxylamine seeding process to form core/shell γ-Fe_2O_3/Au nanoparticles.[53] Those hybrid particles had a highly tunable plasmon resonance in the visible-NIR range, and could be manipulated by using an external magnetic field. Based on the Gd nanoparticles, a new bifunctional $Gd_2O(CO_3)_2{\cdot}H_2O$/silica/gold particles were developed.

Figure 2.4 shows a synthetic procedure for $Gd_2O(CO_3)_2{\cdot}H_2O$-based hybrid particles.[51] The $Gd_2O(CO_3)_2{\cdot}H_2O$/silica/gold hybrid exhibited increasing relaxivity r_1 as the thickness of the Au shell decreased. The optical extinction spectra of the $Gd_2O(CO_3)_2{\cdot}H_2O$/silica/Au hybrid particles with different thicknesses are shown in Fig. 2.4B. The formation of Au shells on $Gd_2O(CO_3)_2{\cdot}H_2O$/silica hybrid particles resulted in the broadened absorption in the region of 600–900 nm. The hybrid particles with 63 nm Au shell had the strongest intensity in 600–900 nm. The thinner Au shell had less absorption. This is due to more Au present in 63 nm Au shell particles, resulting in stronger absorption compared to those of 26 nm and 12 nm Au shell particles. However, the thickness of Au shell influenced the T_1-weighted signal. For 12 nm Au shell, the T_1-weighted signal began to brighten at 0.06 mM Gd^{3+} concentration (Fig. 2.4C). The brightening started at 0.10 mM and 0.30 mM for 26 nm and 63 nm Au shells, respectively (Fig. 2.4C). The longitudinal relaxivities, r_1, were determined to be 8.60 (12 nm), 7.06 (26 nm), and 2.84 (63 nm) $s^{-1}mM^{-1}$. The r_1 relaxivity depends on the thickness of Au shells. The thinner Au shell thickness resulted in higher r_1 value, while thicker Au shell hindered interaction between the protons of water molecules and $Gd_2O(CO_3)_2{\cdot}H_2O$, decreasing the MR contrast effect.

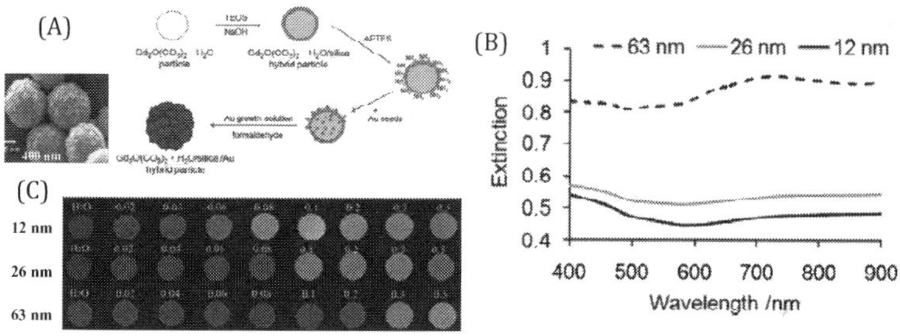

Figure 2.4 (A) Schemes for the fabrication of $Gd_2O(CO_3)_2{\cdot}H_2O$/silica/gold hybrid particles. Inset shows the SEM image of the $Gd_2O(CO_3)_2{\cdot}H_2O$/silica spherical particles embedded in 63 nm Au. (B) UV-vis spectra versus the different thicknesses of Au shells on the $Gd_2O(CO_3)_2{\cdot}H_2O$/silica spheres in the same particle number of 7×10^7 per mL. (C) *In vitro* MR assays of $Gd_2O(CO_3)_2{\cdot}H_2O$/silica/gold hybrid particles in 12, 26, and 63 nm Au shells as a function of Gd^{3+} concentration (mM). [Reprinted with permission from ref. 51. Copyright 2009 Royal Society of Chemistry].

Recently, pure noble metallic Au_3Cu_1 with shell-like nanostructures was fabricated through a reaction of copper nanoparticles with $HAuCl_4$ solution. The surface of Au_3Cu_1 nanoshells could be modified with polyelectrolytes (coated with PEI/PAA/PEI) to form Au_3Cu_1 nanocapsules (Fig. 2.5A).[54] X-ray absorption near-edge spectroscopy (XANES) measurements of Au_3Cu_1 nanoshells indicated the edge positions (E_0), being sensitive to the oxidation state of the metals, shifted slightly to lower energy (−0.23 eV) at the Au L_{III} edge and increased significantly (+6.88 eV) at the Cu K edge. The large E_0 change at the Cu edge reflected its high oxidation state. Here, Cu in Au_3Cu_1 can be assigned up to +3, where Cu^{3+} has an electronic configuration of d^8 with two unpaired electrons. Therefore, Au_3Cu_1 nanocapsules are made of significant numbers of paramagnetic Cu^{3+} ions, resulting in bimodal MR contrast agents for T_1 and T_2 contrast enhancement ($r_1 = 3 \times 10^4$ mM^{-1} s^{-1} and $r_2 = 1.82 \times 10^6$ mM^{-1} s^{-1}). For *in vivo* MR imaging, Au_3Cu_1 nanocapsules were examined in a series of MR imaging studies using BALB/c mice (a dosage of 20 mg kg^{-1}) with an injection in the tail vein. Figures 2.5B (T_1-weighted imaging) and 2.5C (T_2-weighted imaging) shows the monitor of pre- and post-contrast images using Au_3Cu_1 nanocapsules. In T_1-weighted images (Fig. 2.5B), immediately after the injection (post 0 h), the region of the cardiac chamber was brighter in axial and coronal views. After 2 h of circulation, the heart area appeared brighter. Color mapping of the identical MR images also provided evidence of MR signal changes: the light blue color in the cardiac region expanded 2 h after the injection. Taking anatomic T_2-weighted images of mice (Fig. 2.5C), the T_2-weighted imaging

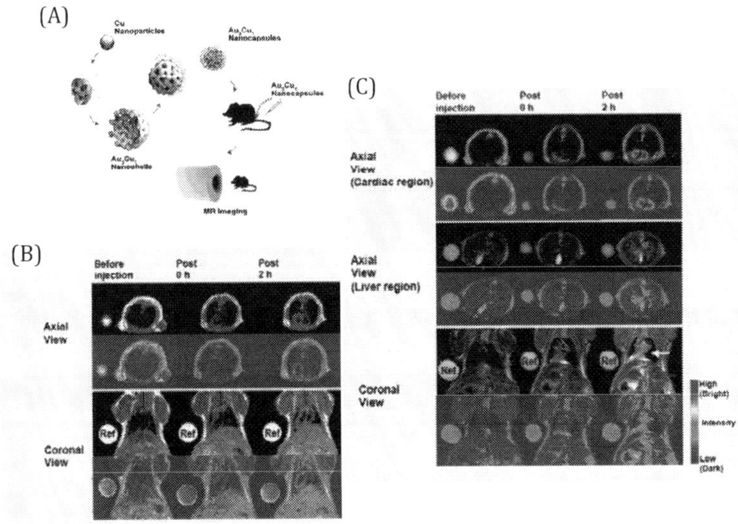

Figure 2.5 (A) Au_3Cu_1 nanocapsules as contrast agents in animal MR imaging. *In vivo* progressive MRI events and color maps. (B) T_1-weighted and (C) T_2-weighted images of male BALB/c mice at the indicated temporal points (pre-injection, immediately postinjection, and 2 h postinjection) in this experiment with Au_3Cu_1 nanocapsules. The arrows in (C) indicate the increase in signal intensity and show visualized vessels for the thorax and liver regions in T_2-weighted images (coronal view). [Reprinted with permission from ref. 54. Copyright 2007 American Chemical Society]. See also Color Insert.

showed that the Au_3Cu_1 nanocapsules brightly lit the cardiac region and the blood vessels of the liver and that the signal level increased for 2 h after the injection. Au_3Cu_1 nanocapsules enhanced the heart chamber images immediately and increasingly enhanced the images of the cardiac region for 2 h. In the liver region, the images of the vessels were significantly enhanced as well, and the vessel branches appeared clearly 2 h post-injection. The coronal views also showed that Au_3Cu_1 nanocapsules provided positive contrast images. Once again, color maps of the T_2-weighted images displayed the imaging difference: the signal intensity and vessel visualization increased for 2 h in the thorax region (white arrow) and liver area (red arrow). The *in vivo* experiments Au_3Cu_1 nanocontrast agents enhanced the contrast of blood vessels and suggested their potential use in MR angiography as blood pool agents.

2.3.3 Optical Imaging

Optical contrast modalities involve absorption, fluorescence, scattering, and vibration (Raman and IR) spectroscopy. In contrast to MRI and CT modalities, optical imaging for biological tracking is versatile with color display, easy approach, and low manufacturing cost of the imaging equipment. Optical instruments include light sources (lasers and lamps), optical equipments (fibers and mirrors), microscopes, and detectors, which are relatively inexpensive in comparison to MRI and X-ray machines. Metallic nanoparticle contrast agents for optical imaging possess greater absorption cross-section or scattering effects and may produce enhance luminescence.[5,55,56] Noble metallic nanomaterials can generate high optical signals from multi-photon luminescence[57,58] and SERS.[59] This amplification is due to resonance coupling with LSPR, particularly with anisotropic gold and silver nanostructures.

Noble metallic nanoparticles have been greatly used as light scattering agents for bio-labeling.[5,55,60–62] As the nanoparticle size increases up to 80 nm, the light scattering ratio is promoted. To collect the peak scattering intensities of nanoparticles, the dark-field microscopy was employed[60,61] in Ag nanomaterials[63], Au nanocages[62], and Au nanorods.[5,55] Using the antibody-modified gold nanoagents, the microstructures of the cell shapes were obtained by recording the scattering images from the labeling cell membranes.[64] Similar result was also reported for the antibody-modified gold nanorods, where not only provided high quality in imaging enhancement to quantify the targeting efficiency but also distinguished malignant cancerous cells from nonmalignant epithelial cell lines (HaCat).[5] Recently, the Au–Fe_3O_4 heterostructures were fabricated as platform for a dual-modelity bio-probe. The dumbbell structures were formed based on the Au nanoparticles (3 nm or 8 nm) grown with Fe_3O_4 nanoparticles (20 nm).[64] Magnetic measurements (M–H curves) showed the Au–Fe_3O_4 heterostructures with superparamagnetic behavior for MR imaging. Reflection spectra of Au–Fe_3O_4 heterostructures exhibited characteristic reflectance in the 590–650 nm range. Once conjugation with epidermal growth factor receptor antibody (anti-EGFR), the Au–Fe_3O_4 showed higher specificity targeting to A431 cells (overexpressed EGFR) than those without anti-EGFR. The dark-field microscope based on Au–Fe_3O_4 reflection provided long-term cell tracking reflection images.

Fluorescent contrast agents such as QDs and organic dyes have been widely used for cell and intracellular imaging. However, photobleaching occurs after a long time exposure for organic dyes. The nonlinear optical effect of gold nanomaterials has attracted much attention because of its excellent anti-photobleaching properties. Multi-photon fluorescence is an optical process, which is strongly depended on the laser flux. For example, two-photon fluorescence (TPF) occurs when the fluorophores are excited by simultaneous absorption of two photons followed by a light emission from a relaxation of a single photon. The LSPR of Au nanorods can locally augment the field of incident electromagnetic waves, increasing the yield of nonlinear optical processes. Au nanorods are ideally suited for nonlinear optical contrast agents in cell imaging using two-photon-excited luminescence.[3] The TPF from a single Au nanorod is 58 times that of a single rhodamine 6G molecule[65] and provides cancer cell images to a depth of 75 μm.[66] Biofunctional Fe_3O_4–Ag nanoparticles were used for TPF labeling of macrophage cells with femtosecond infrared laser pulses (900 nm) as well.[63]

2.4 Conclusion and Outlook

The bioconjugation of noble metal nanoparticles *via* covalent bonds or electrostatic interactions is important for *in vitro* biolabeling and bioimaging. The most important advantage is the selective and specific targeting of molecules, cells, or regions of interest, and observes them through images. Bioconjugation of noble metal nanoparticles also determines their biomedical application depending on what biomolecules are conjugated on the particle surface and which functions are provided, e.g., DNA for DNA detection assays and biolabeling markers, antibodies for specific and selective targeting. Each imaging modality has its own merits and demerits, but by combining different modalities into an all-in-one single system, multimodal imaging nanoagents may provide complementary information for biologically motivated studies. All these imaging methods using noble nanoagents present multiple imaging and are promising to achieve single-molecule or multifunctional detections, either *in vivo* or *in vitro*, for early diagnostics.

References

1. L. J. Sherry, R. Jin, C. A. Mirkin, G. C. Schatz, and R. P Van Duyne, *Nano. Lett.*, **6**, 2020 (2006).
2. X. Zheng, D. Guo, Y. Shao, S. Jia, S. Xu, B. Zhao, W. Xu, C. Corredor, and J. R. Lombardi, *Langmuir*, **24**, 4394 (2008).
3. J. Zhao, X. Zhang, C. R. Youzon, A. J. Haes, and R. P. Van Duyne, *Nano. Lett.*, **1**, 219 (2006).
4. B. Wiley, Z. Wang, J. Wei, Y. Yin, D. H. Cobden, and Y. Xia, *Nano. Lett.*, **6**, 2273 (2006).
5. X. Huang, I. H. El-Sayed, W. Qian, and M. A. El-Sayed, *J. Am. Chem. Soc.*, **128**, 2115 (2006).
6. D. Kim, S. Park, J. H. Lee, Y. Y. Jeong, and S. Jon, *J. Am. Chem. Soc.*, **129**, 7661 (2007).
7. P. Nativo, I. A. Prior, and M. Brust, *ACS Nano*, **2**, 1639 (2008).
8. S. Connolly and D. Fitzmaurice, *Adv. Mater.*, **11**, 1202 (1999).
9. W. Shenton, S. A. Davis, and S. Mann, *Adv. Mater.*, **11**, 449 (1999).
10. S. R.Whaley, D. S. English, E. L. Hu, P. F. Barbara, and A. M. Belcher, *Nature*, **405**, 665 (2000).
11. G. T. Hermanson, *Bioconjugate techniques*; Academic Press: NewYork, 1996.
12. A. Gole and C. J. Murphy, *Langmuir*, **24**, 266 (2008).
13. N. Brandes, P. B. Welzel, C. Werner, and L. W. Kroh, *J. Colloid Interface Sci.*, **299**, 56 (2006).
14. K. A. Hultborn, *et al.*, *Acta. Radiol.*, **43**, 52 (1955).

15. W. Faulk and G. Taylor, *Immunochemistry*, **8**, 1081 (1971).
16. M. A. Hayat, Colloidal Gold: Principles, Methods, and Applications, Academic Press, San Diego, **1** (1989).
17. C. J. Murphy, A. M. Gole, J. W. Stone, P. N. Sisco, A. M. Alkilany, E. C. Goldsmith, and S. C. Baxter, *Acc. Chem. Res.*, **41**, 1721 (2008).
18. P. K. Jain, X. Huang, I. H. El-Sayed, and M. A. El-Sayed, *Acc. Chem. Res.*, **41**, 1578 (2008).
19. C. A. Lin, T. Y. Yang, C. H. Lee, S. H. Huang, R. A. Sperling, M. Znaella, J. K. Li, J. L. Shen, H. H. Wang, H. I. Yeh, W. J. Park, and W. H. Chang, *ACS Nano,* **3**, 395 (2009).
20. C. C. Huang, Z. Yang, K. H. Lee, and H. T. Chang, *Angew. Chem. Int. Ed.*, **46**, 6824 (2007).
21. J. M. Slocik, J. S. Zabinski D. M. Phillips, and R. R. Naik, *Small,* **4**, 548 (2008).
22. J. Xie, Q. Zhang, J. Y. Lee, and D. I. C. Wang, *ACS Nano,* **3**, 2473(2009).
23. S. Lee, S. Kim, J. Choo, S. Y. Shin, Y. H. Lee, H. Y. Choi, S. Ha, K. Kang, and C. H. Oh, *Anal. Chem.*, **79**, 916 (2007).
24. X. Yang, S. E. Skrabalak, Z. Y. Li, Y. Xia, and L. V. Wang, *Nano Lett.*, **7**, 3798 (2007).
25. D. Pan, M. Pramanil, A. Senpan, X. Yang, K. H. Song, M. J. Scott, H. Zhang, P. J. Gaffney, S. A. Wickline, L. V. Wang, and G. M. Lanza, *Angew. Chem. Int. Ed.*, **48**, 4170 (2009).
26. M. Giersig and P. Mulvaney, *Langmuir*, **9**, 3408 (1993).
27. M. C. Daniel and D. Astruc, *Chem. Rev.*, **104**, 293 (2004).
28. C. Burda, X. Chen, R. Narayanan, and M. A. El-Sayed, *Chem. Rev.*, **105**, 1025 (2005).
29. D. A. Stuart, J. M. Yuen, N. Shah, O. Lyandres, C. R. Yonzon, M. R. Glucksberg, J. T. Walsh, and R. P. Van Duyne, *Anal. Chem.*, **78**, 7211 (2006).
30. J. F. Hainfeld, D. N. Slatkin, T. M. Focella, and H. M. Smilowitz, *Brit. J. Radiol.*, **79**, 248 (2006).
31. N. J. Durr, T. Larson, D. K. Smith, B. A. Korgel, K. Sokolov, and A. B. Yakar, *Nano Lett.*, **7**, 941 (2007).
32. C. M. Niemeyer and C. A. Mirkin, *Nanobiotechnology: Concepts, Applications, and Perspectives*; Eds.; Wiley-VCH: Weinheim, Germany (2004).
33. D. S. Ginger, H. Zhang, and C. A. Mirkin, *Angew. Chem., Int. Ed.*, **43**, 30 (2004).

34. Y. Yin, Y. Lu, B. Gates, and Y. Xia, *J. Am. Chem. Soc.*, **123**, 8718 (2001).
35. C. J Ackerson, M. T. Sykes, and R. D. Kornberg, *Proc. Nat. Acad. Sci.*, **102**, 13383 (2005).
36. R. Jin, Y. Cao, C. A. Mirkin, K. L. Kelly, G. C. Schatz, and J. G. Zheng, *Science*, **294**, 1901 (2001).
37. T. A. Taton, G. Lu, C. A. Mirkin, *J. Am. Chem. Soc.*, **123**, 5164 (2001).
38. J. L. Brennan, N. S. Hatzakis, T. Robert Tshikhudo, N. Dirvianskyte, V. Razumas, S. Parkar, J. Vind, A. Svendsen, R. J. M. Nolte, A. E. Rowan, and M. Brust, *Bioconjugate Chem.*, **17**, 1373 (2006).
39. H. Liao and J. H. Hafner, *Chem. Mater..* **17**, 4636 (2005).
40. T. Sen, K. K. Haldar, and A. Patra, *J. Phys. Chem. C*, **112**, 17945 (2008).
41. L. Maus, J. P. Spatz, and R. Fiammengo, *Langmuir*, in press.
42. A. H. Beth, T. E. Conturo, S. D. Venkataramu, and J. V. Satros, *Biochemistry*, **25**, 3824 (1986).
43. X. Huang, D. Du, X. Gong, J. Cai, H. Tu, X. Xu, and A. Zhang, *Electroanalytica*, **20**, 402 (2008).
44. Y. Weizmann, F. Patolsky, and I. Willner, *Anal. Sci.*, **17**, i351 (2001).
45. J. M. Abad, S. F. L. Mertens, M. Pita, V. M. Fernandez, and D. J. Schiffrin, *J. Am. Chem. Soc.*, **127**, 5689 (2005).
46. C. Xu, K. Xu, H. Gu, X, Zhong, Z. Guo, R. Zheng, X. Zhang, and B. Xu, *J. Am. Chem. Soc.*, **126**, 3392 (2004).
47. V. Kattumuri, K. Katti, S. Bhaskaran, E. J. Boote, S. W. Casteel, G. M. Fent, D. J. Robertson, M. Chandrasekhar, R. Kannan, and K. V. Katti, *Small*, **3**, 333 (2007).
48. C.Xu, G. A. Tung, and S. Sun, *Chem. Mater.*, **20**, 4167 (2008).
49. P. J. Debouttière, S. Roux, F. Vocanson, C. Billotey, O. Beuf, A. Favre-Réguillon, Y. Lin, S. Pellet-Rostaing, R. Lamartine, P. Perriat, and O. Tillement, *Adv. Funct. Mater.*, **16**, 2330 (2006).
50. C. Wang, J. Chen, T. Talavage, and J. Irudayaraj, *Angew. Chem. Int. Ed.*, **48**, 2759 (2009).
51. K. W. Hu, Y.Y. Jhang, C. H. Su, and C. S Yeh, *J. Mater. Chem.*, **19**, 2147 (2009).
52. J. Kim, S. Park, J. E. Lee, S. M. Jin, J. H. Lee, I. S. Lee, I. Yang, J. S.. Kim, S. K. Kim, M. H. Cho, and T. Hyeon, *Angew. Chem. Int. Ed.*, **45**, 7754 (2006).
53. J. Xiaojun, S. Ruping, A. M. Elliott, R. J. Stafford, E. Esparza-Coss, J. A. Bamkson, G. Liang, Z.-P. Luo, K. Park, J. T. Markert, and C. Li, *J. Phys. Chem. C*, **111**, 6245(2007).

54. C. H. Su, H. S. Sheu, C. Y. Lin, C. C. Huang, Y. W. Lo, Y. C. Pu, J. C. Weng, D. B. Shieh, J. H. Chen, and C. S. Yeh, *J. Am. Chem. Soc.*, **129**, 2139 (2007).

55. S. E. Skrabalak, J. Chen, Y. Sun, X. Lu, L. Au, C. Cobley, and Y. Xia, *Acc. Chem. Res.*, **41**, 1587 (2008).

56. R. Bardhan, N. K. Grady, and N. J. Halas, *Small*, **4**, 1716 (2008).

57. J. Chen, F. Saeki, B. J. Wiley, H. Cang, M. J. Cobb, Z. Y. Li, L. Au, H. Zhang, M B. Kimmey, X. Li, and Y. Xia, *Nano Lett.*, **5**, 473 (2005).

58. S. P. Tai, Y. Wu, D. B. Shieh, L. J. Chen, K. J., Lin, J. H. Yu, S. W. Chu, C. H. Chang, X. Y. Shi, Y. C. Wen, K. H. Lin, T. M. Liu, and C. K. Sun, *Adv. Mater.*, **19**, 4520 (2007).

59. N. J. Durr, T. Larson, S. D. Smith, B. A. Korgel, K. Sokolov, and A. Ben-Yakar, *Nano Lett.*, **7**, 941 (2007).

60. J. Kneipp, H, Kneipp, B. Wittig, and K. Kneipp, *Nano Lett.*, **7**, 2819 (2007).

61. C. W. Lee, M. J. Chen, J. Y. Cheng, and P. K. Wei, *J. Biomed. Opt.* **14**, 034016 (2009).

62. M. Hu, C. Novo, A. Funston, H. Wang, H. Petrova, S. Zou, P. Mulvaney, Y. Xia, and G. V. Hartland, *J. Mater. Chem.*, **18**, 1949 (2008).

63. J. Jiang, H. Gu, H. Shao, E. Devlin, G. C. Papaefthymiou, and J. Y. Ying, *Adv. Mater.*, **20**, 4403 (2008).

64. C. Xu, J. Xie, D. Ho, C. Wang, N. Kohler, E. G. Walsh, J. R. Morgan, Y. E. Chin, and S. Sun, *Angew. Chem., Int. Ed.*, **47**, 173 (2008).

65. H. Wang, T. B. Huff, D. A. Zweifel, W. He, P. S. Low, A. Wei, and J. X. Cheng, *Proc. Natl. Acad. Sci. U. S. A.*, **102**, 15752 (2005).

66. N. J. Durr, T. Larson, D. K. Smith, B. A. Korgel, K. Sokolov, and A. Ben-Yakar, *Nano Lett.*, **7**, 941 (2007).

Chapter 3

Colorimetric Bioassay Using Noble Metal Nanoparticles

Ming-Feng Huang[a], Yang-Wei Lin[b], and Huan-Tsung Chang[a,*]

[a]*Department of Chemistry, National Taiwan University,*
1, Section 4, Roosevelt Road, Taipei, Taiwan
[b]*Department of Chemistry, National Changhua University of Education,*
1, Jin-De Road, Changhua City 500, Taiwan
*changht@ntu.edu.tw

In this chapter, we attempt to present the development and applications of metal nanoparticle-based colorimetric assays. The sensing strategies are based on analyte-induced nanoparticle (NP) aggregation and dispersion. We begin with the preparation, stabilization, and surface functionalization of Au and Ag NPs. A general introduction of the optical properties of Au and Ag NPs briefly follows. After providing a general background, we concentrate on their applications of sensing analytes, including DNA, proteins, and small solutes, through interparticle crosslinking and non-crosslinking aggregation events.

From Bioimaging to Biosensors: Noble Metal Nanoparticles in Biodetection
Edited by Lai-Kwan Chau and Huan-Tsung Chang

ISBN 978-981-4267-24-3 (Hardcover), 978-981-4303-10-1 (eBook)
www.panstanford.com

3.1 Introduction

The development of simple, rapid, sensitive, selective, and cost-effective approaches to detection of biomolecules is important because of their potential applications in the diagnosis of diseases.[1–3] Radioactive, fluorescent, chemiluminescent, electrochemical, and colorimetric probes are common.[4–6] Colorimetric assays are especially attractive because they allow the observation of results by the naked eye. For example, pH indicators are widely used to determine the concentrations of analytes such as urea and ammonia. However, when compared to other detection formats, colorimetric detection possesses relatively poor sensitivity. Thus, probes with extremely high molar extinction coefficients are highly desirable for the detection of trace amounts of analytes of interest.

The past few years have witnessed significant progress in bioassays using nanomaterials. Gold nanoparticles (Au NPs) are the most widely used nanomaterials in developing colorimetric bioassays, mainly because of their unique size-, shape-, composition-, and distance-dependent optical properties.[7] In addition, Au NPs are stable, simple to prepare and to bioconjugate, and biocompatibile.[8–10] Researchers have realized a variety of colorimetric sensors using Au NPs for different analytes, including DNA, proteins, and small molecules such as metal ions and carbohydrates. Most of the assays take advantage of the localized surface plasmon resonance (LSPR) of Au NPs as sensing elements; the dispersed Au NP solution is red whereas the aggregated Au NP solution is purple.[8,10] Au NPs, with an interparticle distance greater than their average particle diameter, appear red as a consequence of their SPR absorption band centered around 516 nm (for 13 nm Au NPs). As the interparticle distance decreases to a length shorter than the diameter of the particles, coupling interactions result in a broadening and a shift to longer wavelengths of their SPR absorption band, leading to the change in the solution color from red to purple.

Colorimetric NP-based assays for the detection of DNA using Au NPs have created much attention for their practical applications.[11,12] Subsequently, researchers have prepared other Au NP probes for the detection of lectins,[13,14] metal ions,[15–19] antibodies,[20] and other analytes.[21–23] In each instance, the self assembly of a monolayer of a molecular recognition molecule on the NP surface is responsible for the colorimetric assays; controlled aggregation of the NPs occurs with specific recognition and binding of the target species.

Although not frequently reported, Ag NPs can also be used in bioassays, for example biotinylated Ag NPs for detecting avidin through high affinity biotin–avidin interactions.[24] In fact, Ag NPs are the second most useful novel metal nanomaterials for bioassays.[25–29] Monodisperse spherical Ag NPs have LSPR absorption bands around 400 nm. Once aggregation occurs, an Ag NP solution changes its color from yellow to orange. For colorimetric assays, Ag NPs have some advantages over Au NPs to a certain degree, including their higher extinction coefficients and relatively lower costs.[30] However, Ag NPs are not as stable as Au NPs; oxidation and chemical degradation during functionalization may occur. In addition, when Ag NPs are prepared by standard chemical reductions, their size distributions are usually broad. Thus, little attention has been paid to Ag NP based colorimetric assays.[31–34]

When compared to common organic chromophores, Au and Ag NPs have extremely large molar coefficients, leading to the high sensitivity of NP-based colorimetric assays. The molar extinction coefficients for 30 nm Au NPs and 80 nm Ag NPs are 7.1×10^{12} M^{-1} cm^{-1} at 526 nm and 9.5×10^{12} M^{-1} cm^{-1} at 430 nm, respectively, which are much larger than those (10^4 to 10^5 M^{-1} cm^{-1}) for more common chromophores.

To develop sensitive colorimetric assays, the preparation of monodisperse and stable Au and Ag NPs is important. Thus, this chapter focuses on strategies for the preparation and stabilization of Au and Ag NPs. Most Au NPs and Ag NPs that are prepared by chemical reduction approaches lack selectivity for most biomolecules of interest; functionalization of the NPs to provide selective recognition sites on their surfaces is necessary after their preparation. We briefly discuss conjugation approaches to functionalization of Au NPs below. To understand the sensing strategies of colorimetric assays using Au and Ag NPs, the optical properties of these nanomaterials are emphasized. Finally, applications of Au NPs and Ag NPs are provided to show their potential roles in the detection of biomolecules and in cell imaging.

3.2 Synthesis of Au and Ag NPs

Because of their potential uses in many fields, such as catalysis, sensing, and electronics, there are many strategies for the preparation of Au and Ag NPs, including wet chemical, photochemical, and mechanical (top-down) approaches.[35,36] From the view point of green chemistry, the synthesis of Au and Ag NPs in aqueous solutions (wet chemical approaches) is more interesting. In addition, the as-prepared NPs are usually readily bioconjugated and more biocompatible. In this section, we discuss preparation and stabilization of Au and Ag NPs in aqueous solutions. Functionalization of these NPs for the selective sensing of analytes of interest is emphasized as well.

3.2.1 Wet Chemical Approaches

A typical synthesis of spherical Au NPs involves the reduction of gold salts (e.g., $NaAuCl_4$) in solution by reducing agents. Two of the most common reducing agents are citrate and $NaBH_4$. Citrate is usually used to prepare Au NPs with diameters >3 nm because of its weaker reducing strength when compared to that of $NaBH_4$. On the other hand, $NaBH_4$ is used for the preparation of small Au NPs (1–3 nm). Citrate provides one advantage over $NaBH_4$ as it also acts as a capping reagent to stabilize Au NPs. Usually, the growth of Au NPs proceeds via three stages.[37–39] In the first stage (typically complete within a few seconds), a reducing agent reduces metal ions to metal atoms, which then undergo rapid collisions to form stable icosahedral nuclei of 1–2 nm in size. The initial concentration of nuclei depends on the concentration and reducing strength of the reducing agent, the solvent, the temperature, and the reduction potential of the reaction. This stage is important because it determines the heterogeneity of the size and shape of the NPs. Further growth of the NPs occurs, in the second stage, via the reduction of metal ions on the surface of the nuclei until all the metal ions are consumed. The third and final stage involves the prevention of the aggregation of the Au NPs, which is typically achieved by the addition of stabilizing agents. For example, electrostatic repulsions due to the adsorbed citrate ions on the Au NPs' surfaces, which impart negative charge to the NPs, stabilize them. Similarly, Ag NPs are prepared by using $AgNO_3$ as the precursor and citrate or $NaBH_4$ as the reducing agents. Ultimately, polymers such as poly(vinylpyrollidone) are more common capping reagents, used to stabilize the Ag NPs.[40]

Varying the ratio of the reducing agents to the metal salts controls the size of the NPs. Increasing the molar ratio of reductant to metal salt causes rapid formation of a large number of nuclei and leads to smaller, monodisperse Au and Ag NPs. In contrast, decreasing the molar ratio leads to slow formation of a few nuclei and results in larger NPs with a broad size distribution. The nature (reducing strength) of the reductant is an important parameter for controlling the size of NPs. For example, sodium citrate and white phosphorus are used to prepare Au NPs with diameters of 12–100 and 5–12 nm, respectively.[41] Smaller Au NPs (<3 nm in diameter) can be synthesized by the reduction of $HAuCl_4$ in aqueous solution in the presence of $NaBH_4$ or in an organic solvent in the presence of a thiol-capping agent.[42] The nature of the capping agent is also important in determining the size of the NPs. For instance, Ag NPs prepared from the reduction of silver nitrate by $NaBH_4$ in the presence of bis(*p*-sulfonatophenyl)-phenylphosphine and poly(vinylpyrollidone) have diameters of 25–33 nm and 15–36 nm, respectively.[40,43]

Researchers have devoted substantial efforts to the syntheses of anisotropic Au and Ag NPs, which display different optical properties from those of their corresponding spherical NPs. For example, Au nanorods possess traverse and longitudinal SPR bands centered at 520 and 700 nm, respectively. Other interesting anisotropic NPs include Ag nanorods,[44] Ag/Au multimetal micrometer rods,[45] dumbbell-like and peanut-like Au–Ag nanomaterials,[46] Ag nanoprisms,[47] Ag and Au nanocubes,[35] Ag nanoflowers,[48] and Au nanowires.[49] Several factors that control the nuclei and growth rates and the stability of certain sides of the surfaces are important in determining the growth of certain shapes and sizes of anisotropic Au and Ag NPs, including the nature and concentration of the reducing agent, the nature and concentration of the capping agents, the pH and ionic strength of the solution, and the temperature. For example, by controlling the pH, the concentration, and the nature of the amino acids, differently sized and shaped Au–Ag nanorods can be prepared.[50] By controlling the concentration of cetyl trimethylammonium bromide and the pH values, Au nanowires can be prepared from Te nanowires.[51] Two excellent papers summarize many different synthetic strategies for the preparation of anisotropic Au and Ag nanomaterials.[44,52]

3.2.2 Stabilization

Owing to Brownian diffusion and attraction between NPs, Au and Ag NPs are usually unstable in aqueous solutions unless their surfaces are capped with suitable molecules and/or ions. It is extremely important to have monodisperse and stable Au and Ag NPs for bioassays because poor and irreproducible sensitivity results can occur when they are unstable. Increasing the hydrophilicity and/or charge density on the NPs surfaces against van der Waals attraction-induced aggregation is a common way to stabilize NPs.[53] For instance, Au NPs prepared by the classic citrate reduction method are stable due to the existence of charged citrate ions on their surfaces. The stability of Au NPs can be further controlled to an exceptional degree through the introduction of other chemicals or polymers by chemical grafting methods (e.g., Au–thiol and Au–amine), electrostatic adsorption and physical adsorption, and several other methods. Common capping agents for Au and Ag NPs include small organic ions, polymers, and polyelectrolytes, which stabilize the NPs through electrostatic, steric, and electrosteric (a combination of electrostatic and steric) interactions, respectively (see Fig. 3.1).[53,54] Mercaptoundecanoic acid and citrate are common anions for stabilizing Au NPs, mainly because they can form strong Au–S and Au–O bonds, leaving charged parts facing the bulk solution, resulting in increased repulsion forces among the NPs. Common polymers used to stabilize Au and Ag NPs are hydrophilic polymers such as poly(vinylpyrollidone), poly(ethylene oxide), and poly(ethylene glycol). Proteins such as bovine serum albumin and DNA (a negatively charged polymer) are typical polyelectrolytes used to stabilize Au and Ag NPs.

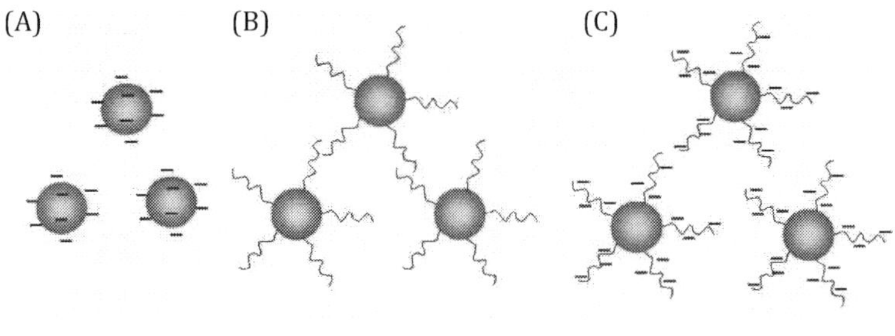

Figure 3.1 Schematic representation of colloidal stabilization through (A) small charged molecules on the Au NP surface (electrostatic stabilization), (B) surface-grafted polymers (steric stabilization), and (C) surface-grafted, charged polymers (electrosteric stabilization).

With respect to electrostatic stabilization (see Fig. 3.1A), the surface charges, together with the counter ions in the medium, form a repulsive electric double layer that stabilizes the NPs against van der Waals attractive forces.[54] A characteristic feature of electrostatic repulsion among NPs is the high sensitivity to the bulk ionic strength. The force of electrostatic repulsion diminishes significantly at high salt concentrations when the electric double layer is highly suppressed, explaining why citrate-capped Au NPs are stabilized in water but aggregate at elevated salt concentrations (e.g., 50 mM NaCl).[55] In the case of steric stabilization (see Fig. 3.1B), macromolecules grafted on colloidal surfaces in a "good solvent" — that is, a solvent in which steric stabilization diminishes with decreasing solubility — impart a polymeric barrier that prevents collision among NPs. Usually, van der Waals attractive forces are dominant in this case. The penetration of polymer chains on the NP surfaces when they approach each other results in a loss of polymer configurational entropy, which is unfavorable to the aggregation process. Steric stabilization is much less sensitive toward ionic strength than electrostatic stabilization. Rather, the molecular weight of the macromolecule and surface graft density are more important factors. In general, thicker polymer layers (ones with longer polymer chains) and higher graft densities lead to more effective steric stabilization. Electrosteric stabilization is probably the most effective strategy to stabilize Au and Ag NPs (see Fig. 3.1C). Bovine serum albumin-stabilized Au NPs are stable in phosphate solution (pH 7.0) at ionic strengths up to 0.1 M NaCl,[56] which is much more stable than mercaptoundecanoic acid-stabilized Au NPs (which aggregate at >50 mM NaCl). DNA-modified Au NPs with high DNA graft densities are stable even at very high salt concentrations (e.g., 300 mM $MgCl_2$). Steric factors are expected to play a major role in stabilizing Au NPs at salt concentrations in which the electrostatic repulsion is significantly diminished.[57]

3.2.3 Functionalization

Most prepared Au and Ag NPs, such as those capped with citrates, are not selective for most biomolecules of interest. Thus, functionalization of Au and Ag NPs is extremely important for providing recognition sites for specific (selective) interactions with target analytes such as DNA and proteins. Bifunctional chemicals, in which a moiety is used for anchorage to the NPs while the other is directed to the outer surface for a specific interaction with biomolecules or for further conjugation, are attractive. Bifunctional chemicals containing SH or NH_2 groups at one of their ends are favorable because they can form strong Au–S and Au–N bonds on the surfaces of Au NPs. For example, thiol-modified oligonucleotides are used to functionalize Au NPs for the specific detection of nucleic acid sequences in biological samples. When the functionalization of Au NPs with biomolecules such as proteins, peptides, and amino acids is necessary, bifunctional chemical such as thiols, imides, and biotin are more favorable. For example, Au NPs functionalized with sulfo-*N*-hydroxysuccinimide can react with primary amines, allowing any protein bearing a primary amine to be linked to Au NPs. Biotin can also be conjugated to Au NPs to detect streptavidin through specific interactions of biotin–streptavidin.[58,59] Figure 3.2 displays one representative example for the functionalization of Au NPs with biotin.[60] The surface of Au NPs is first modified with a layer of poly(acrylic acid). A biotin molecule in biotin–amine, which has an amine group at one end, anchors to the carboxylic acid group of the polyelectrolyte through the well-known carbodiimide chemistry.

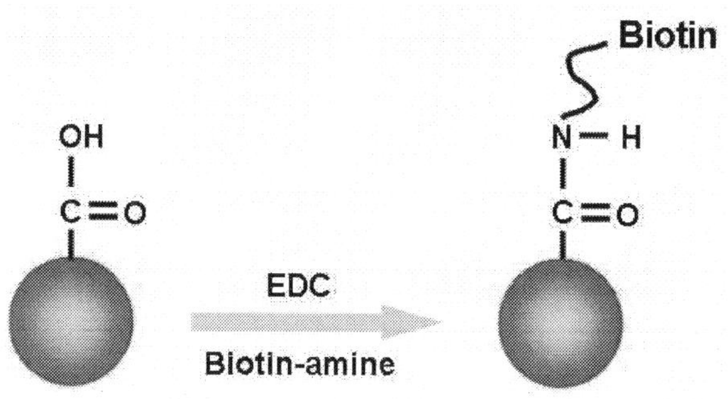

Figure 3.2 Functionalization of Au NPs with biotin–amine.

When compared to Au NPs, Ag NPs are more unstable, and their bioconjugation is not as straightforward, limiting their application in DNA assays. One way to overcome this limitation is the preparation of Ag NPs in the presence of bifunctional chemicals such as hydrazone-functionalized (pyridyldithiopropionyl) dextran.[61] The hydrazone-functionalized (pyridyldithiopropionyl) dextran then reacted with an excess of oligonucleotide that terminates in an aromatic aldehyde group.

3.3 Localized Surface Plasmon Resonance of Au and Ag NPs

Electromagnetic surface waves can propagate along the interface between conducting materials and a dielectric over a broad range of frequencies, ranging from radio frequencies to the visible range. The oscillation modes comprise an electromagnetic field coupled to the oscillations of conduction electrons and are called surface plasmons, which are characterized by strong field enhancement at the interface, while the electric field vector decays exponentially away from the surface (in the nanometer range). Gold and silver belong to a family of free electron metals that have a filled valence shell but an unfilled conduction band; thus, they display strong surface plasmons. When the dimensions of the conductor are reduced, boundary and surface effects become very important, and for this reason, the optical properties of small Au and Ag NPs are dominated by the collective oscillation (LSPR absorption) of the conduction electrons in resonance with incident electromagnetic radiation. Au and Ag NPs display unique optical properties as a result of this LSPR absorption. The LSPR absorptions of Au and Ag NPs are dependent on their size, shape, and composition. For example, aqueous solutions of Au and Ag NPs of 20 nm diameters appear brilliant red and yellow, respectively. The solution colors of Au–Ag nanorods (45 nm in length and 28 nm in width) and boat-like nanomaterials (50 nm in length and 30 nm in width) are red and green, respectively. In addition, the dielectric properties of the medium and the distance between NPs are important parameters when considering their optical properties.[62,63] The influence of the surrounding medium is usually related to its refractive index; Mie theory predicts resonance to occur when $\varepsilon_1(\omega) = -2\varepsilon_m$ (where $\varepsilon_1(\omega)$ is the real component of the metal dielectric function at angular frequency ω and ε_m is the medium dielectric constant), but this equation is only valid for dilute NP dispersions in nonabsorbing media. However, when concentrated systems are considered, the NPs become closer to each other, and interactions between neighboring particles can arise, and the models for isolated particles do not hold any longer. The theoretical modeling of concentrated systems requires the use of effective medium theories, such as those derived in the early 20th century by Maxwell-Garnett and Bruggemann, which allow for the calculation of the average dielectric function for composite media with varying concentrations of an infiltrated material.

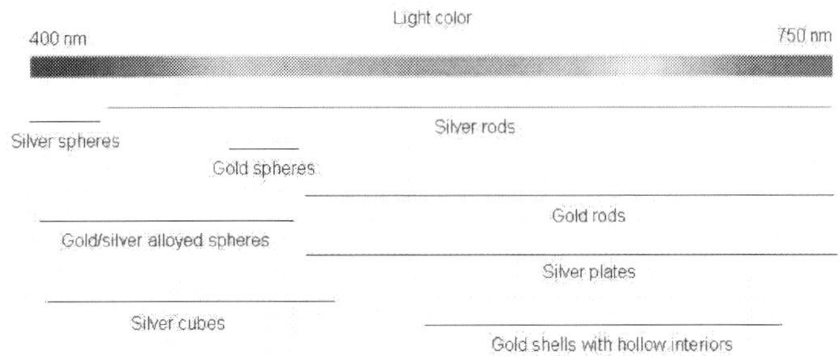

Figure 3.3 A list of silver and gold nanomaterials having various morphologies, compositions, and structures together with the typical locations of their LSPR bands in the visible regime. Reprinted with permission from ref. 62. See also Color Insert.

Figure 3.3 displays that the LSPR absorption bands of Au and Ag NPs can be tuned in the spectral range from 400 to 750 nm.[64] For instance, small Au NPs (e.g., 13 nm in diameter) absorb green light, corresponding to a strong LSPR absorption band at ~520 nm in the visible light spectrum. For small Au NPs, incoming light in a dipole mode oscillates the surface electrons. As the size of the Au NP increases, light can no longer polarize the NPs homogeneously, and then higher order modes at lower energy dominate, causing a red shift and broadening of the SPR absorption band upon increasing the size of the Au NPs.[64] This phenomenon also explains the corresponding LSPR absorption band shifts (redshift) and color changes (red to purple) when the aggregation of small Au NPs occur. When Au NPs aggregate, their surface plasmons combine. Thus, Au NP aggregates can be considered as a single large particle although the detailed interparticle plasmon coupling is rather complex and dependent on many factors, such as aggregate morphology and NP density.

Also displayed in Fig. 3.3 is the fact that different shapes of Au and Ag materials have different colors. The LSPR peaks of Ag/Au alloy nanomaterials are between 405 nm and 516 nm and can be tuned from 405 to 516 nm by simply changing the content of Au with the color changing from yellow to red. The linear relationship between the peak position (λ_{max}) and the molar fraction of Au (x_{Au}) is fitted with $\lambda_{max} = 412 + 1.13\, x_{Au}$. The color of Ag triangular nanoplates with edge lengths varied from ~30 to ~90 nm is greenish blue. These Ag nanoplates exhibit three distinctive peaks located at 690, 485, and 335 nm. These peaks are assigned to the in-plane dipole, in-plane quadrupole, and out-of-plane quadrupole plasmon resonance bands, respectively. The anisotropic, cubic Ag NPs with a mean edge length of 80 nm exhibit three LSPR bands (located at 350, 400, and 470 nm), while the isotropic, spherical Ag NPs with 80 nm diameters display a strong LSPR band around 430 nm. As the size of Ag nanocubes increases from 80 to 175 nm, these three SPR peaks undergo redshifts to 370, 440, and 560 nm. Au nanoshells with hollow interiors have a LSPR peak at 720 nm rather than 520 nm. As more Au atoms are plated onto the surfaces of these shells, their LSPR peak continuously shifts to the blue side (from 720 to 560 nm). The color of these aqueous suspensions of Au nanoshells also changes from dark blue through purple to pink.

3.4 Applications

Possessing high extinction coefficients, size-dependent optical properties, and biocompatibility, Au and Ag NPs have become popular nanomaterials for bioassays. Most colorimetric bioassays in the nanoscale are based on analyte-induced aggregation of Au and Ag NPs through crosslinking or non-crosslinking. Interparticle crosslinking aggregation assays are those that function via interparticle bond formation, while non-crosslinking aggregation assays are those that work through the removal of colloidal stabilization effects, which we discuss in more detail later in this section. Other interesting colorimetric assays based on the analyte-induced redispersion of Au NPs aggregates have also been realized.[65,66] Because of possessing high extinction coefficients, Au and Ag NPs can act as superquenchers in fluorescence quenching-based assays for the analysis of Hg^{2+}, platelet-derived growth factor (PDGF), and so on.[23,67]

3.4.1 Crosslinking Aggregation-Based Assays

A crosslinking aggregation-based assay is the most common type of colorimetric bioassays when using Au NPs. Crosslinking occurs either by using crosslinker molecules that have multiple binding sites for the receptor molecules on Au NPs or by the direct interaction (without crosslinkers) between receptors on Au NPs to which complementary (or antireceptor) molecules are attached. When interparticle bond formation (e.g., H-bonding, electrostatic attraction, hydrophobic interaction, and metal–ligand coordination) associated with interparticle biological recognition overcome the interparticle repulsive forces, interparticle crosslinking initiates aggregation of the NPs. Typical biological recognition events include DNA hybridization; aptamer–target, antibody–antigen, streptavidin–biotin, and lectin–sugar interactions; and metal–ligand coordination. Furthermore, biologically relevant organic molecules (such as peptides) containing residues, such as thiol and guanidine, can directly induce crosslinking aggregation of Au NPs by chemical interactions (e.g., Au–S).

3.4.1.1 Protein assays

Crosslinking-based colorimetric assays have been applied to the determination of a number of target proteins, including streptavidin, concanavalin (Con A), protein A, and PDGF. In these assays, recognition molecules are anchored to the Au NP directly or through coupling reactions as shown in Fig. 3.2. Common recognition molecules for proteins include biotin, mannose, aptamers, antibodies, and others. Once specific interactions between the recognition molecules and target proteins occur, the aggregation of Au NPs leads to color changes. Representative examples of crosslinking-based assays using Au NPs are for the determination of human chorionic gonadotrophin in urine and serum.[68–70] Au NPs conjugated to antibodies are crosslinked (agglutinated) by multivalent binding to the target molecules (see Fig. 3.4). In the aggregates, the distances between Au NPs are ~25 nm, which is smaller than the size (60 nm) of the Au NPs themselves. At high concentrations (>0.1 nM) of target molecule, there is a visible color change from red to blue, but at lower concentrations, this change can only be detected with a spectrophotometer.

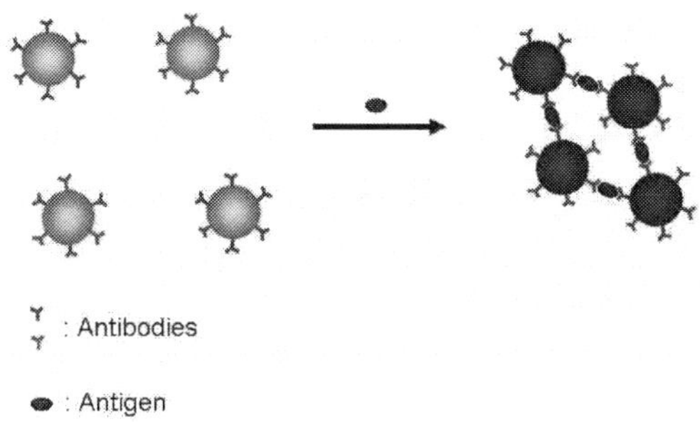

Figure 3.4 A schematic diagram of a distance-dependent sandwich assay for high-molecular-weight polyvalent antigen (green ovals) leading to agglutination of Au NPs and a redshift in their extinction spectrum. See also Color Insert.

Another interesting example is the use of Au nanoshells for protein assays. Each nanoshell consists of a silica core surrounded by a thin shell of Au atoms. By tuning the relative dimensions of the core and shell, the extinction maximum can be systematically varied from 700 to 1300 nm. One advantage of this property is that the extinction maximum can be tuned to a wavelength at which interference from absorbing molecules in blood and other matrices is minimal. Researchers have used Au nanoshells consisting of a 96 nm diameter core surrounded by a 22 nm shell for distance-dependent immunoassays for immunoglobulins in dilute serum.[71]

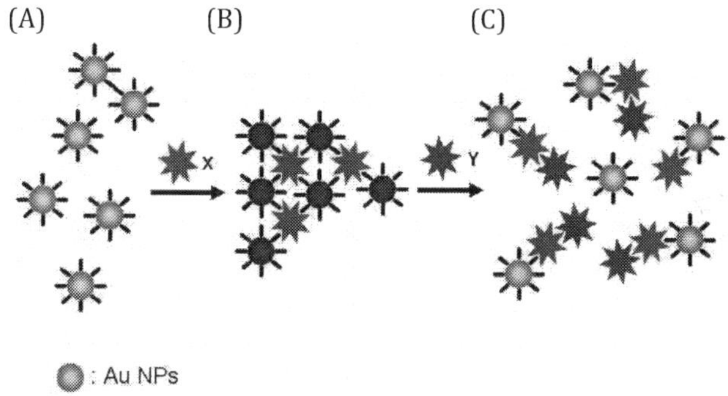

Figure 3.5 A schematic illustration for the colorimetric detection of protein–protein interactions. See also Color Insert.

Au NP-based competitive colorimetric assays are useful for the identification of proteins and the determination of the binding constants between recognition molecules and target proteins. Mannopyranoside-encapsulated Au NPs (Man-Au NPs) are used for the identification of Con A and the determination of the interaction between Con A and thyroglobulin by the naked eye.[72] In the absence of thyroglobulin, Con A-induced aggregation of the Man-Au NPs results in a color change from red to purple. In the presence of thyroglobulin, interaction of Con A and Man decreases as a result of a competitive reaction between Con A and thyroglobulin, leading to decreased aggregation. Figure 3.5 illustrates a representative detection scheme for protein–protein interactions. A protein, denoted by X, binds the ligands protruding from the Au NP surface and promotes agglomeration of the particles via multivalent ligand–protein interactions giving rise to a blue colored solution. However, the addition of a putative protein, denoted by Y, capable of interacting with protein X, influences the binding between X and

Au NPs, causing the disruption of Au NP aggregates. As a result, the color of the solution changes from purple to the original red color.

Similarly, a colorimetric bioassay using Ag NPs conjugated with 2-mercaptoethyl α-d-mannopyranoside has been used for the analysis of Con A.[34,73] Con A induces aggregation of the Man-Ag NPs, leading to color changes from yellow to brown. The color changes correspond to the changes in the LSPR absorption wavelength from 400 to 480 nm. The spectra show an isosbestic point at 440 nm upon addition of the Con A, demonstrating that the aggregation of Man-Ag NPs is directly related to the concentration of Con A. Man-Ag NPs at a concentration of 3 nM provide an assay for Con A with the largest linear range. One beneficial feature of assays using Ag NPs are their faster kinetic rates of aggregation than those using Au NPs. Self-assembled monolayers on Ag and Au surfaces have different surface orientations.[74] However, this may account for the significant difference in the rate of aggregation between the Man-Ag and Au NPs.

Protein assays based on DNA-protein interactions are common in the life sciences. Recently, DNA-conjugated Au NPs have become interesting nanomaterials for protein assays. Aptamers are especially interesting because they are easily synthesized by using an automatic DNA synthesizer and are extremely stable. Aptamers are nucleic acid macromolecules (DNA and RNA) that bind tightly to a specific molecular target (proteins and small molecules). Like all nucleic acids, a particular aptamer is described by a linear sequence of nucleotides (A, U, T, C, and G), typically 15–40 nucleotides long. In solution, the chain of nucleotides forms intramolecular interactions to fold the molecule into a complex three-dimensional shape. The shape of the aptamer allows it to bind tightly to the surface of its target molecule.

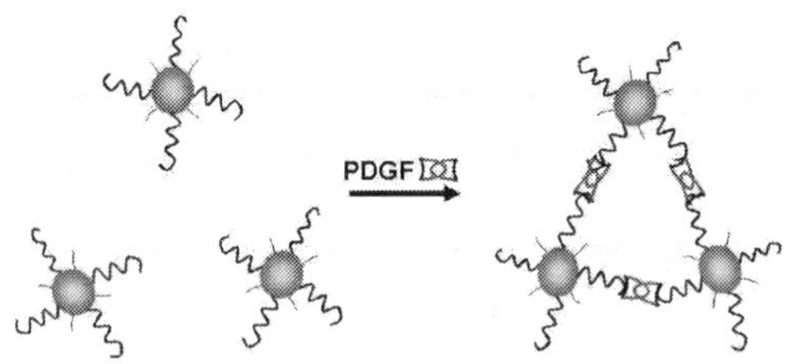

Figure 3.6 Schematics of aptamer-directed Au NP-based colorimetric sensors. Assembly of aptamer-functionalized Au NPs by a target protein (PDGF). Each PDGF can bind two aptamer molecules.

Aptamer-modified Au NPs (Apt-Au NPs) are useful for the detection of PDGF.[23] Since each PDGF can bind two aptamers, the color of Apt-Au NPs changes from red to purple at low concentrations (<400 nM) as a result of aggregation with crosslinking between the Au NPs. Interestingly, the color is reversed to red at very high PDGF concentrations (>400 nM) due to the repulsion and steric effects because the surface of the Apt-Au NPs quickly becomes saturated with PDGF molecules through aptamer-PDGF binding (see Fig. 3.6).

By plotting the ratios of the extinction coefficients of the Apt-Au NPs at 650 and 530 nm against the concentrations of PDGF–AA, the linear ranges of the increases and decreases in this extinction ratio are 25–75 and 75–200 nM, respectively. This assay can be applied to detect the PDGF receptor-β (PDGFR-β) at concentrations as low as 3.2 nM on the basis of the competition between the Apt-Au NPs and PDGFR-β for PDGF-BB. In the presence of PDGFR-β, the interaction between PDGF and Apt-Au NPs decreases, leading to a lesser extent of aggregation. Similar strategies have been demonstrated for the determination of other proteins such as thrombin, β-lactamase, and phosphatase.[75-77]

3.4.1.2 DNA and RNA assays

The first reported DNA-Au NPs for the detection of target DNA based on the aggregation of Au NPs through hybridization of two complementary DNA strands was reported in 1996.[11] Two noncomplementary DNA oligonucleotides each containing thiol groups in one end were bound to the surfaces of two batches of 13 nm Au NPs. When DNA, which is complementary to the two grafted sequences, was added to the solution, a polymer network formed (see Fig. 3.7). This condensed network causes the conjugated Au NPs to self-assemble into aggregates with a concomitant red-to-purple color change. Because of significant changes in color, this approach can detect DNA in concentrations as low as 10 fM. The sensitivity can be further improved by placing the DNA–Au NP aggregates on solid substrates such as a C18 reversed-phase thin-layer chromatography plate. The blue color can be observed by the naked eye after the plate dries.

For a given sequence, the temperature at which the reverse color change (melting) takes place depends primarily on the salt concentration but is also influenced by the distance between the particles and the density of the oligonucleotides attached to them.[78]

This temperature is always greater than the melting temperature of the corresponding duplex without Au NPs. The exact temperature at which the color change occurs is thought to depend on a mechanism in which the melting of one linker sequence promotes the melting of others.[78] Interestingly, the melting profile of the DNA-Au NP aggregation is extraordinarily sharp, occurring over a temperature range much narrower than that of the original DNA. By controlling the temperature, this approach provides a limit of detection (LOD) down to the nanomolar level for DNA with a single base mismatch resolution.

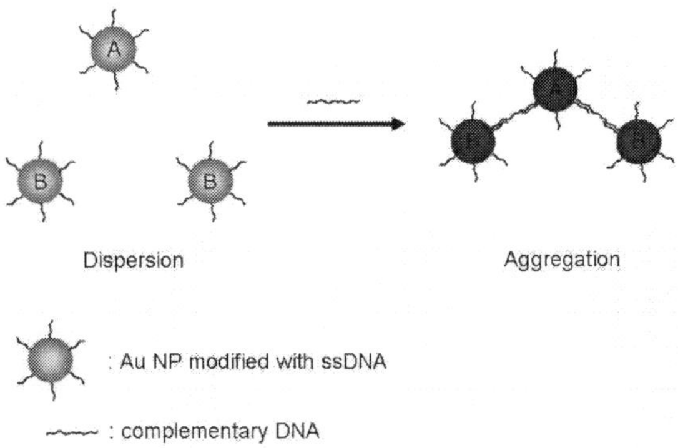

Figure 3.7 Aggregation of ssDNA-modified Au NPs by the addition of the DNA complementary to the DNA on the Au surface.

In order to further improve the sensitivity, researchers have demonstrated bio-barcode amplification approaches, using Au NPs and magnetic microparticles.[79–81] Each magnetic microparticle that has a magnetic iron oxide core with an amine-modified silane coating is functionalized with alkanethiol-capped oligonucleotides that are complementary to one 12-mer portion (5′-ATTGATAAGGAT-3′) of a target sequence using a sulfosuccinimidyl 4-*N*-maleimidomethyl cyclohexane-1-carboxylate linker. The second probe is a 30 nm Au NP modified with two types of oligonucleotides; one is complementary to the target sequence of interest (5′-GGATTATTGTTAAAT-3′), and the other is complementary to a barcode sequence that is a unique identification tag for the target sequence. After hybridization, the signal can be detected by using a spectrophotometer or a scanometric detection system after further amplification by using silver enhancement. The LODs for the two detection modes are 100 fM and 500 zM, respectively. The last detection approach provides sensitivity that is comparable to PCR-based approaches.

3.4.1.3 Small analyte assays

Colorimetric assays using conjugated Apt-Au NPs are sensitive and selective for the determination of a number of small analytes, including metal ions such as Hg^{2+} and K^+.[82,83] Selective and sensitive (LOD = 100 nM) detection of Hg^{2+} ions in aqueous solutions in the presence of 2,6-pyridinedicarboxylic acid has been realized by using 3-mercaptopropionic acid functionalized Au NPs (MPA-Au NPs), based on aggregation-induced color changes. Figure 3.8A shows the UV-visible absorption response to Hg^{2+} of a 3.0 nM suspension of MPA-Au NPs in 50 mM Tris-borate buffer at pH 9.0. The dispersed MPA-Au NPs display a LSPR band at 520 nm, which undergoes redshifts with decreased extinction (the extinction at 650 nm increases) upon aggregation. The extinctions at 520 and 650 nm are related separately to the quantities of the dispersed and aggregated MPA-Au NPs. The inset A to Fig. 3.8A displays the color changes from red to purple following the addition of 1.0 mM $Hg(NO)_3$ (100 μL) to the MPA-Au NP solution (900 μL), and the aggregated MPA-Au NPs precipitate after 1 h. As shown in inset B of Fig 3.8A, the Hg^{2+} induced aggregation of the MPA-Au NPs reaches completion within 60 min according to the monitoring of the extinction ratios ($Ex_{650/520}$) in the time frame of these measurements. Figure 3.8B,C displays the transmission electron microscopy and optical dark-field scattering images of the MPA-Au NP solutions in the absence and presence of Hg^{2+}, respectively. Owing to low scattering intensity and faster diffusion of the Au NPs (13.3 nm), the scattering light from single MPA-Au NPs is not easily observed by the dark field spectroscopy system. It is important to highlight that strong scattering occurs once the MPA-Au NPs aggregate; the orange and red spots correspond to the scattering images of the MPA-Au NP aggregates.

Apt-Au NPs have also been developed for the detection of small solutes such as adenosine and cocaine based on reversed sensing mechanisms (from aggregation to suspension).[84,85] The NP aggregates contain Apt-Au NPs (3′- and 5′-thiol-modified DNA) and a linker DNA molecule that is divided into two segments, including hybridized and recognized sites. In the presence of adenosine, the aptamer changes its structure to bind adenosine, leading to the disruption of the aggregates and thus a change in the solution color from purple to red at room temperature. Under optimized conditions, the approach provides an LOD of 20 μM for the adenosine by the naked eye.

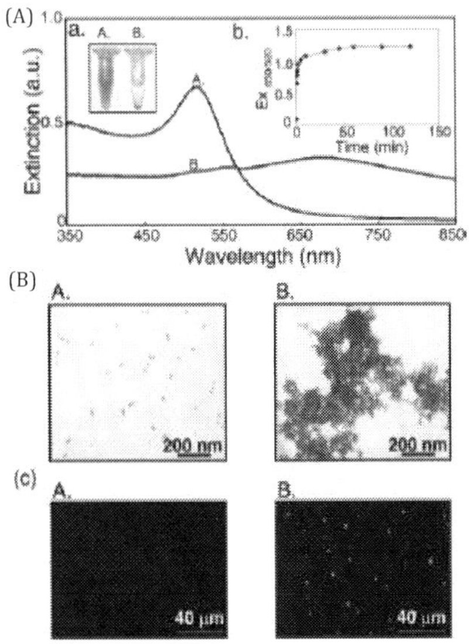

Figure 3.8 (A) UV-Vis absorbance spectra, (B) TEM, and (C) scattering images of solutions containing MPA-Au NPs in the (A) absence and (B) presence (100 mM) of Hg^{2+}. Reprinted with permission from ref. 82.

3.4.2 Non-Crosslinking Aggregation-Based Assays

In non-crosslinking aggregation-based assays, the controlled loss of electrostatic, steric, or electrosteric stabilizations without the formation of interparticle bonds induces the aggregation of Au NPs. The non-crosslinking aggregation process is much more rapid than that of the crosslinking systems, which takes several tens of minutes to hours at room temperature. In non-crosslinking systems, aggregation is driven by the London–van der Waals attractive force between NPs. On the other hand, in crosslinking systems, the kinetics of the aggregation is dominated by random collisions between the NPs with relatively slow Brownian motion. However, non-crosslinking detection systems suffer from poor sensitivity and selectivity since many factors, such as changes in the pH, ionic strength, and nonspecific adsorption of the solutes from the samples, may cause instability of the Au NPs to various extents.

3.4.2.1 DNA assays

Poly(*N*-isopropylacrylamide)-DNA-conjugated Au NPs are useful for the detection of single-stranded DNA above the physiological temperature. The conjugated Au NPs are stable at 1.5 M NaCl. Because of the great negative charge density from the conjugated DNA on the Au NP surface, the repulsion force is dominant. In the presence of the target DNA that is perfectly complementary to the probe, in sequence as well as in chain length, the conjugated Au NPs aggregate, leading to a change in color. When DNA hybridization occurs, the charge density on the Au NP surface decreases. Similar phenomena also occurred using bare Au NPs (without capping with the probe DNA) for detection of DNA.[86,87] Bare Au NPs immediately aggregate at 0.1 M NaCl while they do not exhibit any visible change in solutions with concentrations up to 2.5 M NaCl in the presence of DNA because DNA molecules assemble around the Au NP surfaces through electrostatic interactions (see Fig. 3.9). In the presence of a target DNA molecule with complementary sequences to the probe DNA, a clear colorimetric change from red to purple immediately occurs (<3 min) at NaCl concentrations greater than 0.5 M. Similar strategies have been applied to the studies of eukaryotic gene expression, *Mycobacterium tuberculosis* DNA, and single nucleotide polymorphism in clinical samples.[88–90]

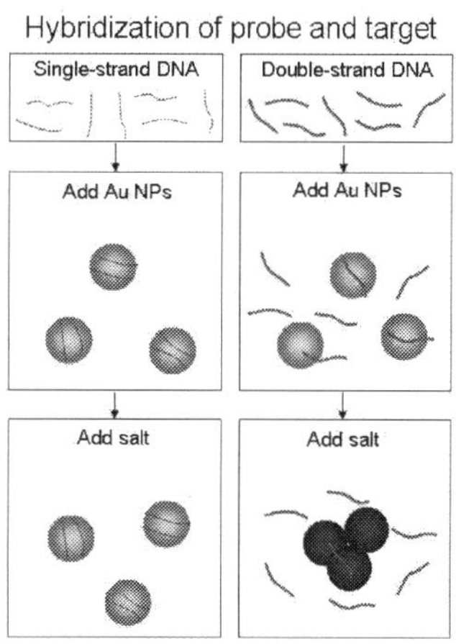

Figure 3.9 Pictorial representation of the colorimetric method for differentiating between single- and double-stranded oligonucleotides. The circles represent colloidal gold nanoparticles.

3.4.2.2 Protein and small analyte assays

Apt-Au NPs are useful for the analysis of small molecules such as adenosine triphosphate (ATP), cocaine, DNase I, and Pb^{2+}.[91–93] Similar to protein assays, the small analytes induced aggregation of Apt-Au NPs through their specific interactions with the aptamers. Figure 3.10 illustrates a representative colorimetric assay for ATP.[94] Aliquots of salt (e.g., 300.0 mM NaCl) are added to Apt-Au NPs in solutions with and without ATP. The solution without ATP changes color from wine red to purple as a result of aggregation while the one containing ATP retains its original color. A decreased zeta potential due to salt screening is the main cause of the instability of the Apt-Au NP solutions without ATP. Once ATP binds to the Apt-Au NPs, the aptamer on the Au NP surfaces folds into a four-stranded tetraplex structure (G-quartet).[95] In addition, the negatively charged density on the Apt-Au NP surfaces increases. Polyethylene glycol promotes the structural rigidity of the G-quartet, and TOTO-3 stabilizes the stem structure of the aptamer. The linear range and LOD of this sensing system for ATP are 20.0–100.0 nM and 10.0 nM, respectively.

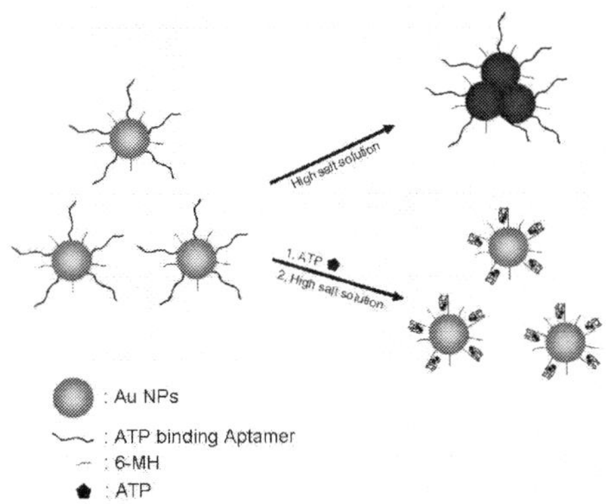

Figure 3.10 A schematic representation of the sensing mechanism of Apt-Au NPs for the colorimetric determination of ATP.

Similarly, Apt-Au NPs are useful for the detection of thrombin.[96] When thrombin interacts with its aptamer (29 base single-stranded DNA), the aptamer is much more inclined to fold into a G-quadruplex/duplex structure. Unfolded ssDNA can stabilize the Au NPs in the presence of a given high concentration of salt while the quadruplex/duplex structure can destroy this protecting function, leading to the aggregation of the Au NPs.[87] This approach provides an LOD of 500 nM for thrombin.

The detection of Pb^{2+} ions is of great importance to human health and for environmental monitoring. Recently, researchers have developed several varieties of DNAzyme-based analytical methods for Pb^{2+} detection. DNAzymes are small catalytic DNA molecules that efficiently cleave target RNA molecules. The catalytic activity of some DNAzymes is specific toward divalent metal ions — just as the catalytic activity of some protein enzymes is dependent on metal ion cofactors.[97] Taking advantage of the high specificity of 17E DNAzyme for Pb^{2+}, highly sensitive and selective colorimetric sensors have been developed for Pb^{2+}. Lu and coworkers recently developed a strategy based on 17E DNAzyme, involving Au NPs as the sensing elements.[98,99] The DNAzyme molecules are modified onto the Au NPs and then hybridize with the substrate to form duplex DNA. The dissociation of DNA strands from the Au NP surfaces results in Au NP aggregation at a high salt concentration because the unfolded single-stranded DNA can be adsorbed on the citrate-protected Au NPs while double-stranded DNA (dsDNA) cannot. Thus, unfolded ssDNA stabilizes the Au NPs in the presence of a given high concentration of salt while dsDNA cannot, and the Au NPs aggregate in the presence of the same concentration of salt. A similar strategy has been developed for Pb^{2+} using unmodified Au NPs.[100] Initially, 17E DNAzyme is hybridized with its substrate to form the duplex. In the presence of Pb^{2+}, the substrate strand is cleaved, resulting in the release of fragments that are adsorbed on the Au NP probes, leading to stable Au NPs in the presence of a given high concentration of salt (the red solution appears). In the absence of Pb^{2+}, however, the remaining duplex cannot be adsorbed on the Au NP probes, leading to the formation of Au NP aggregates (see Fig. 3.11). The detection of Pb^{2+} can be realized within 20 min with a detection limit of 500 nM.

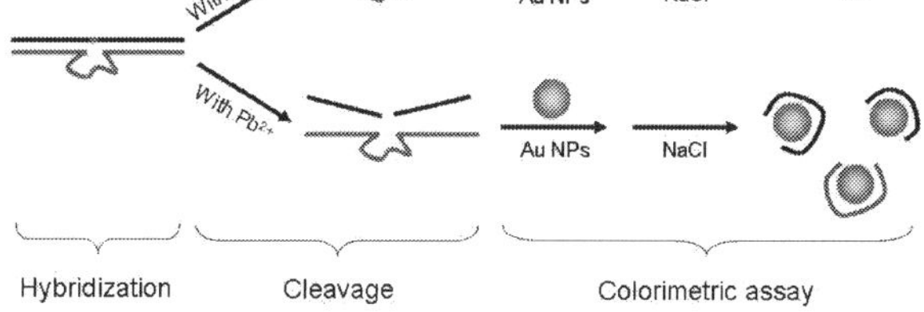

Figure 3.11 Strategy for Pb^{2+} detection using Au NP colorimetry.

Selective sensing of Hg^{2+} using DNA-conjugated Au NPs is practical via thymine–Hg–thymine (T–Hg^{2+}–T) coordinatination.[101] Poly-T_n ssDNA (n = 33, 50, or 80) and Au NPs (13 nm diameter) in the presence of salt are used for the detection of Hg^{2+} ions based on Hg^{2+}-DNA complexes inducing the aggregation of Au NPs (see Fig. 3.12). Random coil DNA molecules adsorb onto Au NP surfaces through electrostatic attraction. In the presence of salt, poly-T_n ssDNA on the surface of Au NPs remains in a random coil structure as a result of the electrostatic repulsion between DNA molecules. Owing to the high negative charge density of DNA on each Au NP surface, monodisperse Au NPs exist in the salt solution. Upon formation of Hg^{2+}–DNA complexes through T–Hg^{2+}–T coordination, the conformation of the poly-T_n ssDNA changes to folded structures. As a result of the decreased zeta potential on each Au NP and the reduced degree of electrostatic repulsion between Au NPs, aggregation of the Au NPs occurs, and hence, the color of the solution changes from red to purple in a process that is detectable by the naked eye. The LOD for Hg^{2+} at a signal-to-noise ratio of 3 is about 250 nM.

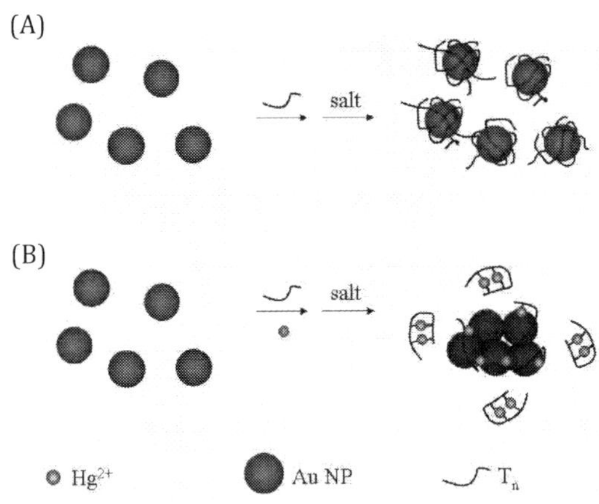

Figure 3.12 Schematic representation of Hg^{2+} nanosensors. Reprinted with permission from ref. 101.

A label-free, sensitive, selective, and simple enzyme colorimetric assay using unmodified Ag NPs is practical for the determination of the activity of enzymes,[102] based on the fact that the dispersed Ag NP solution is yellow whereas the aggregated Ag NPs solution is pale red (or brown). Enzymatic reactions concerning ATP dephosphorylation by calf intestine alkaline phosphatase (CIAP) and peptide phosphorylation by protein kinase A (PKA) are representative. In the absence of the enzymes, unreacted ATP protects Ag NPs from salt-induced aggregation whereas in the presence of the enzymes, the reaction product of ATP (i.e., adenosine for CIAP and ADP for PKA) cannot (see Fig. 3.13). The colors of Ag colloidal solutions containing ATP in the absence and presence of CIAP are yellow and pale red, respectively, after the addition of 15 μL of 0.5 M NaCl. A similar strategy is also useful for the determination of PKA activity using a phosphorylation of the PKA substrate H-Leu-Arg-Arg-Ala-Ser-Leu-Gly-OH (peptide 1) (see Fig. 3.13). When PKA phosphorylates 1 mol of peptide 1, 1 mol of ATP is consumed to form 1 mol of ADP. As a result, the color of the Ag NP solution changes from yellow to yellowish brown in the presence of PKA. This approach provides LODs of 1 and 0.022 unit/mL for CIAP and PKA, respectively.

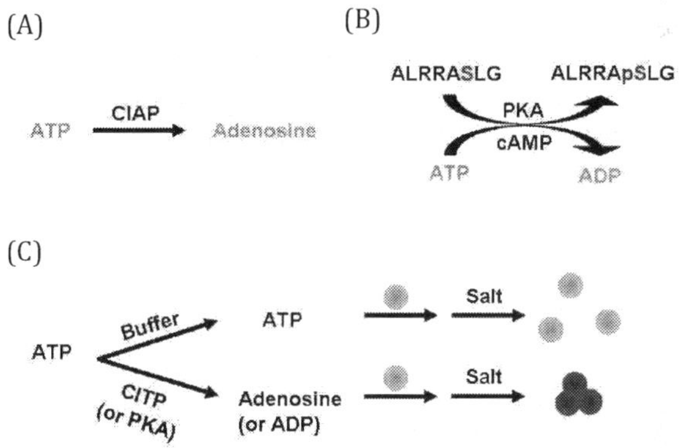

Figure 3.13 Enzymatic reactions with (A) CIAP and (B) PKA and (C) an Ag NP-based enzyme colorimetric assay.

3.5 Summary

In this chapter, we present Au and Ag NP-based colorimetric assays for the determination of various analytes, including DNA, antigens, and proteins. Au NPs offer advantages such as high molar extinction coefficients, simple preparation and bioconjugation, and biocompatibility and thus are the most popular nanomaterials for colorimetric assays. After suitable bioconjugation, functionalized Au NPs provide high sensitivity and selectivity for many biomolecules.

The key factor in these assays is to control aggregation and dispersion stages of NPs that are guided by interparticle attractive and repulsive forces. Thus, control of the charge densities on the NP surfaces through capping, functionalization, and selection of suitable media is extremely important to provide highly selective and sensitive colorimetric assays. Adding hydrophilic polymers and polyelectrolytes is practical for minimal nonspecific interactions, which decrease errors that usually occur when NPs are applied to biological samples. In order to realize this advantage, functionalization and stabilization strategies for improving the selectivity of NPs are required. Because anisotropic Au and Ag NPs possess high molar absorptivility in the near infrared region, they also hold great potential for colorimetric bioassays. However, more advanced functionalization approaches are required.

Acknowledgments

This work was supported by the National Science Council of Taiwan under contracts NSC 98-2113-M-002-011-MY3 and NSC 99-2113-M-018-005-MY2. We would like to thank those who provided preprints that were used in this article.

References

1. D. H. Charych, J. O. Nagy, W. Spevak, and M. Bednarski, *Science*, **261**, 585. (1993).
2. A. Reichert, J. O. Nagy, W. Spevak, and D. H. Charych, *J. Am. Chem. Soc.*, **117**, 829 (1995).
3. Z. F. Ma, J. R. Li, M. H. Liu, J. Cao, Z. Y. Zou, J. Tu, and L. Jiang, *J. Am. Chem. Soc.*, **120**, 12678 (1998).
4. T. A. Byassee, W. C. W. Chan, and S. M. Nie, *Anal. Chem.*, **72**, 5606 (2000).
5. W. E. Moerner and M. Orrit, *Science*, **283**, 1670 (1999).
6. S. Tyagi and F. R. Kramer, *Nat. Biotechnol.*, **14**, 303 (1996).
7. M. A. El-Sayed, *Acc. Chem. Res.*, **34**, 257 (2001).
8. N. L. Rosi and C. A. Mirkin, *Chem. Rev.*, **105**, 1547 (2005).
9. E. Katz and I. Willner, *Angew. Chem., Int. Ed.*, **43**, 6042 (2004).
10. M. C. Daniel and D. Astruc. *Chem. Rev.*, **104**, 293–346 (2004).
11. C. A. Mirkin, R. L. Letsinger, R. C. Mucic, and J. J. Storhoff, *Nature*, **382**, 607 (1996).

12. J. J. Storhoff, A. A. Lazarides, R. C. Mucic, C. A. Mirkin, R. L. Letsinger, and G. C. Schatz, *J. Am. Chem. Soc.*, **122**, 4640 (2000).

13. H. Otsuka, Y. Akiyama, Y. Nagasaki, and K. Kataoka, *J. Am. Chem. Soc.*, **123**, 8226 (2001).

14. D. C. Hone, A. H. Haines, and D. A. Russell, *Langmuir*, **19**, 7141 (2003).

15. S. Lin, S. Liu, C. Lin, and C. Chen, *Anal. Chem.*, **74**, 330 (2002).

16. Y. Kim, R. C. Johnson, and J. T. Hupp, *Nano Lett.*, **1**, 165 (2001).

17. S. O. Obare, R. E. Hollowell, and C. J. Murphy, *Langmuir*, **18**, 10407 (2002).

18. A. J. Reynolds, A. H. Haines, and D. A. Russell, *Langmuir*, **22**, 1156 (2006).

19. S.-Y. Lin, C.-H. Chen, M.-C. Lin, and H.-F. Hsu, *Anal. Chem.*, **77**, 4821 (2005).

20. N. T. K. Thanh and Z. Rosenzweig, *Anal. Chem.*, **74**, 1624 (2002).

21. J. Liu and Y. Lu, *Angew. Chem. Int. Ed.*, **45**, 90 (2006).

22. C. Guarise, L. Pasquato, V. de Fillippis, and P. Scrimin, *Proc. Natl. Acad. Sci.*, **103**, 3978 (2006).

23. C.-C. Huang, Y.-F. Huang, Z. Cao, W. Tan, and H.-T. Chang, *Anal. Chem.*, **77**, 5735 (2005).

24. M. Sastry, N. Lala, V. Patil, S. P. Chavan, and A. G. Chittiboyina, *Langmuir*, **14**, 4138 (1998).

25. Y. W. Cao, R. Jin, and C. A. Mirkin, *J. Am. Chem. Soc.*, **123**, 7961 (2001).

26. R. C. Jin, Y. W. Cao, C. A. Mirkin, K. L. Kelly, G. C. Schatz, and J. G. Zheng, *Science*, **294**, 1901 (2001).

27. L. J. Sherry, R. C. Jin, C. A. Mirkin, G. C. Schatz, R. P., and Van Duyne, *Nano Lett.*, **6**, 2060 (2006).

28. H. Wei, J. Li, T. L. Wang, and E. K. Wang, *Nanotechnology*, **18**, 295603 (2007).

29. G. Braun, S. J. Lee, M. Dante, T. Q. Nguyen, M. Moskovits, and N. Reich, *J. Am. Chem. Soc.*, **129**, 6378 (2007).

30. J. S. Lee, A. K. R. Lytton-Jean, S. J. Hurst, and C. A. Mirkin, *Nan. Lett.*, **7**, 2112 (2007).

31. Y. Chen, J. Aveyard, and R. Wilson, *Chem. Commun.*, 2804 (2004).

32. S. H. Liu, Z. H. Zhang, and M. Y. Han, *Anal. Chem.*, **77**, 2595 (2005).

33. K. Yoosaf, B. I. Ipe, C. H. Suresh, and K. G. Thomas, *J. Phys. Chem. C*, **111**, 12839 (2007).

34. C. L. Schofield, A. H. Haines, R. A. Field, and D. A. Russell, *Langmuir*, **22**, 6707 (2006).

35. Y. Sun and Y. Xia, *Science*, **298**, 2176 (2002).

36. P. Baptista, E. Pereira, P. Eaton, G. Doria, A. Miranda, I. Gomes, P. Quaresma, and R. Franco, *Anal. Bioanal. Chem.*, **391**, 943 (2008).
37. J. Turkevich, *Gold Bulletin*, **18**, 86 (1985).
38. D. V. Goia, and E. Matijevic, *New J. Chem.*, **22**, 1203 (1988).
39. D. V. Goia and E. Matijevic, *Colloids Surf. A-Physicochem. Eng. Aspects*, **146**, 139 (1999).
40. P. Y. Silvert, R. HerreraUrbina, N. Duvauchelle, V. Vijayakrishnan, and K. T. Elhsissen, *J. Mater. Chem.*, **6**, 573 (1996).
41. D. A. Handley, *Colloidal Gold: Principles, Methods, and Applications* (Vol. 1), Academic Press, San Diego, CA, pp. 13 (1989).
42. M. Brust, M. Walker, D. Bethell, D. J. Schiffrin, and R. Whyman, *J. Chem. Soc., Chem. Commun.*, **7**, 801 (1994).
43. Y. Cao, R. Jin, and C. A. Mirkin, *J. Am. Chem. Soc.*, **123**, 7961 (2001).
44. C. J. Murphy and N. R. Jana, *Adv. Mater.*, **14**, 80 (2002).
45. S. R. Nicewarner-Pena, R. G. Freeman, B. D. Reiss, L. He, D. J. Pena, I. D. Walton, R. Cromer, C. D. Keating, and M. J. Natan, *Science*, **294**, 137 (2001).
46. Y.-F. Huang, Y.-W. Lin, and H.-T. Chang, *Nanotechnology*, **17**, 4885 (2006).
47. R. C. Jin, Y. W. Cao, C. A. Mirkin, K. L. Kelly, G. C. Schatz, and J. G. Zheng, *Science*, **294**, 1901 (2001).
48. Z. Yang, T.-C. Chiu, and H.-T. Chang, *Open Nanosci. J.*, **1**, 5 (2007).
49. Z. Yang and H.-T. Chang, *Nanotechnology*, **17**, 2304 (2006).
50. Y.-F. Huang, Y.-W. Lin, and H.-T. Chang, *Nanotechnology*, **17**, 4885 (2006).
51. Z.-H. Lin, Y.-W. Lin, K.-H. Lee, and H.-T. Chang, *J. Mater. Chem.*, **18**, 2569 (2008).
52. N. R. Jana, L. Gearheart, and C. J. Murphy, *Adv. Mater.*, **13**, 1389 (2001).
53. D. H. Napper, *Polymeric Stabilization of Colloidal Dispersions*, Academic Press, London (1983).
54. H. W. Walker and S. B. Grant, *Langmuir*, **12**, 3151 (1996).
55. J. Turkevich, P. C. Stevenson, and J. Hillier, *Discuss. Faraday Soc.*, **11**, 55 (1951).
56. T.-C. Chiu, S.-H. Chiou, M.-M. Hsieh, Y.-T. Chen, and H.-T. Chang, *J. Nanosci. Nanotech.*, **5**, 1 (2005).
57. R. J. Hunter, *Foundations of Colloid Science*, Oxford University Press, New York, (2004).
58. A. Gole, C. J. Murphy, *Langmuir*, **21**, 10756 (2005).

59. R. Gref, P. Couvreur, G. Barratt, E. Mysiakine, *Biomaterials*, **24**, 4529 (2003).
60. A. Gole and C. J. Murphy, *Langmuir*, **21**, 10756 (2005).
61. R. Wilson, Y. Chen, and J. Aveyard, *Chem. Commun.*, 1156 (2004).
62. Y. Sun and Y. Xia, *Analyst*, **128**, 686 (2003).
63. K. Aslan, J. R. Lakowicz, and C. D. Geddes, *Anal. Biochem.*, **330**, 145 (2004).
64. S. K. Ghosh and T. Pal, *Chem. Rev.*, **107**, 4797 (2007).
65. K. Aslan, J. R. Lakowicz, and C. D. Geddes, *Anal. Chim. Acta*, **517**, 139 (2004).
66. K. Aslan, J. R. Lakowicz, and C. D. Geddes, *Anal. Biochem.*, **330**, 145 (2004).
67. C.-C. Huang and H.-T. Chang, *Anal. Chem.*, **78**, 8332 (2006).
68. J. H. W. Leuvering, P. J. H. M. Thal, M. V. D. van der Waart, and A. H. W. M. Schuurs, *Fresenius' J. Anal. Chem.*, **301**, 132 (1980).
69. J. H. W. Leuvering, P. J. H. M. Thal, M. V. D. van der Waart, and A. H. W. M. Schuurs *J. Immunol. Methods*, **45**, 183 (1981).
70. J. H. W. Leuvering, B. C. Goverde, P. J. H. M. Thal, and A. H. W. M. Schuurs., *J. Immunol. Methods*, **60**, 9 (1983).
71. L. R. Hirsch, J. B. Jackson, A. Lee, N. J. Halas and J. West, *Anal. Chem.*, **75**, 2377 (2003).
72. C.-S. Tsai, T.-B. Yu, and C.-T. Chen, *Chem. Commun.*, 4273 (2005).
73. T. K. Dam and C. F. Brewer, *Chem. Rev.*, **102**, 387 (2002).
74. P. Harder, M. Grunze, R. Dahint, G. M. Whitesides, and P. E. Laibinis, *J. Phys. Chem. B*, **102**, 426 (1998).
75. R. Stoltenburg, C. Reinemann, and B. Strehlitz, *Biomol. Eng.*, **24**, 381 (2007).
76. Z. Wu, S. Zhang, M. Guo, C. Chen, G. Shen, and R. Yu, *Anal. Chim. Acta*, **584**, 122 (2007).
77. R. Liu, R. Liew, J. Zhou, and B. Xing, *Angew. Chem.*, **119**, 2069 (2007).
78. R. C. Jin, G. S. Wu, Z. Li, C. A. Mirkin, and G. C. Schatz, *J. Am. Chem. Soc.*, **125**, 1643 (2003).
79. J.-M. Nam, C. S. Thaxton, and C. A. Mirkin, *Science*, **301**, 1884 (2003).
80. J.-M. Nam, S. I. Stoeva, and C. A. Mirkin, *J. Am. Chem. Soc.*, **126**, 5932 (2004).
81. E. D. Goluch, J.-M. Nam, D. G. Georganopoulou, T. N. Chiesl, K. A. Shaikh, K. S. Ryu, A. E. Barron, C. A. Mirkin, and C. Liu, *Lab Chip*, **6**, 1293 (2006).

82. C.-C. Huang and H.-T. Chang, *Chem. Commun.*, 1215 (2007).
83. S.-Y. Lin, S.-W. Liu, C.-M. Lin, and C-H. Chen *Anal. Chem.*, **74**, 330 (2002).
84. J. Liu, and Y. Lu, *Org. Biomol. Chem.*, **4**, 3435 (2006).
85. J. Liu, and Y. Lu, *Adv. Mater.*, **18**, 1667 (2006).
86. K. Sato, K. Hosokawa, and M. Maeda, *J. Am. Chem. Soc.*, **125**, 8102 (2003).
87. H. Li, L. Rothberg, *Proc. Natl. Acad. Sci. U. S. A.*, **101**, 14036 (2004).
88. P. V. Baptista, G. Doria, D. Henriques, E. Pereira, and R. Franco, *J. Biotechnol.*, **119**, 111 (2005).
89. P. V. Baptista, M. Koziol-Montewka, J. Paluch-Oles, G. Doria, and R. Franco, *Clin. Chem.*, **52**, 1433 (2006).
90. G. Doria, R. Franco, and P. V. Baptista, *Nanobiotechnology*, **1**, 53 (2007).
91. J. Liu, and Y. Lu, *Angew. Chem. Int. Ed.*, **45**, 90 (2006).
92. W. Zhao, W. Chiuman, M. A. Brook, and Y. Li, *Chem. Bio. Chem.*, **8**, 727 (2007).
93. W. Zhao, J. C. F. Lam, W. Chiuman, M. A. Brook, and Y. Li, *small*, **4**, 810 (2008).
94. S.-J. Chen, Y.-F. Huang, C.-C. Huang, K.-H. Lee, Z.-H. Lin, and H.-T. Chang, *Biosensors and Bioelectronics*, **23**, 1749 (2008).
95. J. Wang, Y. Jiang, C. Zhou, and X. Fang, *Anal. Chem.*, **77**, 3542 (2005).
96. D. M. Tasset, M. F. Kubik, and W. Steiner, *J. Mol. Biol.*, **272**, 688 (1997).
97. K. E. Nelson, P. F. Bruesehoff, and Y. Lu, *J. Mol. Evol.*, **61** 216 (2005).
98. J. W. Liu, and Y. Lu, *J. Am. Chem. Soc.*, **125**, 6642 (2003).
99. J. W. Liu, and Y. Lu, *J. Am. Chem. Soc.*, **126**, 12298 (2004).
100. H. Wei, B. Li, J. Li, S. Dong, and E. Wang, *Nanotechnology*, **19**, 095501 (2008).
101. C.-W. Liu, Y.-T. Hsieh, C.-C. Huang, Z.-H. Lin and H.-T. Chang, *Chem. Commun.*, 2242 (2008).
102. H. Wei, C. Chen, B. Han, and E. Wang, *Anal. Chem.*, **80**, 7051 (2008).

Chapter 4

Slide- and Micoarray-Based Biosensors Using Noble Metal Nanoparticles

Ping-Ji Huang[a,c] **and Lai-Kwan Chau**[a,b,*]

[a]*Department of Chemistry and Biochemistry, National Chung Cheng University, 168 University Road, Min-Hsiung, Chia-Yi 621, Taiwan*
[b]*Center for Nano Bio-Detection, National Chung Cheng University, 168 University Road, Min-Hsiung, Chia-Yi 621, Taiwan*
[c]*Institute of Nuclear Energy Research, Atomic Energy Council, 1000 Wenhua Road, Chiaan Village, Lungtan, Taoyuan 325, Taiwan*
[*]chelkc@ccu.edu.tw

Localized surface plasmon resonance (LSPR) excitation in noble metal nanoparticles (NMNPs) produces strong extinction spectra that in recent years have been used for chemical and biological sensing. This chapter describes recent developments in LSPR sensing that utilize key relationships governing the LSPR spectra, particularly wavelength shift, and their sensitivity to the local environment, including particle size and shape. Since the detection process is based on the change of refractive index of the surrounding medium when the analyte interacts with a molecular group on the nanoparticle surface, the sensor is label free.

From Bioimaging to Biosensors: Noble Metal Nanoparticles in Biodetection
Edited by Lai-Kwan Chau and Huan-Tsung Chang

ISBN 978-981-4267-24-3 (Hardcover), 978-981-4303-10-1 (eBook)
www.panstanford.com

4.1 Introduction

The development of biosensors for the analysis of biomolecular recognition and biomolecular interactions, such as diagnosis and monitoring of diseases, drug discovery, proteomics, and environmental detection of biological agents, is in progress to find methods that enable simple but efficient and sensitive affinity-based detection schemes. Some methods required labeling of the target analyte with fluorescent dyes or radioactive markers often interfere with the biorecognition reactions under investigation (see Fig. 4.1A). Moreover, the labeling process is a time-consuming step during the analysis process and it is difficult to homogeneously label multiple targets in a complex biological sample. Enzyme-linked immunosorbent assay (ELISA) is an attractive and well-established approach to avoid this problem by using some kind of labeled secondary recognition element which binds specifically to already captured target molecules in a subsequent step of the analysis (see Fig. 4.1B).[1] However, this assay does not allow for real-time analysis of the biomolecular interactions and cannot obtain essential information for the determination of reaction rate, affinity constants, and kinetic pathways.

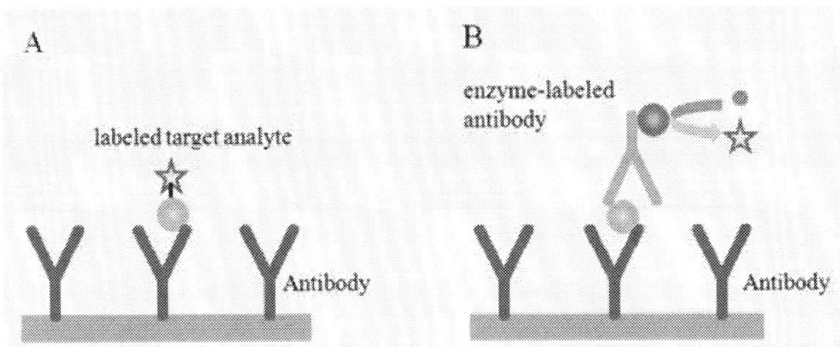

Figure 4.1 Illustration of two different schemes for biosensing: (A) target analytes are labeled with fluorescent dyes or radioactive markers; (B) secondary recognition elements with enzyme-labeled are used for detection of target analyte.

Fundamentally, a biosensor is derived from the coupling of a ligand–receptor binding reaction to a signal transducer. A large number of transducer principles are currently being utilized in affinity-based, label-free signal transduction of biomolecular recognition events, and most of them provide real-time information about interfacial binding reactions. Some examples of those are mechanical,[2,3] magnetic,[4,5] electric,[6] and optical methods[7]. Optical techniques, in particular noble metal film-based surface plasmon resonance (SPR),[8,9] are the most common among these methods (see Fig. 4.2). There are some reasons for this. First, since they all rely on changes in refractive index induced by biomolecular binding reactions confined to the interface, there is, in principle, no limitation on the nature of the interactions that can be probed. Second, because there is a linear relationship between refractive index increment and the concentration of biomolecule, the changes in signal are generally proportional to the number of bound molecules, and it is possible to translate the signal into absolute mass uptake. Third, the readout process does not affect the molecules, and many of the optical techniques are compatible with miniaturization and microfluidics.

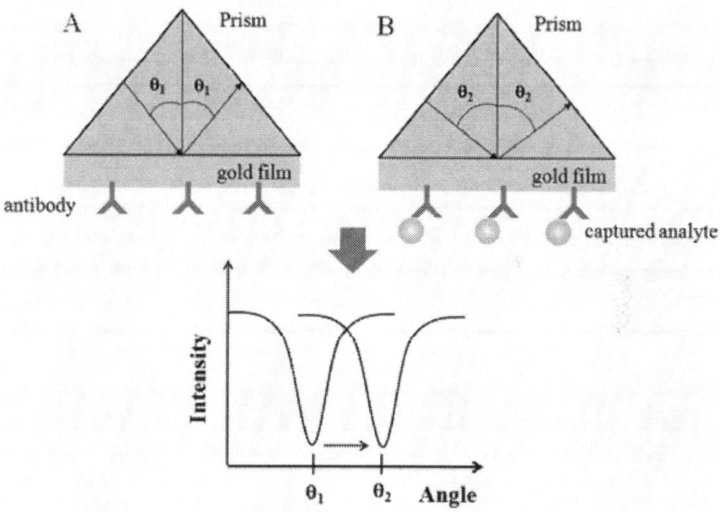

Figure 4.2 Schematic illustration of propagating surface plasmon resonance. The sensor surface is deposited with gold thin film and attached with antibodies. (A) The sensor surface is gold with antibodies attached to it. (B) As the target analyte binds to the antibodies, the refractive index shifts and the reflected light moves from original angle (θ_1) to larger angle (θ_2).

4.2 Localized Surface Plasmon Resonance

For the development of integrated lab-on-a-chip and array-based biosensors,[10] the LSPR phenomenon[11–13] associated with nanoscale structures of noble metals appears to be especially attractive. This is due to a change in interfacial refractive index upon biomolecular binding induces a change in the color of the sensor substrate, thus providing an easily detectable optical signal. Moreover, since LSPR excitations are confined to the nanostructures, miniaturization down to the scale of single nanoparticle can be accomplished. This is a strong contrast to conventional SPR, also call propagating surface plasmon resonance (PSPR), in which the laterally propagating nature of the surface plasmon polaritons[14] limits the lateral resolution to tens of micrometers.[15] In PSPR, bulk plasmons cannot be excited by freely propagating light owing to the longitudinal nature of the oscillating charges in the plasmon and the transverse nature of the electric field of light. As such, a momentum matching scheme such as prism coupling or Bragg scattering is required for excitation of PSPR.[16] On the contrary, LSPR is attributed to the collective oscillations of surface electrons in a nanostructure excited directly by an incident optical wave, resulting in peaks in the extinction (absorption and

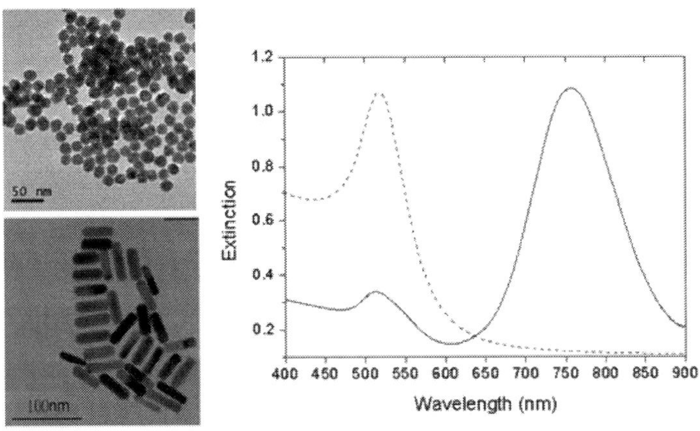

Figure 4.3 (Left) Transmission electron micrographs of Au nanospheres (upper left) and Au nanorods (lower left) and (Right) UV-vis absorption spectra of a sample of Au nanorods having an aspect ratio of 3.2 (solid line) compared to that of 16 nm Au nanospheres (dot line).

scattering) spectrum at wavelengths determined by the size,[17] shape,[18] or arrangement[19,20] of the nanostructures. An example of various morphologies and their corresponding LSPR spectra are shown in Fig. 4.3. The sensitivity of LSPR-based sensors in terms of the changes in peak position and peak magnitude upon variations in bulk or interfacial refractive index varies with these parameters.[17,18] This interfacial phenomenon is analogous to conventional PSPR, and has been utilized to determine biomolecular binding on the surface of a colloid in suspension.[21,22]

4.3 Slide-Based LSPR Biosensors

For the development of a LSPR biosensor fabricated in a planar, slide-based format using immobilized NMNPs on an optically transparent substrate, there are, in general, three advantages for this purpose. First, because most of, NMNPs permit the transmission of light in the visible region of the electromagnetic spectrum, in principle, a slide-based LSPR sensor should enable LSPR to be performed in transmission mode or reflection mode by a UV-visible spectrophotometer. Second, LSPR biosensing can be performed with nanostructures on solid surfaces to avoid the need to control the delicate balance between keeping the biofunctionalized particles in aqueous solution for measurements and aggregation of particles due to biomolecular interactions since extensive biomolecular interactions may cause gradual sedimentation of the particles over time. Third, slide-based sensor can be designed in an array format for rapid, high-throughput screening of biomolecular interactions.

A biorecognition couple, biotin–streptavidin, was the model couple for creating a ligand–receptor binding reaction in a LSPR-based biosensor. In one of these examples, biotin was attached to 13 nm diameter Au nanospheres (AuNPs) which were previously immobilized on a glass substrate through an amino or mercapto functionalized silane linker (see Fig. 4.4).[23] Local refractive index changes induced by the binding of streptavidin were monitored via the UV-vis spectral changes in transmission mode. This spectrophotometric sensor shows concentration-dependent binding and a detection limit of 16 nM for streptavidin. Upon optimization of the size of AuNP, it has been found that the LSPR sensor fabricated from 39 nm diameter AuNPs exhibits maximum sensitivity to the change of the bulk refractive index. The detection limit (DL) for streptavidin–biotin binding by a sensor fabricated from 39 nm diameter AuNPs is 20-fold better than a sensor fabricated from 13 nm diameter AuNPs.[17] Moreover, Au and Ag nanoparticles functionalized with bovine or human serum albumin and attached to glass substrates were also used to detect the respective antibody and a detection limit of about 10 nM was achieved.[24,25]

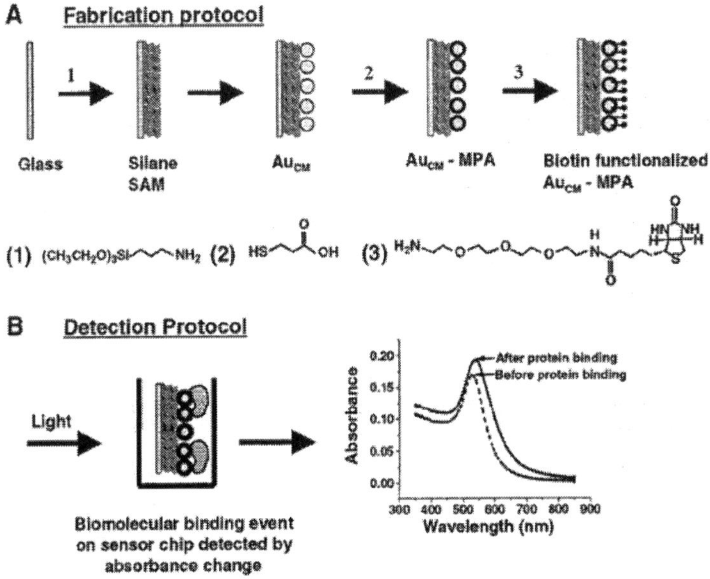

Figure 4.4 (A) Schematic of the steps involved in the fabrication of the immobilized colloidal gold sensor chip on glass. Glass substrate was functionalized with APTES (1) to provide an amine-terminated surface for formation of a monolayer of gold nanoparticles. Self-assembled monolayer of MPA (2) on gold nanoparticles provides a reactive carboxyl group that can be further modified by biotin (3) to study specific binding of streptavidin. (B) Biomolecular binding at the surface of the functionalized gold monolayer results in a shift in peak wavelength as well as an increase in intensity. Reprinted with permission from ref. 23, Copyright 2002, American Chemical Society.

The refractive index sensitivity (RIS) of LSPR-based sensors in terms of wavelength-shift can be largely influenced by the size or shape of NMNPs. The change in the LSPR band position as a function of the bulk refractive index around the nanoparticles has been reported for nanorods,[26] hollow nanoshells,[27] nanorings,[28] nanodisk,[29] nanocubes,[30] triangular nanoprisms,[31] nanodecahedra,[32] nanobipyramids,[33] crescent-shaped nanoparticles,[34] and nanobranches,[35] and those nanostructures provide a chance to be used in biosensor development. Using electrodynamic simulations of gold nanoparticle spectra, Miller and Lazarides demonstrate that the sensitivity of a plasmon peak wavelength to a variation in RI of the environment is determined by the location of the peak wavelength and the dielectric properties of the material.[36] Later, Wang and coworkers[35] have carried out a systematic study on the sensitivity of AuNPs of various shapes, including nanospheres, nanocubes, nanobranches, nanorods, and nanobipyramids toward bulk RI changes by using both RISs and figures of merits as performance indicators. They have found that the sensitivities generally increased as AuNPs became elongated and their apexes became sharper.

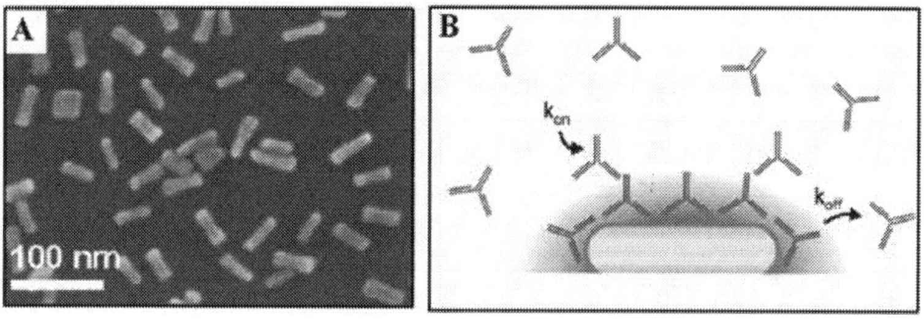

Figure 4.5 (A) Scanning electron microscopy of films of gold nanorods. (B) Schematic of the nanorod-based immunoassay. The nanorods were fixed to a glass surface via an APTES monolayer, and then coated with a self-assembled monolayer to which the capture antibody is coupled by carbodiimide cross-linking. The substrate was exposed to antigen (in this case secondary antibodies) and the binding was monitored via real-time absorption spectra. Reprinted with permission from ref. 39, Copyright 2008, American Chemical Society.

Although gold nanospheres are popular since they can be easily prepared, gold nanorods display a much higher sensitivity toward bulk refractive index changes than AuNPs (366 nm/RIU for Au nanorods with a mean aspect ratio of 5.2 and 76.4 nm/RIU for AuNPs).[37] Such a biosensing material was further modified to demonstrate its effectiveness in quantitative detection for selective binding events, such as the biotin–streptavidin pair interaction, through a process in which the biotin molecules were chemically attached to the Au nanorod's surface prior to detection measurements. Results showed that the peak wavelength of the LSPR band shifts linearly to the concentration of streptavidin, and detection limits of 0.42 nM for solutions prepared in buffer[37] and 19 nM for solutions prepared in serum[38] were achieved. As illustrated in Fig. 4.5, the detection of various anti-IgG has been also reported using Au nanorods.[39,40]

Hollow gold nanoshells have also been synthesized by reacting aqueous $HAuCl_4$ solutions with solid templates such as silver nanoparticles.[27] The surface plasmon peaks of these gold nanoshells are considerably red-shifted as compared with solid gold nanospheres. Comparing gold nanoshells with a mean diameter of 50 nm and shell thickness of 4.5 nm, gold solid nanospheres of 50 nm in diameter, and gold solid nanospheres of 30 nm in diameter, the RISs are 409, 60, and 71 nm/RIU, respectively. When the gold nanoshells were modified on poly(methyl methacrylate) and functionalized with anti-transferrin, a detection limit of 5.9 nM for transferrin was achieved.[41] Because the LSPR of gold nanoshells can be controlled in the near-infrared region of the spectrum, where the optical transmission through tissue and whole blood is optimal, gold nanoshells with a silica core have also been applied to monitor biomolecular interactions in diluted whole blood.[42]

Besides using self-assembly of NMNPs on substrates to prepare chemical and biochemical sensors, nanosphere lithography (NSL) has been employed to fabricate nanostructures with highly tunable localized surface plasmons.[43] Biotinylated Ag triangular nanoparticles were first used to detection of anti-biotin, and reached a detection limit of 0.7 nM (see Fig. 4.6).[44] Modification of the particle surface with mannose monosaccharide then illustrated the real time detection of the binding of concanavalin A to the particle surface.[45] These nanostructures were also used to detect the biomolecules possibly involved in Alzheimer disease. In the first experiment, amyloid-β-derived diffusible ligand (ADDL) was attached to the surface of Ag triangles to detect the specific antibody anti-ADDL.[46] In the second experiment, the anti-ADDL antibodies were first immobilized onto the surfaces of nanoparticles, and then the interaction of ADDL with its antibody via a sandwich immunoassay was analyzed.[47] The detection of anti-ADDL was both carried out on synthetic and clinical samples.

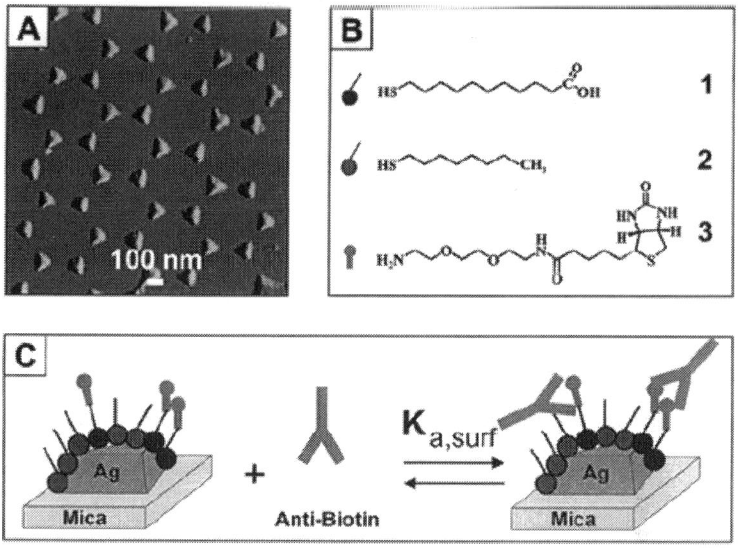

Figure 4.6 LSPR nanobiosensor. (A) Tapping mode AFM image of the Ag nanoparticles (nanosphere diameter, D = 390 nm; mass thickness, d_m = 50.0 nm Ag on a mica substrate). Scan area, 3.0 μm^2. Scan rate between 1 and 2 Hz. After solvent annealing, the resulting nanoparticles have in-plane widths of ~100 nm and out-of-plane heights of ~51 nm. (B) Surface chemistry of the Ag nanobiosensor. A mixed monolayer of (1) 11-MUA and (2) 1-OT is formed on the exposed surfaces of the Ag nanoparticles followed by the covalent linking of (3) biotin (B) to the carboxyl groups of (1) 11-MUA. (C) Schematic representation of anti-biotin (AB) binding to a biotinylated Ag nanobiosensor fabricated by NSL on a mica substrate. Reprint with permission from ref. 44, Copyright 2003, American Chemical Society.

The biosensing capability of the nanostructures fabricated by NSL has been compared with the conventional PSPR sensor.[45] Although the PSPR sensors exhibit significantly higher RIS, the shorter electromagnetic field decay length associated with NMNPs provides the LSPR sensors with enhanced sensitivity in surface binding.[48] As a result, their overall sensitivities in biosensing are approximately equivalent.[49]

Alternatively, Tamiya and coworkers focused their attention on the fabrication of gold-capped nanoparticle layer substrates (see

Fig. 4.7) for LSPR sensing.[50] The optical characteristics of the gold-capped nanoparticle layer substrate depend on the diameter of the dielectric nanoparticles to form a layer and the thickness of the gold layer on the dielectric nanoparticle layer, and may be attributed to a similar phenomenon described for the plasmon resonance spectra of the nanoshell-structured nanoparticles.[51] Such gold-capped nanoparticle layer substrates have been used to detect DNA hybridization[50] and antigen–antibody immunoreactions.[52]

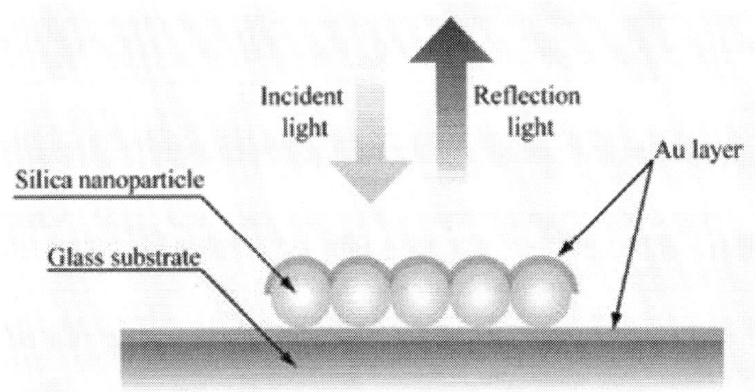

Figure 4.7 Construction of the multiarray LSPR-based nanochip. The surface-modified silica nanoparticles were aligned onto the gold-deposited glass substrate surface. Subsequently, the gold layer was deposited onto the silica nanoparticle layer. Reprinted with permission from ref. 69, Copyright 2006, American Chemical Society.

Gold nanoholes in metal films are other attractive metal nanostructures for biosensing. Taking the advantage of its dual optical properties, which combine the LSPR created by the nanostructures with the surface plasmon polaritons in metal films,[53] nanoholes fabricated with colloidal lithography on thin gold films have been reported for biosensing (see Fig. 4.8).[54,55] As a notable aspect, the preferential occurrence of spontaneous-supported phospholipid bilayers (SPB) formation on silicon-based substrates, but not on bare noble metal surfaces, was found to induce the rupture of phospholipid vesicles at the bottom of the nanoholes. This self-assembly process allows the detection of biochemical interactions confining exclusively inside the nanoholes, where the electromagnetic field enhancement induced by LSPR is maximized. These experiments show that the sensitivity toward the detection of biomolecules in the SPB patches is 16 times higher than on a bare gold surface.

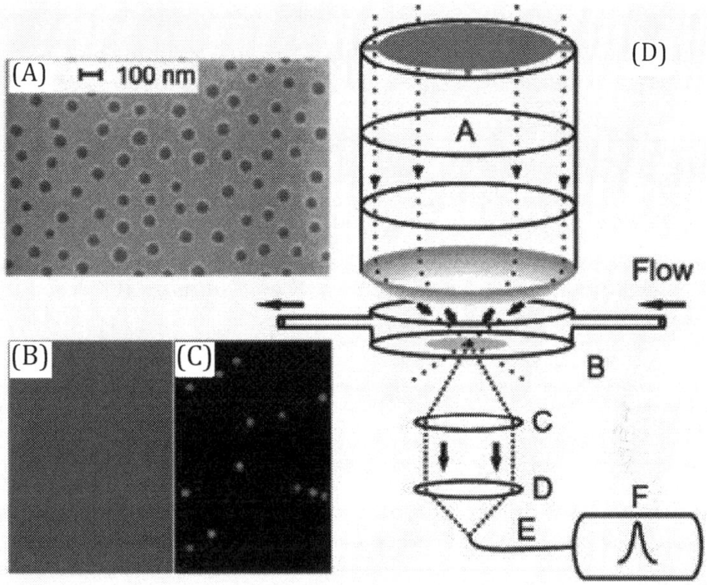

Figure 4.8 (A) Representative SEM image of $D \sim 60$ nm holes in a gold film (h = 20 nm) at a density of ~60 holes/μm^2. Dark-field microscopy images of (B) dense and (C) isolated nanoholes, respectively. (D) Schematics of the experimental setup. Reprinted with permission from ref. 55, Copyright 2005, American Chemical Society.

Due to the laterally propagating nature of the surface plasmon polaritions, the lateral resolution of the PSPR sensors is limited to tens of micrometers. On the contrary, LSPR nano-sensor arrays will provide pixel sizes 20–50 times smaller than the PSPR sensor arrays.[56] In principle, the smallest possible pixel size is the size of one nanoparticle. Taking this ideal case in mind, single AuNPs[57] and single Au nanorods[58] were used to detect biotin and a detection limit of 1 nM was achieved by using Au nanorods,[58] while single Ag nanoparticles were used to detect thiol adsorption and a zeptomole sensitivity was achieved.[59] Moreover, the method used to immobilize the single Au triangular nanoprism on the substrate can strongly affect the sensitivity toward refractive index changes.[60] The study shows that the LSPR resonance is not as sensitive to the medium when the particle is adsorbed to a substrate.

The NMNPs can also be applied to biosensing in a dry-reagent dipstick format. The dry-reagent dipstick test has been widely used for pregnancy test, which is essentially an immunochromatographic assay for human chorionic gonadotropin, with all required reagents deposited in a dry form on a suitable strip. Test strips based on gold nanoparticle as the visual indicator have already been commercialized for pregnancy diagnosis. Ioannou and coworkers have extended the assay to detection of genetically modified organisms (GMO)[61] and genotyping.[62] The principle of the visual detection of amplified DNA fragments, by using the nanoparticle-based DNA biosensor, is illustrated in Fig. 4.9 (Left). Typical photographs of two dry-reagent dipsticks for the hybridization analysis of amplified lectin DNA is shown in Fig. 4.9 (Right).

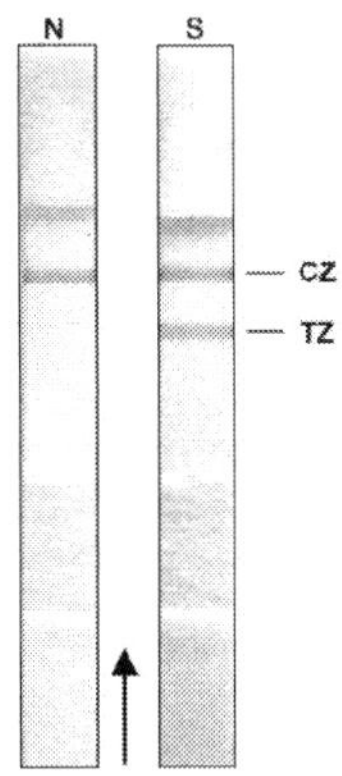

Figure 4.9 (Left) Schematic illustration of the principle of the nanoparticle-based DNA biosensor for visual detection of GMO. Biotinylated PCR product is hybridized to a specific oligo(dA)-tailed probe and loaded on the sample application area (S) of the sensor. As the buffer migrates upward (direction of the arrow), it rehydrates the oligo(dT)-conjugated gold nanoparticles, which are then coupled with the DNA target through poly(dA/dT) hybridization. The first red line is formed in the test zone (TZ), as the immobilized streptavidin captures the hybrids. The second red line is developed on the control zone (CZ), when the excess of conjugated gold nanoparticles hybridize with immobilized oligo(dA) probe. Au, conjugated gold nanoparticles; B, biotin; SA, streptavidin. (Right) Hybridization assay of amplified lectin DNA by using the dry-reagent dipsticks. A PCR negative (N) and a positive samples (S) are shown. TZ, test zone and CZ, control zone. Reprinted with permission from Ref. 61, Copyright 2006, Elsevier.

The biosensor has been applied to the screening of a number of real samples derived from sausages, soybeans, soy flour, and fish meal that contain GMO.[61] Genotyping of single-nucleotide polymorphisms (SNP) in the mannose-binding lectin (MBL2) gene has also been demonstrated.[62] The dipstick test can be completed within 10 min and does not require specialized instrumentation or highly trained technical personnel. However, the sensitivity of immunochromatographic assay is significantly lower than ELISA. Tamiya and coworkers have reported a gold nanoparticle-based enhancement method for obtaining a better sensitivity in immunochromatographic test strips.[63] In this method, AuNP-conjugated primary antibody and the antigen are used as a sensitizer. The antigen is captured by the secondary antibody at the test line on the strip. As a result, gold nanoparticles accumulate at the test line, resulting in sensitivity almost at the same level of the ELISA assay.

A simple portable system for the detection of bioanalytes would be of high demand for a wide range of applications such as point-of-care diagnostics as well as field detection of pathogens.[64] Recently, Neuzil and Rebound[65] integrated the LSPR detection process into a complete, simple, palm-sized device. This system does not require any external power supply or personal computer. The spectrum analyzer is replaced by four pulse-powered light-emitting diodes (LED), each with different emission spectra. The reflected light beams from all LEDs are detected by a single photodiode. Its composite output current is demultiplexed by a four-channel lock-in amplifier. Device performance has been demonstrated through characterization of solutions with various RIs in real time. Due to its small size and portability, the system may be useful for field and point-of-care applications.

In recent years, compact biosensors combined with microfluidic technologies have received increasing interest because they have been shown capable to provide faster and less expensive approaches to detect chemical and biochemical entities comparing with existing approaches in macro scale.[66,67] Huang and coworkers have integrated a slide-based LSPR sensor with a microfluidic chip.[68] Using a green LED as a light source and a novel quadrant detection scheme, the sensitivity of this low-cost biosensor is comparable to conventional slide-based LSPR biosensors. Besides that, the high surface to volume ratio of the microfluidic chip enhances mass transport, resulting in shorter assay time and lower consumption of samples and reagents.

It brought a promising example of a low-cost and portable biosensor candidate compared to the larger and more expensive commercial instruments.

4.4 Microarray-Based LSPR Biosensors

In the development of multiplexed sensing and high throughput LSPR assays, Nath and Chilkoti[23] first demonstrated that the colorimetric LSPR sensor can be performed in an array format for end-point assays by using a low-cost optical scanner. As shown in Fig. 4.10, the color difference between the four sensor chips could be discerned visually and was quantitatively confirmed by conversion of the images to gray scale and calculation of the average intensity.

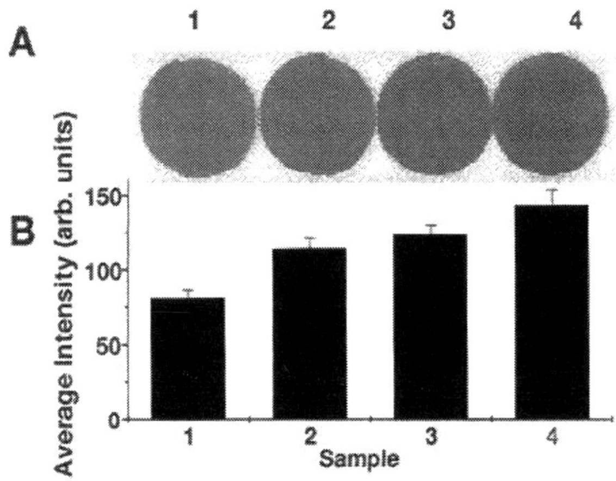

Figure 4.10 (A) Scanned images of AuNPs on glass functionalized with APTES (1), after formation of MPA monolayer (2), and after 30 min incubation with 10 (3), and 1000 μg/mL (4) fibrinogen. (B) Histogram of the average intensity of each chip. Error bar represents standard deviation of the intensity distribution of each chip. Reprinted with permission from ref. 23, Copyright 2002, American Chemical Society. See also Color Insert.

The gold-capped nanoparticle layer substrates have also been used to develop a multiarray LSPR-based nanochip (see Fig. 4.7) composed of 300 sensing spots, for the label-free detection of antigen–antibody reactions.[69] Antibodies were immobilized onto the nanospots and the interaction with different concentrations of their corresponding antigens was analyzed through the changes in the extinction spectra (see Fig. 4.11). The detection limit of this biosensor was 100 pg/mL.

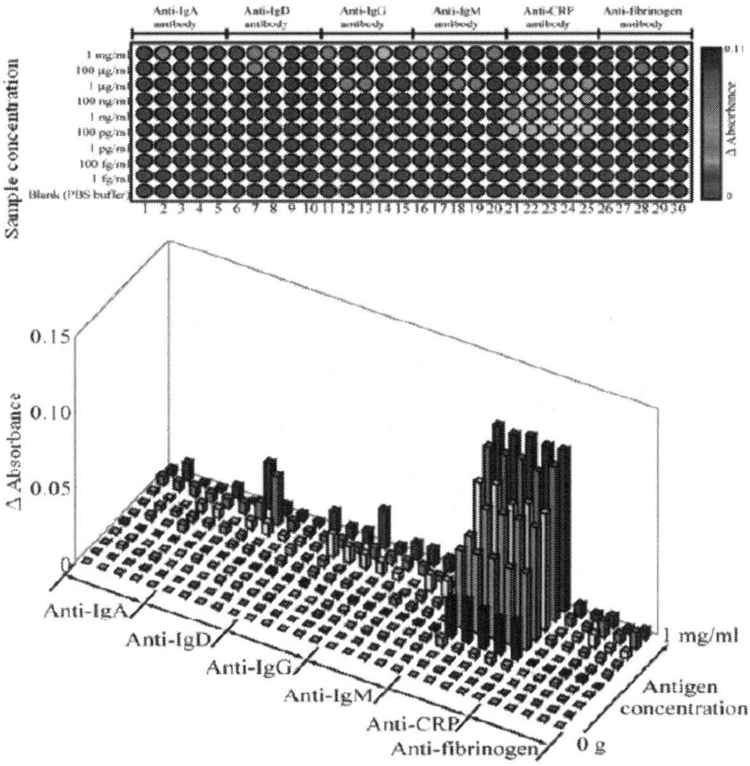

Figure 4.11 Absorbance measurements at each spot using the multiarray LSPR-based nanochip. After the introduction of antigens at different concentrations using the nanoliter dispensing system, the LSPR spectra were recorded for C-reactive protein (CRP). Reprinted with permission from ref. 69, Copyright 2006, American Chemical Society. See also Color Insert.

Gold nanorods posses two plasmon bands: one is transverse plasmon wavelength (TPW) and another is longitudinal plasmon wavelength (LPW) appearing in visible or near-infrared range. Because the LPW of gold nanorods can be fine-tuned by the length-to-diameter aspect ratio of the nanorods, a significant multi-throughput for simultaneous detection of multiple targets could be achieved if various gold nanorods with different LPWs are carefully designed and then assembled on chips. In 2009, Huang and coworkers demonstrated the use of five kinds of gold nanorods to construct the multi-throughput LSPR biosensor for simultaneous detection of antigen–antibody interactions in the wavelength range from 530 to 940 nm.[70] Thus, the broad tunability of the LPW of gold nanorods and other NMNPs open a door for multiplex LSPR biosensing.

4.5 Conclusions and Outlook

In conclusion, LSPR sensing offers many promising features and potential applications (Table 4.1) and has been demonstrated by the development of LSPR-based biosensors in this chapter. However, there are still many challenges before they can be used in practice. These include the improvements in the detection capability, sensitivity[71,72] or combination with other identification techniques.[73] A combined multidisciplinary research effort is still necessary to collect all these features to develop highly sensitive and reliable biosensing platforms.

Table 4.1 Summary of the LSPR-based biosensing assays with various nanostructures

Nanostructure	Target
Au nanospheres	Streptavidin[17,23]
Au or Ag nanospheres	Anti-BSA[24] or anti-HSA[25]
Au nanorods	Various anti-IgG[39,40]
Au nanoring	Neutravidin[28]
Au nanohole	Neutravidin[54,55]
Ag triangles	Anti-biotin,[44] ConA,[45] anti-ADDL,[46] anti-ADDL (sandwich)[47]
Au-capped nanoparticles layer substrate	Nucleic acids,[50] anti-IgA, IgD, IgG, IgM,[52] C-reactive protein and fibrinogen[69]

References

1. A. Voller, A. Bartlett, and D. E. Bidwell, *J. Clin. Pathol.*, **31**, 507 (1978).
2. A. Janshoff, H. J. Galla, and C. Steinem, *Angew. Chem., Int. Ed.*, **39**, 4004 (2000).
3. N. Backmann, C. Zahnd, F. Huber, A. Bietsch, A. Pluckthun, H. P. Lang, H. J. Guntherodt, M. Hegner, and C. Gerber, *Proc. Natl. Acad. Sci. U. S. A.*, **102**, 14587 (2005).
4. Y. R. Chemla, H. L. Crossman, Y. Poon, R. McDermott, R. Stevens, M. D. Alper, and J. Clarke, *Proc. Natl. Acad. Sci. U. S. A.*, **97**, 14268 (2000).
5. S. Tanaka, Z. Aspanut, H. Kurita, C. Toriyabe, Y. Hatsukade, and S. Katsura, *IEEE Trans. Appl. Supercond.*, **15**, 664 (2005).
6. Y. Cui, Q. Q. Wei, H. K. Park, and C. M. Lieber, *Science*, **293**, 1289 (2001).
7. G. Gauglitz, *Anal. Bioanal. Chem.*, **381**,141 (2005).
8. B. Liedberg, C. Nylander, and I. Lundstrom, *Biosens. Bioelectron.*, **10**, i (1995).
9. J. Homola, *Chem. Rev.*, **108**, 462 (2008).
10. B. Sepulveda, P. C. Angelome, L. M. Lechuga, and L. M. Liz-Marzan, *Nano Today*, **4**, 244 (2009).
11. W. L. Barnes, A. Dereux, and T. W. Ebbesen, *Nature*, **424**, 824 (2003).
12. E. Hutter and J. H. Fendler, *Adv. Mater.*, **16**, 1685 (2004).
13. S. G. Penn, L. He, and M. J. Natan, *Curr. Opin. Chem. Biol.*, **7**, 609 (2003).
14. J. Homola, S. S. Lee, and G. Gauglitz, *Sens. Actuators B*, **54**, 3 (1999).
15. A. J. Haes and R. P. Van Duyne, *Anal. Bioanal. Chem.*, **379**, 920 (2004).
16. W. A. Murray and W. L. Barnes, *Adv. Mater.*, **19**, 3771 (2007).
17. N. Nath and A. Chilkoti, *Anal. Chem.*, **76**, 5370 (2004).
18. A. Haes, S. L. Zou, G. C. Schatz, and R. P. Van Duyne, *J. Phys. Chem. B*, **108**, 6961 (2004).
19. S. Lee, and V. H. Perez-Luna, *Anal. Chem.*, **77**, 7204 (2005).
20. W. Rechberger, A. Hohenau, A. Leitner, J. R. Krenn, B. Lamprecht, and F. R. Aussenegg, *Opt. Commun.*, **220**, 137 (2003).
21. P. Englebienne, *Analyst*, **123**, 1599 (1998).
22. D. Eck, C. A. Helm, N. J. Wagner, and K. A. Vaynberg, *Langmuir*, **17**, 957 (2001).
23. N. Nath and A. Chilkoti, *Anal. Chem.*, **74**, 504 (2002).

24. F. Frederix, J.-M. Friedt, K.H. Choi, W. Laureyn, A. Campitelli, D. Mondelaers, G. Maes, and G. Borghs, *Anal. Chem.*, **75**, 6894 (2003).

25. K. Fujiwara, H. Watarai, H. Itoh, E. Nakahama, and N. Ogawa, *Anal. Bioanal. Chem.*, **386**, 639 (2006).

26. K. S. Lee and M. A. El-Sayed, *J. Phys. Chem. B*, **110**, 19220 (2006).

27. Y. Sun and Y. Xia, *Anal. Chem.*, **74**, 5297 (2002).

28. E. M. Larsson, J. Alegret, M. Kall, and D. S. Sutherland, *Nano Lett.*, **7**, 1256 (2007).

29. P. Hanarp, M. Kall, and D. S. Sutherland, *J. Phys. Chem. B*, **107**, 5768 (2003).

30. L. J. Sherry, S.-H. Chang, G. C. Schatz, R. P. Van Duyne, B. J. Wiley, and Y. Xia, *Nano Lett.*, **5**, 2034 (2005).

31. L. J. Sherry, R. Jin, C. A. Mirkin, G. C. Schatz, and R. P. Van Duyne, *Nano Lett.*, **6**, 2060 (2006).

32. I. Pastoriza-Santos, A. Sanchez-Iglesias, F. J. Garcia de Abajo, and L. M. Liz-Marzán, *Adv. Funct. Mater.*, **17**, 1443 (2007).

33. J. Burgin, M. Liu, and P. Guyot-Sionnest, *J. Phys. Chem. C*, **112,** 19279 (2008).

34. N. L. Bocchio, A. Unger, M. Alvarez, and M. Kreiter, *J. Phys. Chem. C*, **112**, 14355 (2008).

35. H. Chen, X. Kou, Z. Yang, W. Ni, and J. Wang, *Langmuir*, **24**, 5233 (2008).

36. M. M. Miller and A. A. Lazarides, *J. Phys. Chem. B*, **109**, 21556 (2005).

37. C.-D. Chen, S.-F. Chen, L.-K. Chua, and C. R. C. Wang, *Biosens. Bioelectron.*, **22**, 926 (2007).

38. S. M. Marinakos, S. Chen, and A. Chilkoti, *Anal. Chem.*, **79**, 5278 (2007).

39. K. M. Mayer, S. Lee, H. Liao, B. C. Rostro, A. Fuentes, P. T. Scully, C. L. Nehl, and J. H. Hafner, *ACS Nano*, **2**, 687 (2008).

40. H. Huang, C. He, Y. Zeng, X. Xia, X. Yu, P. Yi, and Z. Chen, *Biosens. Bioelectron.*, **24**, 2255 (2009).

41. S.-F. Cheng, L.-K. Chau, and K.-C. Pao, *J. Biomed. Nanotechnol.*, **1**, 143 (2005).

42. Y.Wang, W. Qian, Y. Tan, and S. Ding, *Biosens. Bioelectron.*, **23**, 1166 (2008).

43. C. L. Haynes and R. P. Van Duyne, *J. Phys. Chem. B*, **105**, 5599 (2001).

44. J. C. Riboh, A. J. Haes, A. D. McFarland, C. R. Yonzon, and R. P. Van Duyne, *J. Phys. Chem. B*, **107**, 1772 (2003).

45. C. R. Yonzon, E. Jeoung, S. Zou, G. C. Schatz, M. Mrksich, and R. P. Van Duyne, *J. Am. Chem. Soc.*, **126**, 12669 (2004).

46. A. J. Haes, W. P. Hall, L. Chang, W. L. Klein, and R. P. Van Duyne, *Nano Lett.*, **4**, 1029 (2004).

47. A. J. Haes, L. Chang, W. L. Klein, and R. P. Van Duyne, *J. Am. Chem. Soc.*, **127**, 2264 (2005).

48. A. J. Haes, S. Zou, G. C. Schatz, and R. P. Van Duyne, *J. Phys. Chem. B*, **108**, 6961 (2004).

49. A. J. Haes, S. Zou, G. C. Schatz, and R. P. Van Duyne, *J. Phys. Chem. B*, **108**, 109 (2004).

50. T. Endo, K. Kerman, N. Nagatani, Y, Takamura, and E. Tamiya, *Anal. Chem.*, **77**, 6976 (2005).

51. E. Prodan, P. Nordlander, and N. J. Halas, *Nano Lett.*, **3**, 1411 (2003).

52. T. Endo, S. Yamamura, N. Nagatani, Y. Morita, Y. Takamura, and E. Tamiya, *Sci. Technol. Adv. Mater.*, **6**, 491 (2005).

53. Y. Alaverdyan, B. Sepulveda, L. Eurenius, E. Olsson, and M. Kall, *Nat. Phys.*, **3**, 884 (2007).

54. A. Dahlin, M. Zach, T. Rindzevicius, M. Kall, D. S. Sutherland, and F. Hook, *J. Am. Chem. Soc.*, **127**, 5043 (2005).

55. T. Rindzevicius, Y. Alaverdyan, A. Dahlin, F. Hook, D. S. Sutherland, and M. Kall, *Nano Lett.*, **5**, 2335 (2005).

56. M. D. Malinsky, K. L. Kelly, G. C. Schatz, and R. P. Van Duyne, *J. Am. Chem. Soc.*, **123**, 1471 (2001).

57. G. Raschke, S. Kowarik, T. Franzl, C. Sonnichsen, T. A. Klar, and J. Feldmann, *Nano Lett.*, **3**, 935 (2003).

58. G. J. Nusz, S. M. Marinakos, A. C. Curry, A. Dahlin, F. Hook, A. Wax, and A. Chilkoti, *Anal. Chem.*, **80**, 984 (2008).

59. A. D. McFarland and R. P. Van Duyne, *Nano Lett.*, **3**, 1057 (2003).

60. C. Novo, A. M. Funston, I. Pastoriza-Santos, L. M. Liz-Marzan, and P. Mulvaney, *J. Phys. Chem. C*, **112**, 3 (2008).

61. D. P. Kalogianni, T. Koraki, T. K. Christopoulos, and P. C. Ioannou, *Biosens. Bioelectron.*, **21**, 1069 (2006).

62. I. K. Litos, P. C. Ioannou, T. K. Christopoulos, J. Traeger-Synodinos, and E. Kanavakis, *Anal. Chem.*, **79**, 395 (2007).

63. N. Nagatani, R. Tanaka, T. Yuhi, T. Endo, K. Kerman, Y. Takamura, and E. Tamiya, *Sci. Technol. Adv. Mater.*, **7**, 270 (2006).

64. J. Comley, *Drug Discovery World Winter*, **5**, 63 (2004).

65. P. Neuzil and J. Reboud, *Anal. Chem.*, **80**, 6100 (2008).

66. G. H. W. Sanders and A. Manz, *Trends Anal. Chem.*, **19**, 364 (2000).
67. K. Sato, A. Hibara, M. Tokeshi, H. Hisamoto, and T. Kitamori, *Adv. Drug Delivery Rev.*, **55**, 379 (2003).
68. C. Huang, K. Bonroy, G. Reekmans, W. Laureyn, K. Verhaegen, I. De Vlaminck, L. Lagae, and G. Borghs, *Biomed. Microdevices*, **11**, 893 (2009).
69. T. Endo, K. Kerman, N. Nagatani, H. M. Hiepa, D.-K. Kim, Y. Yonezawa, K. Nakano, and E. Tamiya, *Anal. Chem.*, **78**, 6465 (2006).
70. H. Huang, C. He, Y. Zeng, X. Xia, X. Yu, P. Yi, and Z. Chen, *Biosens. Bioelectron.*, **24**, 2255 (2009).
71. A. B. Dahlin, J. O. Tegenfeldt, and F. Hook, *Anal. Chem.*, **78**, 4416 (2006).
72. J. N. Anker, W. P. Hall, O. Lyandres, N. C. Shah, J. Zhao, and R. P. Van Duyne, *Nat. Mater.*, **7**, 442 (2008).
73. J. A. McLean, K. A. Stumpo, and D. H. Russell, *J. Am. Chem. Soc.*, **127**, 5304 (2005).

Chapter 5

Optical Waveguide-Based Biosensors Using Noble Metal Nanoparticles

Lai-Kwan Chau,[a,b,*] Chang-Yue Chiang,[a] Wei-Ting Hsu,[a] Shin-Huei Chen,[a] and Shu-Fang Cheng[a]

[a]*Department of Chemistry and Biochemistry, National Chung Cheng University, 168 University Road, Min-Hsiung, Chia-Yi 621, Taiwan*
[b]*Center for Nano Bio-Detection, National Chung Cheng University, 168 University Road, Min-Hsiung, Chia-Yi 621, Taiwan*
[*]chelkc@ccu.edu.tw

The particle plasmon resonance (PPR) property of noble metal nanoparticles allows label-free and real-time detection of biomolecules. To enhance the signal derived from this property, the use of optical waveguide sensing technology further increases the sensitivity of the PPR biosensing technique. The optical waveguides described in this chapter include optical fiber, planar waveguide, and tubular waveguide. The principle for this improvement is discussed.

5.1 Introduction

The development of biosensors for medical diagnostics,[1] drug discovery,[2] monitoring of food safety,[3] agricultural diagnostics,[4] bioprocess monitoring,[5] environmental monitoring,[6] and detection

From Bioimaging to Biosensors: Noble Metal Nanoparticles in Biodetection
Edited by Lai-Kwan Chau and Huan-Tsung Chang

ISBN 978-981-4267-24-3 (Hardcover), 978-981-4303-10-1 (eBook)
www.panstanford.com

of biological warfare agents[7] is an extremely significant problem. For many biosensing techniques, the analyte must wear an electrochemical or spectroscopic signature. Unfortunately, a lot of biochemical species do not wear such signatures. Hence, labeling of the analyte is then required. However, the labeling procedures are often tedious and sometimes may lead to errors. Alternatively, a second recognition biomolecule (e.g., use of second antibody in enzyme-linked immunosorbent assay, ELISA) which can produce an electrochemical or spectroscopic signature will be used. Nevertheless, the use of a second recognition molecule not only lengthens the analysis time and complicates the procedures but also increases cost. Furthermore, both approaches do not allow real-time detection of the analyte. Hence, development of label-free and real-time biosensors with additional characteristics such as high sensitivity and selectivity, portable for point-of-care, easy to use, and cost-effective is extremely necessary.

Much biosensor research has been devoted to the evaluation of the relative merits of various label-free signal transduction methods including optical, piezoelectric, and impedimetric. Although each of these methods has its individual strengths and weaknesses, a strong case has been made that optical sensors, in particular those based on evanescent electromagnetic fields such as surface plasmon resonance (SPR) at planar gold surfaces, are the methods of choice in many biosensing applications today.[8] Unfortunately, SPR sensors require bulky and expensive optical equipment and hence are difficult to be miniaturized.

The development of portable biosensors composed of a highly miniaturized signal transducer element that enables point-of-care applications is one of the important driving forces in biosensor research.[1] Also important are their potential capabilities for on-site, *in situ*, *in vivo*, remote sensing, and disposable use. In these situations, it is necessary to utilize sensor platforms that have as many of the desirable characteristics of SPR sensors as possible, but also can be easily configured in a miniaturized format, and minimize the time required to achieve measurable signals, and the volume of sample required.

Recently, scientific community has begun to explore alternative strategies for the development of new optical sensing platforms based on the extraordinary optical properties of noble metal nanoparticles (NMNP).[9–11] These nanoparticles characteristically exhibit a strong extinction band that is not present in the spectrum of the bulk metal. The extinction band results when the incident photon frequency is resonant with the collective oscillation of the conduction electrons and is known as PPR, also known as localized surface plasmon resonance (LSPR). The extinction cross-section and peak wavelength of the PPR band is highly dependent on the local environment of the nanoparticle (i.e., refractive index of the surrounding medium),[12–16] and furthermore, the binding events to those functionalized nanoparticles.[17–21] However, the signal-to-noise ratio for slide-based PPR sensors obtained by either the transmission mode with a single pass of light or reflection mode with a double pass of light through a NMNP layer is not so high, as a result of the low absorbance of the NMNP layer. The absorbance of such a NMNP layer can be enhanced by optical waveguide (OW) sensing[22] which is based on the absorption of the evanescent field via multiple total internal reflections. By this approach, we have developed a novel fiber optic particle plasmon resonance (FO-PPR) biosensing platform that exploits PPR of self-assembled NMNPs on the unclad portion of an optical fiber for monitoring the refractive index (RI) of solution bulk and for label-free detection of molecular or biomolecular binding at the surface of NMNPs.[23–25] Other OW-based PPR biosening platforms are also possible and are described later in this chapter. For such OW-PPR biosensing platforms, the nanoparticles act as chromophores, while their interactions with the analytes will result in colorimetric changes. Hence, with a suitable receptor immobilized on the surface of the NMNPs, the resulting OW-PPR sensor can detect the corresponding analyte even if the analyte is spectroscopically silent in the UV-vis region. The FO-PPR sensing platform has been demonstrated to be sensitive to biomolecular binding events at the pico-molar level.[23,24]

In comparison to the SPR sensor, the OW-PPR sensor retains many of the desirable features of the SPR sensor and has at least nine additional advantages. First, without the need of employing a momentum matching scheme by using either a prism or a grating to excite the surface plasmons in SPR sensors,[26] OW-PPR sensors have a simple optical configuration and, hence, a high potential being miniaturized to a portable format. Second, OW-PPR measurement is based on extinction spectroscopy and, hence, the normalization by the relative change of transmission response alleviates the demand on precise optical alignment. Third, sensitivity of SPR sensors cannot benefit from increasing the interaction length of the sensor[27] while OW-PPR sensors can take advantage of multiple total internal reflections (TIR) along the optical waveguide to increase sensitivity.[24] Fourth, the simple wet chemical approach typically used to construct a NMNP layer on an OW element for OW-PPR sensors has a cost advantage and allows a wider choice of the shape of the sensor substrate, while the vacuum-based sputtering method typically used to make a noble metal film for SPR sensors is expensive and difficult to coat substrates with a complicated shape. Fifth, chemically tailorable physically properties such as size, shape, and composition lead to tunable PPR band, allowing the spectroscopic sensing window to be tuned without re-alignment of the optical setup.[28,29] Sixth, because of the lower refractive index sensitivity, the PPR sensor requires little temperature control whereas the SPR sensor (with large refractive index sensitivity) requires stringent temperature control.[30] Seventh, the rate of analyte mass transport to a nanoparticle sensor will be governed by radial diffusion and consequently will be faster than that to the planar format SPR sensor operating under semi-infinite linear diffusion.[18,30,31] Eighth, the smaller electromagnetic field decay length in PPR sensor[32] as compared to that of SPR sensor yields better sensitivity in detecting small molecules,[30,33] and also eliminates the need to trap the interacting molecules of interest in a polymer matrix to enhance the signal.[34] Finally, the most dramatic difference between the OW-PPR and SPR sensors is cost. Commercialized SPR instruments can vary between USD150,000~300,000,[30,35] whereas the prototype FO-PPR system costs less than USD5,000. Thus, the unique optical properties exhibited by NMNPs and the combined benefits with the OW technology have paved the way for the construction of new biosensors. We believe this novel biosensing technology has a high potential of being commercialized.

5.2 Principle of the Biosensors

In this section, we take the FO-PPR biosensor as an example to illustrate the principle of the biosensing platforms. A schematic illustrating the principle and the setup of the FO-PPR biosensor is shown in Fig. 5.1. Optical waveguide formats other than optical fiber generally follow the same principle but some modifications to accommodate the specific optical waveguide mode are needed.

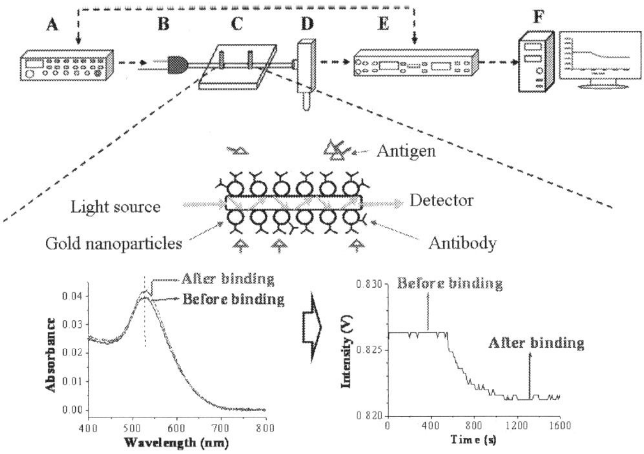

Figure 5.1 A schematic illustration of the principle and experimental setup for the FO-PPR biosensor to make measurements. The setup consists of A, function generator; B, light emitting diode (530 nm); C, FO-PPR sensing chip; D, photodiode; E, lock-in amplifier; F, computer. Biomolecular binding at the surface of the functionalized gold nanoparticle layer results in an increase in absorbance and hence a decrease in light intensity exiting the optical fiber.

Optical fiber evanescent wave absorption sensors are based on attenuated total reflection (ATR) spectroscopy. This technique relies on the penetration of the evanescent wave (EW) in the absorbing medium outside the fiber core and interacts with the analyte, whose distance from the fiber surface is generally smaller than the wavelength of the traveling light.[36] Since light propagates in optical fiber by virtue of multiple TIR, the summation of each local evanescent field results in a continuous evanescent field at the waveguide surface immediately adjacent to the region occupied by a propagating mode. As a result, the overall sensitivity of the structure depends on the modes of light propagation in the fiber,[37] the length of the fiber core exposed to the chromophore,[38] and the chemical interaction between the analyte and the immobilized binding sites.[39] Hence, the low absorbance of a NMNP layer can be enhanced by a fiber optic EW sensing scheme.[23]

Fiber optic EW absorbance measurements typically are performed by comparing the light intensity of a sensor immersed in an analyte solution (I_S) to the intensity of the sensor in a blank

(I_0), where the refractive index of a sample, n_S, differs from that of a blank, n_R. At a nonabsorbing wavelength, a change in critical angle, ϕ_c, for internal reflection will cause a change in numerical aperture (NA),[40] where NA is related to the core RI, n_1, and cladding RI, n_2, by the following equation:

$$NA = (n_1^2 - n_2^2)^{1/2} \tag{5.1}$$

and the resulting transmittance signal, $T = I_S/I_0$, is given by

$$T = \frac{I_S}{I_0} = \frac{NA_S^2}{NA_0^2} \tag{5.2}$$

$$NA_0 = (n_1^2 - n_0^2)^{1/2} \tag{5.3}$$

$$NA_S = (n_1^2 - n_S^2)^{1/2} \tag{5.4}$$

Refractive index sensing based on Eq. 5.2 has been demonstrated.[41] However, because of the long penetration depth of the evanescent wave which leads to lower biosensing sensitivity[42] and the need for thin monomode waveguides with a large difference of RI between the waveguide and substrate materials to have high sensitivity,[43] biosensing applications based on this concept are not much explored.

At an absorbing wavelength, the resulting absorbance signal, A, can be described by a relationship given by Degrandpre and Burgess:[40]

$$A = -\log\frac{I_S}{I_0} = \gamma \cdot L - \log\left(\frac{NA_S^2}{NA_0^2}\right) \tag{5.5}$$

where γ is the evanescent absorption coefficient and L is the sensor length. For a weakly guiding fiber, the evanescent absorption coefficient is related to the bulk absorption coefficient by the expression

$$\gamma = \eta \cdot \alpha \tag{5.6}$$

where the power distribution, η, is the fraction of total light intensity in the evanescent field and α is the bulk absorption coefficient of the NMNP layer.[44] The power distribution can be calculated from[22]

$$\eta = \frac{k}{V} \tag{5.7}$$

$$V = \frac{2\pi \cdot \rho \cdot NA}{\lambda} \tag{5.8}$$

where k is a constant, V is a normalized frequency (also called V-number), λ is the wavelength of light in the fiber core, and ρ is the core radius. After correcting an error in Gloge's original paper,[45] k is given by a value of 4/3.[46] However, in evanescent wave spectroscopy using a fiber, the cladding material is often partially removed and replaced with, in general, a material having a much lower RI. Thus, only some of the possible bound modes of the sensing region propagate and the evanescent absorption coefficient can be described by an expression given by Ruddy:[44]

$$\gamma = \frac{\alpha \cdot \lambda}{2 \cdot \rho \cdot n_1 \cdot (1 + \sin\phi_c)} \tag{5.9}$$

For a NMNP layer, the absorbance of the NMNP layer changes when it is immersed in a sample of refractive index n_S different from that of a blank, n_R.[19] Previous study indicates that at a long enough L, the change in NA_S with respect to the change in n_S is negligible as compared to the change of α with respect to the change of n_S.[24] In other words, the second term in Eq. 5.5 is negligible when $\gamma \cdot L$ is large enough. Under this condition, substituting Eq. 5.9 into Eq. 5.5 yields

$$A = -\log\left(\frac{I_S}{I_0}\right) = \frac{\alpha \cdot \lambda \cdot L}{2 \cdot \rho \cdot n_1 \cdot (1 + \sin\phi_c)} \tag{5.10}$$

For the PPR sensors, the NMNP acts as a reporter chromophore and its interaction with an analyte will result in a change in its bulk absorption coefficient and absorbance. As such, the FO-PPR measurements actually reflect the change in absorbance. When I_R is defined as the sensor response of a NMNPs-modified optical fiber in a blank, I_S is the sensor response of a NMNPs-modified optical fiber in a sample, and I_0 is the sensor response of the same optical fiber without NMNPs and is in the blank, then Eq. 5.10 can be rewritten as

$$\Delta A = -\log\left(\frac{I_S}{I_R}\right) = \frac{\Delta\alpha \cdot \lambda \cdot L}{2 \cdot \rho \cdot n_1 \cdot (1 + \sin\phi_c)} \tag{5.11}$$

where ΔA is the absorbance change from A_R (in a blank) to $A_R + \Delta A$ (in a sample) and bulk absorption coefficient changes from α_R (in a blank) to $\alpha_R + \Delta\alpha$ (in a sample) when the RI of the medium surrounding the NMNP layer changes from n_R to n_S.

For multimode EW optical fiber sensors, Payne and Hale[46] showed that the simple Beer's law model overestimated the fiber absorbance and an expression for such sensors at the condition of very strong absorption was derived:

$$\frac{I_S}{I_0} \approx \frac{V}{\alpha \cdot L} = \frac{\pi \cdot \rho \cdot NA_0}{\lambda \cdot \alpha \cdot L} \tag{5.12}$$

Again, the FO-PPR measurements actually reflect the change of light attenuation through the fiber. When I_R is defined as the sensor response of a NMNPs-modified optical fiber in a blank, I_S is the sensor response of a NMNPs-modified optical fiber in a sample, and I_0 is the sensor response of the same optical fiber without NMNPs and is in the blank, then Eq. 5.12 can be rewritten as

$$\frac{I_S}{I_R} \approx \frac{\alpha_R}{\alpha_R + \Delta\alpha} \tag{5.13}$$

where the bulk absorption coefficient changes from α_R (in a blank) to $\alpha_R + \Delta\alpha$ (in a sample) when the RI of the medium surrounding the NMNP layer changes from n_R to n_S.

Further theoretical work is needed to relate the sensor response with respect to the parameters to construct the fiber optic sensor. Nevertheless, both Eqs. 5.10 and 5.12 indicate that the use of a smaller core radius may be beneficial to improve the sensitivity of the sensor. However, a smaller core radius also lead to a lower intensity signal received by the detector and is very fragile. Thus, a trade-off core radius is often employed.

The bulk absorption coefficient of a NMNP is related to the extinction cross-section of a particle. According to Mie's theory, the extinction cross-section of a single spherical particle much smaller than the wavelength of light can be approximately expressed by the following relationship:[12]

$$\sigma_{\text{ext}} = \frac{24\pi^2 r^3 \varepsilon_S^{3/2}}{\lambda} \cdot \frac{\varepsilon_2(\omega)}{(\varepsilon_1(\omega) + 2\varepsilon_S)^2 + \varepsilon_2(\omega)^2} \tag{5.14}$$

where σ_{ext} is the extinction cross-section of the particle, r is the radius of the particle, λ is the wavelength of light, and ε_S and $\varepsilon(\omega) = \varepsilon_1(\omega) + i\varepsilon_2(\omega)$ are the dielectric functions of the surrounding medium and the metal itself, respectively. While the dielectric function of the surrounding medium is assumed to be frequency independent, the dielectric function of metal is complex and depends on the frequency. If ε_2 is small or weakly dependent on ω, the resonance condition is fulfilled roughly when $\varepsilon_1(\omega) = -2\varepsilon_S$, or $\lambda = \sim 500$ nm for gold in air and $\lambda = \sim 350$ nm for silver in air.[47]

Previous study demonstrated that, within a limited RI range, the absorbance of a NMNP layer is linearly dependent on the RI of the surrounding medium.[19] Examination of Eq. 5.5 indicates that the value of the second term is also affected by the medium RI but in a non-linear fashion and, hence, a plot of absorbance versus medium RI is expected to be non-linear. However, the linear sensor response (intensity, transmittance, or absorbance) of the FO-PPR sensor over a range of medium RI indicates that the change of the sensor response due to the change of numerical aperture and V-number at different medium RI is negligible.[23] In other words, the second term in Eq. 5.5 is negligible when the evanescent absorption coefficient of the NMNP layer is large enough. As a result, Eq. 5.5 describes the attenuation caused by the absorption of light in the cladding and shows a pseudo-Beer's dependence of the absorbance on the evanescent absorption coefficient of the NMNP layer, which depends on the length of the fiber core modified with NMNPs, the surface concentration of NMNPs on the fiber core, and the mean extinction cross-section of the NMNPs. Empirically, we found that the plot of I_S (or I_S/I_R) versus n_S has a better linear relationship than the plot of $-\log(I_S/I_R)$ versus n_S,[23] and thus the following expression is used in subsequent sections:

$$I_R - I_S = -k' \cdot (n_R - n_S) + k'' = k' \cdot \Delta n + k'' \qquad (5.15)$$

where k' and k'' are constants depending on the optical setup and the structure of the NMNP layer and $\Delta n = n_S - n_R$.

It is evidence that affinity-based biosensor technology has changed the way we view bio-molecular interactions. The ability to probe complex formation in real time provides detailed insights into the binding process. In the simplest model for the interaction of an immobilized species B (a receptor) and a mobile species X (an analyte), both reactants reversibly form a 1:1 complex BX. The general equilibrium reaction is

$$B + X = BX \qquad (5.16)$$

Considering a Langmuir adsorption model and assuming that the deviation of the equilibrium solution concentration of X from its initial concentration is negligibly small, then the thermodynamic equilibrium association constant, K_a, of the reaction can be expressed as

$$K_a = \frac{\theta}{[X]_0 \cdot (1-0)} \tag{5.17}$$

where θ is the fractional coverage (in molar ratio) of X on a full monolayer of B and $[X]_0$ is the initial concentration of the analyte in solution.

At full coverage of X (i.e., $\theta = 1$), I_S should be at a minimum value, I_{min}, and results in a maximum change in intensity, $\Delta I_{max} = I_R - I_{min}$. If we further assume that the change in intensity signal from a FO-PPR sensor is proportional to the change in θ, then

$$I_R - I_S = \Delta I_{max} \cdot \theta \tag{5.18}$$

Combining Eqs. 5.17 and 5.18 results in the following expression:

$$\frac{1}{I_R - I_S} = \frac{1}{\Delta I_{max}} + \frac{1}{\Delta I_{max} \cdot K_a \cdot [X]_0} \tag{5.19}$$

Hence, a linear plot of $1/(I_R - I_S)$ versus $1/[X]_0$ would allow the calculation of K_a by dividing the y intercept by the slope.

5.3 Optical Fiber-Based PPR Biosensor

The use of optical fibers for sensing has many attractions, in particular the intrinsic freedom from electromagnetic interference, high information capacity (using wavelength discrimination), the relative safety in explosive environments, the ability to be multiplexed in a distributed system, and the low attenuations which make remote measurements feasible. With the addition of label-free and real-time detection capabilities, the scope of fiber optic biosensors could be further extended to *in vivo*, on-line, and on-site applications. In this regard, the FO-PPR biosensor may be one of the ideal candidates.

The development of the FO-PPR sensor was first reported by Cheng and Chau in 2003.[23] The report demonstrated the ability of the FO-PPR sensor to transduce changes in the surrounding RI into ATR spectra and a refractive index resolution (RIR, defined as minimum change in refractive index unit, RIU, that can be resolved by the sensor) of 7.0 × 10^{-5} RIU was achieved. Such a bulk RIR is inferior to that achieved by many SPR sensors.[48] Nevertheless, a surprising low detection limit (DL) of 9.8 × 10^{-11} M for detection of streptavidin was achieved.[23] There must be a reason.

Both PPR and SPR biosensors measure changes in the RI of the surface adlayer. A consequence of the evanescent character of both sensing techniques is that the sensing field strength decays quite markedly with distance from the sensor surface.[30] The SPR response with respect to the dissipating filed strength can be depicted by exponent dependency on distance normal from the surface:[49]

$$\Delta\lambda = m \cdot \Delta n \cdot \left[1 - e^{-2d/l_d}\right] \quad (5.20)$$

where Δλ is the wavelength shift response, *m* is the refractive index sensitivity, Δ*n* is the change in RI induced by an adsorbate, *d* is the effective adsorbate layer thickness, and l_d is the characteristic field decay length. Equation 5.18 is also used in a review article to account for the wavelength shift response in PPR biosensors, but the authors caution that the electromagnetic fields associated with NMNPs is oversimplified.[50]

In biosensor applications, it is common to attach a selective receptor on the sensor surface, and an analyte subsequently binds with the selective receptor from solution. Assuming the thickness of the immobilized receptor is *h*, a simple extension of Eq. (5.20) yields[49]

$$\Delta\lambda = m \cdot \Delta n \cdot \left[1 - e^{-2d/l_d}\right] \cdot e^{-2h/l_d} \quad (5.21)$$

For the PPR biosensor or FO-PPR biosensor which interrogates the binding event via absorbance change, Δ*A*, similar relationships are proposed as following:

$$\Delta A = m \cdot \Delta n \cdot \left[1 - e^{-2d/l_d}\right] \quad (5.22)$$

$$\Delta A = m \cdot \Delta n \cdot \left[1 - e^{-2d/l_d}\right] \cdot e^{-2h/l_d} \quad (5.23)$$

In a review article by Willets and Van Duyne,[51] the authors give the following summary: although SPR spectroscopy provides much higher sensitivity to changes in bulk RI (~3100 to 8800 nm/RIU)[49] than PPR spectroscopy (~70 to 880 nm/RIU),[16,19,52–54] the responses of the two techniques become comparable when measuring short-range changes in RI owing to a molecular adsorption layer. This is a result of the much smaller sensing volume offered by the PPR sensors (20–40 nm),[55,56] as the electromagnetic field decay length is about 10 times shorter than that of the SPR sensors (200–400 nm).[48]

To improve the RIR of the FO-PPR sensor, the key is to lower the noise and baseline drift of the system. Upon improvement of the instrumentation as shown in Fig. 5.1, an optical stability (OS) of 0.0091% in terms of coefficient of variation (CV) was achieved. The OS is calculated by

$$\mathrm{OS} = \frac{e}{I_\mathrm{R}} \times 100\% \tag{5.24}$$

where e is the root-mean-square noise of the system with a blank. Using this system, an RIR of 1.9×10^{-6} RIU can be achieved, as shown in Fig. 5.2. Now, even the bulk RIR by the FO-PPR sensor is comparable to that achieved by many SPR sensors.[48] The figure also shows that the plot of I_S/I_R versus medium RI with a correlation coefficient (R) of 0.9994 is slightly more linear than the plot of $-\log(I_S/I_R)$ versus medium RI (R = 0.9934). The slopes of the plots I_S/I_R versus medium RI and $-\log(I_S/I_R)$ versus medium RI are −7.9 RIU^{-1} and 5.0 absorbance unit (AU)/RIU, respectively. In a previous study, a sensitivity of 4.2 AU/RIU has also been reported.[23] The value of the slope is a useful indicator of the density of NMNPs on the fiber core, although the size of the NMNPs should also be taken into consideration.

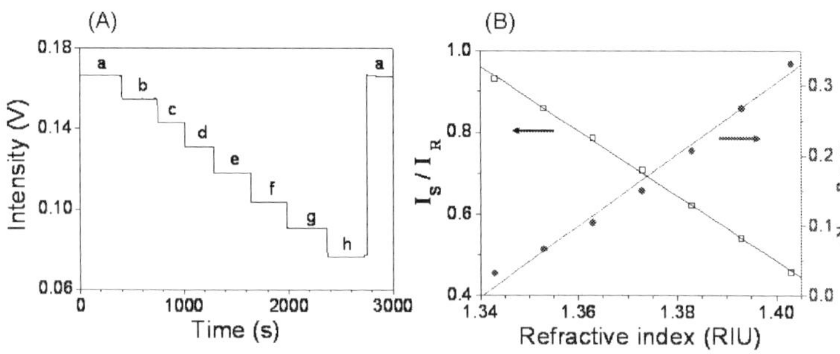

Figure 5.2 (A) Temporal response of a FO-PPR sensor with serial injection of samples with refractive index of (a) 1.333, (b) 1.343, (c) 1.353, (d) 1.363, (e) 1.373, (f) 1.383, (g) 1.393, and (h) 1.403. (B) Dependency of the FO-PPR biosensor signal expressed as I_S/I_R or $-\log(I_S/I_R)$ on the refractive index of the surrounding medium.

As a comparison to the FO-PPR sensor, the sensitivity of the PPR spectroscopy to a layer of spherical NMNPs on a glass slide in terms of absorbance change rather than peak wavelength shift was explored. The slide was immersed in solutions of different refractive indexes and the spectra were measured in a transmission mode, as shown in Fig. 5.3. Over the range of RI studied, the response is linear ($R = 0.9990$) with a slope of 0.12 AU/RIU. In a previous study, a sensitivity of 0.46 AU/RIU has also been reported.[19] The difference is probably due to the variation in size and density of the NMNPs immobilized on the surface. With a noise of 9.0×10^{-5} AU, the RIR by PPR spectroscopy as shown in Fig. 5.3 is 7.5×10^{-4} RIU. Thanks to the sensitivity gain via the OW sensing technology, multiple TIR along the optical fiber yield an absorbance change per RIU about one order of magnitude and a RIR of about two orders of magnitude better than that through a single NMNP layer by the simple transmission spectroscopy.

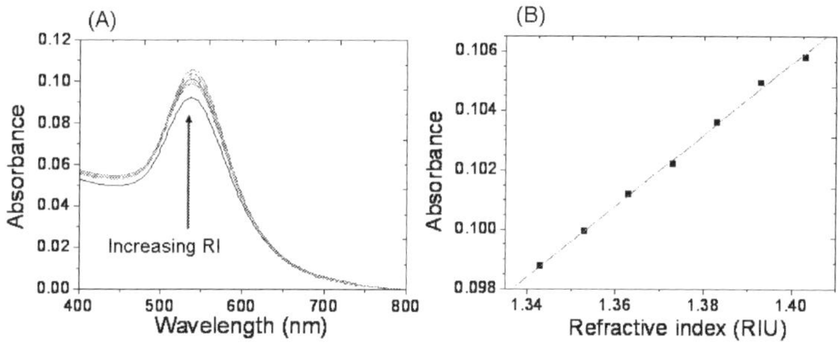

Figure 5.3 (A) Absorbance spectra of a monolayer of immobilized gold nanoparticles on glass in samples of increasing refractive indexes (1.333, 1.343, 1.353, 1.363, 1.373, 1.383, 1.393, 1.403). The spectra were interrogated via transmission mode. (B) Linear dependence of the absorbance at 534 nm on the refractive of the surrounding medium. See also Color Insert.

One of the advantages of a label-free biosensor is its capability of real-time detection of biomolecular interactions. Figure 5.4 shows a FO-PPR sensorgram of an analyte, anti-dinitrophenyl antibody (anti-DNP), with sequential increase in concentration by 10-fold injected over a surface with immobilized DNP as a receptor. The real-time response shows response times (time to reach 90% of the equilibrium signal level) of about 300 s. In this system, a microfluidic chip has been integrated with the FO-PPR sensor, resulting in a significantly reduced response time from several thousand seconds in a conventional liquid cell[25] to several hundred seconds in this microfluidic cell. This reduction in response time can be accounted for by an expression derived from the Fick's Law of Diffusion:[57]

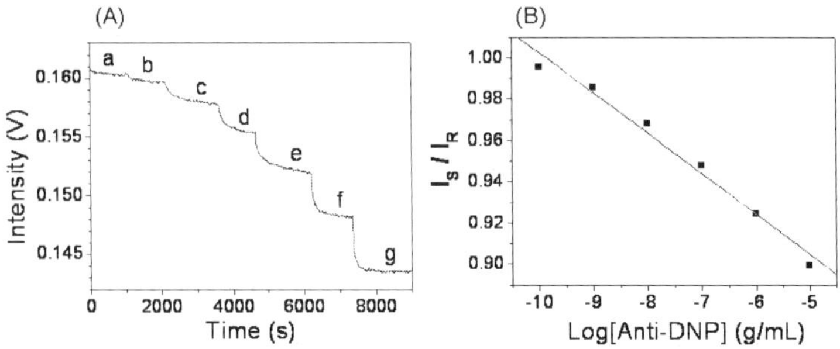

Figure 5.4 (A) Temporal response of a DNP-functionalized FO-PPR sensor with serial injection of (a) a PBS buffer and samples of an anti-DNP solution with concentration of (b) 1×10^{-10} g/mL, (c) 1×10^{-9} g/mL, (d) 1×10^{-8} g/mL, (e) 1×10^{-7} g/mL, (f) 1×10^{-6} g/mL, and (g) 1×10^{-5} g/mL. (B) Calibration graph of I_S/I_R versus log anti-DNP concentration.

$$t = \frac{x^2}{D} \tag{5.25}$$

where t, x, and D are the molecular transportation time, diffusion distance, and diffusion coefficient, respectively. This means that a down-scale to 1/10 of the original size of the sensing cell reduces the molecular transport time to 1/100.[58] Based on this relationship, a decrease in the response time by reducing the width of the microfluidic channel is expected. Further reduction in response time can be achieved by active mass transport, for example, by ac electro-osmosis driven by field-induced polarization.[59] Using this micro-mixer (see Chapter 7 for details), the sensing response time of detecting an orchid Odontoglossum ringspot virus (ORSV) has been reduced from 1000 s to 330 s when the external field is applied to mix for 60 s while detection limit is maintained.[60]

Although in principle a refractive index sensor is almost totally insensitive to volume change of the sensing cell,[55] the performance of a biosensor has been suggested to be limited by the rate at which an analyte molecule is transported to a surface-immobilized recognition molecule.[61,62] When this binding process is diffusion limited, the sensor's DL and response time are limited by analyte mass transport. As compared to the DL (9.8×10^{-11} M) for streptavidin using the FO-PPR sensor in a conventional liquid cell,[23] we have found that the DL (1.1×10^{-11} M) under similar conditions has been improved by about ninefold when the FO-PPR sensor was integrated with a microfluidic cell. Since the invention of the FO-PPR sensor, we have been working on a number of immunoassays with various binding affinities. So far, the DL found is limited to the picomolar level. It has been suggested that nanoscale sensors without active mass transport will be subject to picomolar detection limit for practical time scales.[62] As an example, the inset of Fig. 5.4 shows a calibration graph of the sensor response (I_S/I_R) versus log anti-DNP concentration. From this linear plot ($R = 0.9910$), a DL of 6.2×10^{-13} M for anti-DNP is estimated.

As the refractive index increment induced by an adlayer as shown in Eqs. (18–21) is related to the analyte concentration to be measured, the detection of absolute number quantities of adsorbed analyte becomes more sensitive with increasing mass of adsorbed analyte (with thickness d). On the other hand, the detection of absolute number quantities of adsorbed analyte becomes less sensitive with increasing mass of immobilized receptor (with thickness h). With this in mind, we have carried out of a series of biomolecular interaction studies using various sizes of immobilized receptors and analytes. The results are summarized in Table 5.1. It can be seen that the DL is mainly dependent on K_a as well as the size the analyte.

Table 5.1 Detection limits and equilibrium association constants of different receptor–analyte pairs obtained by the FO-PPR sensor under similar immobilization and detection conditions

Immobilized receptor	Analyte	Detection limit (M)	K_a (M)
DNP	Anti-DNP	2.7×10^{-10}	4.8×10^{8}
HSA	Anti-HSA	1.6×10^{-10}	3.6×10^{8}
Biotin	Anti-biotin	8.5×10^{-8}	1.7×10^{6}
Anti-HSA	HSA	4.6×10^{-7}	1.3×10^{6}

DNP: dinitrophenyl, MW = 297 Da
Anti-DNP: MW = 220 kDa[63]
Biotin: MW = 244 Da
Anti-biotin: MW = 150 kDa[18]
HSA: human serum albumin, MW = 67 kDa[64]
Anti-HSA: MW = 160 kDa[64]

Consider the receptor–analyte pairs, DNP–anti-DNP, and HSA–anti-HSA, that have K_a and analyte size in a similar level, the detection limits are similar although HSA has a much larger molecular weight (MW) than DNP. For the receptor–analyte pairs, biotin–anti-biotin and anti-HSA–HSA, that have K_a in a similar level, the DL by immobilized biotin to detect anti-biotin is better than that by immobilized anti-HSA to detect HSA, suggesting that the size of the analyte is an important factor for determining the DL. Interestingly, with anti-HSA is immobilized as receptor to detect HSA, the K_a decreases by two orders of magnitude as compared to that with HSA as immobilized receptor to detect anti-HSA. Such a decrease in K_a may be attributed to a loss of activity of the coupled antibody, since antibody is an asymmetrical macromolecule which often has a disorder orientation after immobilization on a surface. The study illustrates how important an immobilization step can affect the biosensor performance, whereas the binding affinity can actually be revealed by a FO-PPR biosensor.

The FO-PPR sensors have been applied to detect staphylococcal enterotoxin B (SEB),[24] organophosphorous pesticides,[65] lead ion,[66] cadmium ion,[67] antinuclear antibodies (ANA),[25] orchid Odontoglossum ringspot virus (ORSV)[60], guanosine 3′,5′-cyclic monophosphate (cCMP),[68] and interleukin-1β (IL-1β).[69] In the determination of staphylococcal enterotoxin B (SEB),[24] the DL of the FO-PPR sensor is 0.04 ng/mL (1.4×10^{-12} M), which is the lowest as compared to enzyme-linked immunosorbent assay (ELISA) (3.9 ng/mL)[70] and competing biosensor technologies such as SPR sensors (0.5~10 ng/mL),[71,72] piezoelectric crystal biosensors (0.1 μg/mL),[73] and fiber optic fluorescence biosensor (0.5 ng/mL).[74]

In the determination of organophosphorous pesticides,[65] the gold nanoparticle (GNP) surface was covalently coupled with acetylcholinesterase (AChE) to detect paraoxon. The underlying mechanism is that paraoxon prevents acetylchloline chloride (Ach) reacting with AChE by destroying the OH bond of serine in AChE. The deactivated AChE can be reactivated with dephosphorylation by 2-pyridine-aldoxime methoiodide. The DL of the sensor is 0.23 ppb, which is slightly lower than the DL of 0.3 by an amperometric biosensor.[75] The sensor gave reproducible results after storage in dry state at 4°C for 60 days and remained 94% of its original activity after six cycles of inhibition and reactivation.

In the determination of ANA in sera from patients[25] or IL-1β in synovial fluids from patients with osteoarthritis,[69] the GNP surface was covalently coupled with extractable nuclear antigens or anti-IL-1β, respectively. The results by both sensors agree quantitatively with the clinically accepted ELISA method. Furthermore, the FO-PPR sensor for ANA is more sensitive than ELISA, the gold standard in immunoassay, by at least an order of magnitude, and the analysis time is significantly shorter (<15 min) as compared to ELISA.

The FO-PPR sensor not only works in the transmission mode, but has also been developed into a dip-probe configuration.[24] The dip-probe has been used to detect SEB[24] and lead ion.[66] Moreover, the dip-probe has also been developed to determine RI, nickel ion, streptavidin, and immunoglobulin G (IgG) at high-pressure conditions (up to 20.4 MPa),[76] which provides a basis as a detector for supercritical chromatography.

Different fiber optic probe design including straight, U-bent, D-shape, tapered, and biconical tapers have been employed in development of absorbance-based biosensor. U-bent probes have been demonstrated to have a 10-fold improvement in absorbance sensitivity over straight probes.[77] Mukherji and coworkers combined the advantage of NMNP with U-bent fiber optic probe to develop a U-bent FO-PPR sensor, which showed a RIR of 3.8×10^{-5} RIU and a sensitivity of 35 AU/RIU at 540 nm.[78] With IgG as the immobilized receptor to detect anti-IgG, a DL of 0.8 nM was achieved. D-shape optical fiber fabricated by femotosecond laser micromachining has been used to develop a small-size FO-PPR sensor,[79] which can take advantage of the technologies established by the fiber optic communication industries and also fulfill the need for *in vivo* analysis. The D-shape FO-PPR sensor showed a RIR of 1.4×10^{-4} RIU. Besides using optical fibers of different geometries, FO-PPR sensor based on long-period fiber grating (LPFG) has also been developed.[80] By this approach, when the GNP surface is modified with DNP, the sensor can detect anti-DNP down to 9.5×10^{-10} M.

5.4 Planar Waveguide-Based PPR Biosensor

Cylindrical waveguides show some interesting features because they allow remote measurements and are capable of reaching places hard to access for *in situ* environmental monitoring or *in vivo* bioanalysis.

On the other hand, planar waveguides represent practically the same concept as optical fibers but in a microfabricated planar design. However, planar waveguides offer advantages such as ease of miniaturization in form of an integrated optical sensor and compatibility with microelectronic technology.

Richardson and coworkers[81] used indium tin oxide (ITO) as planar waveguide (PW) and immobilized GNPs on the surface of ITO. The sensing region had a length of 2 cm.[82] A study of the refractive index sensitivity of this sensing configuration showed that the PW-PPR sensor had a sensitivity of 9.2 AU/RIU. Such a high sensitivity is due to the extremely high number of reflections along the waveguide since the thickness of an ITO layer is typically around 50–100 nm, while the FO-PPR sensor as described above typically has a core diameter of 400 nm and sensing length of 2 cm. The optical path length of the PW sensor can be estimated by using a ray optics model to describe light propagation in the guiding layer.[83] The work also demonstrated that the sensor can detect adsorption of fibrinogen on GNP surface and is more sensitive than the PPR sensor employing a single pass transmission measurement.[19] Since ITO is conductive, this sensing configuration also allows spectroelectrochemistry to be performed.

Although a thin film PW can be used to increase the effective pathlength of an ATR measurement and enhance the sensitivity, light coupling into the waveguide is not an easy task. Typically, prism or grating coupling is used. Prism coupling is only practical for benchtop applications since the prisms must be placed on the surface of the thin film and it is difficult to isolate the prisms from the liquid sample. Moreover, coupling efficiency is very sensitive to the input beam alignment and prism contact with the surface. On the other hand, the coupling efficiency with grating is low and sophisticated microfabrication processes are often required to construct the gratings on the sensing chips. An alternative is to use direct coupling but precise alignment of the incident light beam to the end face of the PW is required, especially for thin film PWs.

In an attempt to study the sensitivity of a PW-PPR sensor, a simple optical setup and a thin glass slide (0.1 mm) as shown in Fig. 5.5 were used. GNPs were immobilized on one side of the slide and a PMMA chip with a microfluidic channel (0.4 mm × 3 mm × 30 mm) was placed on top of the glass slide in a manner that the GNPs could be exposed in the microfluidic channel. When I_S/I_R is plotted versus RI of the surrounding medium, a linear fit (R = 0.9940) is observed. From the plot, a RIR of 1.5 $\times 10^{-4}$ RIU and a slope of 4.6 AU/RIU is estimated. To further increase the sensitivity of the PW-PPR sensors, it has been shown that single-mode planar waveguide structures are more sensitive by a few orders of magnitude than their thicker multimode counterparts.[84,85] However, direct coupling is extremely difficult for single-mode planar waveguide structures. Buried grating coupler have been suggested because the beam input and collection optics are located behind the waveguide and are completely isolated from the liquid sample and thus are much more amendable to a sensor format.[86]

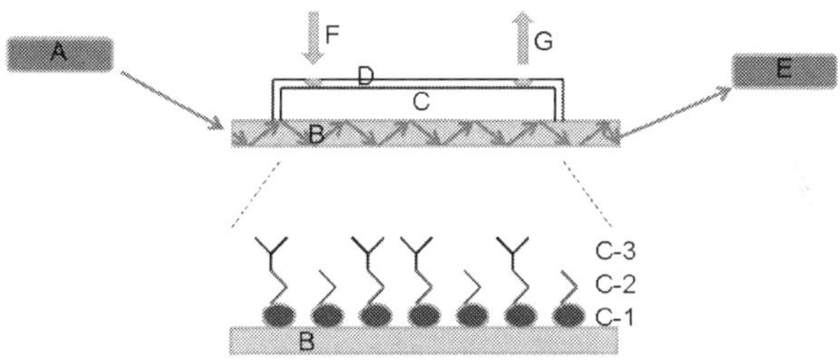

Figure 5.5 Schematic representation of the experimental setup for the PW-PPR biosensor to make measurements: A, laser; B, gold nanoparticles-modified glass slide; C, microfluidic channel; D, top cover; E, photodiode; F, liquid inlet; G, liquid outlet. The biosensing chip (B) consists of gold nanoparticles (C-1) and immobilized receptor molecules (C-2), which bind with analyte molecules (C-3) in the microfluidic channel (C).

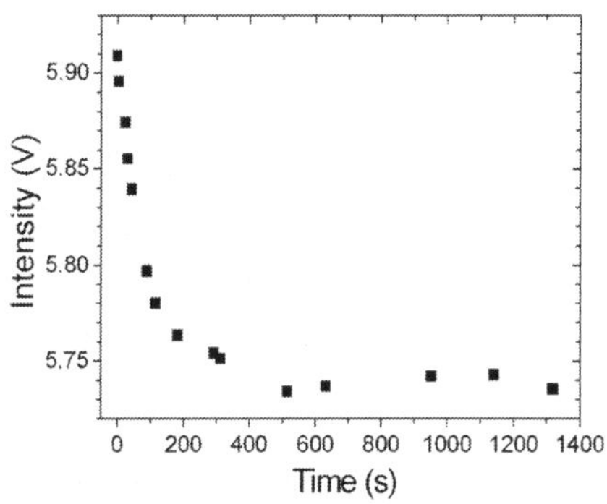

Figure 5.6 Temporal response of a DNP-functionalized PW-PR sensor with injection of a 1 $\times 10^{-4}$ g/mL anti-DNP solution.

As shown in Fig. 5.6, real-time detection of biomolecular interaction of anti-DNP with DNP on the GNP surface shows a response time of 300 s. As suggested by Eq. 5.25, reduced channel height will lead to shorter response time. For this sensing configuration, the height of the microfluidic channel can be easily adjusted. Thus, the integration of a PW-PPR biosensor and a microfluidic chip can be easily optimized.

5.5 Tubular Waveguide-Based PPR Biosensor

A tubular waveguide (TW) can be a light guiding tube or a light guiding capillary. Tubular waveguide sensors typically have a chemically sensitive inner coating in the TW. They are multifunctional devices in being optical waveguides, sample cavities of defined volumes, sampling devices, flow-through cells, mechanical support for sensor coatings, and wavelength discriminators.[87] As a device for direct sampling, samples may be drawn by capillary action, and this is considered to be particularly convenient in the case of blood and other biological fluids. In addition, TWs may be fabricated by simple and inexpensive means and therefore are ideally suited for disposable sensors.

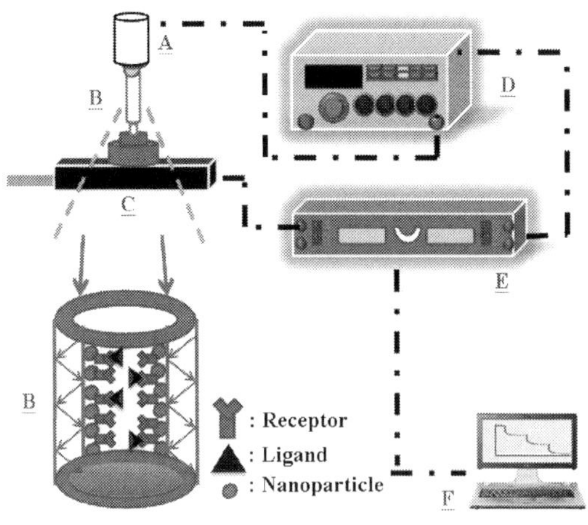

Figure 5.7 Schematic representation of the experimental setup for the TW-PPR biosensor to make measurements: A, light emitting diode; B, gold nanoparticles-modified glass tube; C, photodiode; D, function generator; E, lock-in amplifier; F, computer.

In an attempt to study the sensitivity of a TW-PPR sensor, an integration of a simple optical setup and a glass tube (inner diameter = 4.2 mm, outer diameter = 5.0 mm, length = 31 mm) with one closed end as shown in Fig. 5.7 were used. GNPs were immobilized on the inner wall of the glass tube. When I_S/I_R is plotted versus RI of the surrounding medium, a linear fit (R = 0.9971) is observed. From the plot, a RIR of 5.4 × 10^{-6} RIU and a slope of 8.6 AU/RIU is estimated. Such a high sensitivity is probably due to the long sensor length and the large surface area available for immobilization of NMNPs and their interactions with the sample. It has been demonstrated that a long optical path TW absorbance sensor can be achieved by using a flexible fused-silica capillary.[88] Unfortunately, theoretical models for TW absorbance sensors have not been found in literatures, but models based on fiber optic absorbance sensors should be useful for TW absorbance sensors.

As shown in Fig. 5.8A, upon serial injection of streptavidin samples of increasing concentration, biomolecular interaction of streptavidin with biotin on the GNP surface can be observed in real-time. When I_S/I_R is plotted versus log streptavidin concentration as shown in Fig. 5.8B, a linear fit (R = 0.9964) is observed. From this calibration graph, a DL of 3.3 × 10^{-12} M for streptavidin is estimated. Because of the small size and self-contained sample holding design, the TW-PPR biosensor has a high potential of being developed to be a portable biosensor. Furthermore, when the tubular waveguides are arranged in an array, a high throughput biosensing system is anticipated.

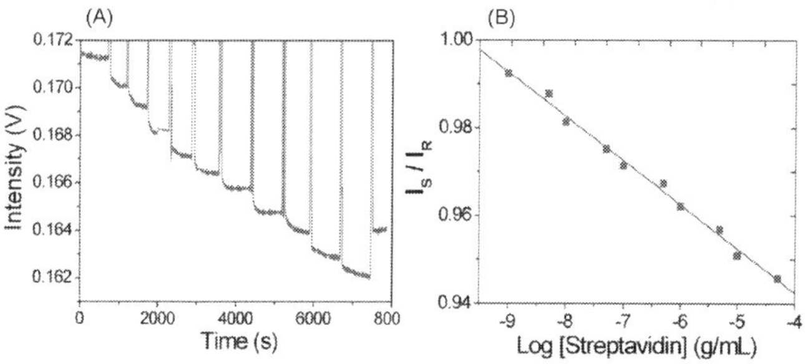

Figure 5.8 (A) Temporal responses of a biotin-functionalized TW-PRR sensor with serial injection of streptavidin samples of increasing concentration. (B) Calibration graph of I_S/I_R versus log streptavidin concentration.

5.6 Conclusions and Outlook

Label-free biosensing systems enable flexibility to the process of assay design with potentially fewer artifacts. Scientists in both academia and industry are using biosensors in areas that encompass almost all areas of the chemical and biological sciences, but the technology remains some way from being accepted as mainstream. This chapter has described studies related both to the fundamentals and applications of OW-PPR biosensors. The results demonstrate that the OW sensing technology enhance the sensitivity of the PPR biosensing technique. Furthermore, OW-PPR measurement is based on extinction spectroscopy and, hence, the normalization by I_S/I_R or $(I_R - I_S)/I_R = \Delta I_S/I_R$, the relative change of transmission response, alleviates the demand on precise optical alignment. In other words, the OW-PPR sensor response presented as I_S/I_R or $\Delta I_S/I_R$ provides a mean of normalization to ensure that some variation of I_R is acceptable. Despite these advantages, many practical challenges remain before OW-PPR biosensors can reach their full potential as analytical tools for chemical quantification, characterization of binding affinities and kinetics, and detection of conformational changes. As technology is developed to improve the instrumentation aspects such as instrumental resolution, instrument stability, easy to operate, user-friendly software, ease of data interpretation, portability, and inexpensive, as mass production techniques mature and nanoparticles become more uniform and stable, and as more diverse and complementary techniques such as mass spectrometry, surface-enhanced Raman scattering, electrochemical techniques, and microfluidics are integrated, future commercialization of PPR biosensors is foreseeable.

Acknowledgment

This work was supported by the Natural Science Council (Taiwan), National Chung Cheng University, and Buddhist Dalin Tzu Chi General Hospital.

References

1 S. A. Soper, K. Brown, A. Ellington, B. Frazier, G. Garcia-Manero, V. Gau, S. I. Gutman, D. F. Hayes, B. Korte, J. L. Landers, D. Larson, F. Ligler, A. Majumdar, M. Mascini, D. Nolte, Z. Rosenzweig, J. Wang, and D. Wilson, *Biosens. Bioelectron.*, **21**, 1932 (2006).

2. M. A. Cooper, *Drug Discovery World*, **68** (Summer 2006).
3. P. D. Patel, *Trends Anal. Chem.*, **21**, 96 (2002).
4. I. E. Tothill, *Comput. Electron. Agric.*, **30**, 205 (2001).
5. L. Olsson, U. Schulze, and J. Nielsen, *Trends Anal. Chem.*, **17**, 88 (1998).
6. S. Rodriguez-Mozaz, M. J. L. De Alda, M.-P. Marco, and D. Barcelo, *Talanta*, **65**, 291 (2005).
7. J. J. Gooding, *Anal. Chim. Acta*, **559**, 137 (2006).
8. F. Comley, *Drug Discovery World*, **28** (Fall 2008).
9. N. L. Rosi, and C. A. Mirkin, *Chem. Rev.*, **105**, 1547 (2005).
10. J. A. Anker, W. P. Hall, Lyandres, N. C. Shan, J. Zhao, and R. P. Van Duyne, *Nat. Mater.*, **7**, 442 (2008).
11. Stewart, C. R. Anderton, L. B. Thompson, J. Maria, S. K. Gray, J. A. Rogers, and R. G. Nuzzo, *Chem. Rev.*, **108**, 494 (2008).
12. P. Mulvaney, *Langmuir*, **12**, 788 (1996).
13. T. R. Jensen, M. L. Duval, K. L. Kelly, A. A. Lazarides, G. C. Schatz, and R. P. Van Duyne, *J. Phys. Chem. B*, **1999**, 103, 9846–9853.
14. Y. Sun, and Y. Xia, *Anal. Chem.*, **74**, 5297 (2002).
15. E. M. Larsson, J. Alegret, M. Kall, and D. S. Sutherland, *Nano Lett.*, **7**, 1256 (2007).
16. H. Chen, X. Kou, Z. Yang, W. Ni, and J. Wang, *Langmuir*, **24**, 5233 (2008).
17. P. Englebienne, *Analyst*, **1998**, 123, 1599–1603.
18. A. J. Haes, and R. P. Van Duyne, *J. Am. Chem. Soc.*, **124**, 10596 (2002).
19. N. Nath, and A. Chilkoti, *Anal. Chem.*, **74**, 504 (2002).
20. S.-F. Cheng, L.-K. Chau, and K.-C. Pao, *J. Biomed. Nanotechnol.*, **1**, 143 (2005).
21. C.-D. Chen, S.-F. Cheng, L.-K. Chau, and C. R. C. Wang, *Biosens. Bioelectron.*, **22**, 926 (2007).
22. M. D. Degrandpre, and L. W. Burgess, *Anal. Chem.*, **60**, 2582 (1988).
23. S.-F. Cheng, and L.-K. Chau, *Anal. Chem.*, **75**, 16 (2003).
24. L.-K. Chau, Y.-F. Lin, S.-F. Cheng, and T.-J. Lin, *Sens. Actuators B*, **113**, 100 (2006).
25. N.-S. Lai, C.-C. Wang, H.-L. Chiang, and L.-K. Chau, *Anal. Bioanal. Chem.*, **388**, 901 (2007).
26. W. A. Murray, and W. L. Barnes, *Adv. Mater.*, **19**, 3771 (2007).
27. J. Homoloa, S. S. Yee, and G. Gauglitz, *Sens. Actuators B*, **54**, 3 (1999).

28. S. Link, and M. A. El-Sayed, *Int. Rev. Phys. Chem.*, **19**, 409 (2000).
29. E. Hao, G. C. Schatz, and J. T. Hupp, *J. Fluorescence*, **14**, 331 (2004).
30. A. J. Haes, and R. P. van Duyne, *Anal. Bioanal. Chem.*, **379**, 920 (2004).
31. C. R. Yonzon, E. Jeoung, S. Zou, G. C. Schatz, M. Mrksich, and R. P. Van Duyne, *J. Am. Chem. Soc.*, **126**, 12669 (2004).
32. A. J. Haes, S. Zou, G. C. Schatz, and R. P. Van Duyne, *J. Phys. Chem. B*, **108**, 109 (2004).
33. A. J. Haes, S. Zou, G. C. Schatz, and R. P. Van Duyne, *J. Phys. Chem. B*, **108**, 6961 (2004).
34. B. Liedberg, I. Lundstrom, and E. Stenberg, *Sens. Actuators B*, **11**, 63 (1993).
35. R. Mukhopadhyay *Anal. Chem.*, **77**, 313A (2005).
36. S. K. Khijwania, and B.G. Gupta, *Opt. Commun.*, **152**, 259 (1998).
37. P. H. Paul, and G. Kychakoff, *Appl. Phys. Lett.*, **51**, 12 (1987).
38. H. Tai, H. Tanaka, and T. Toshino, *Opt. Lett.*, **12**, 437 (1987).
39. S. A. Merschman, and D. C. Tilotta, *Appl. Spectrosc.*, **52**, 106 (1998).
40. M. D. Degrandpre, and L. W. Burgess, *Appl. Spectrosc.*, **44**, 273 (1990).
41. M. Archenault, H. Gagnaire, J. P. Goure, and N. Jaffrezic-Renault, *Sens. Actuat. B*, **5**, 173 (1991).
42. R. Cush, J. M. Cronin, W. J. Stewart, C. H. Maule, J. Molloy, and N. J. Goddard, *Biosens. Bioelectron.*, **8**, 347 (1993).
43. W. Lukosz, *Biosens. Bioelectron.*, **6**, 215 (1991).
44. V. Ruddy, *Fiber Integr. Opt.*, **9**, 142 (1990).
45. D. Gloge, *Appl. Opt.*, **10**, 2252 (1971).
46. F. P. Payne, and Z. M. Hale, *Int. J. Optoelectron.*, **8**, 743 (1993).
47. J. A. Creighton, and D. G. Eadon, *J. Chem. Soc. Faraday Trans.*, **87**, 3881 (1991).
48. J. Homola, S. S. Yee, and G. Gauglitz, *Sens. Actuat. B*, **54**, 3 (1999).
49. L. S. Jung, C. T. Campbell, T. M. Chinowsky, M. N. Mar, and S. S. Yee, *Langmuir*, **14**, 5636 (1998).
50. A. J. Haes, C. L. Haynes, A. D. McFarland, G. C. Schatz, R. P. Van Duyne, and S. Zou, *MRS Bull.*, **30**, 368 (2005).
51. K. A. Willets, and R. P. Van Duyne, *Annu. Rev. Phys. Chem.*, **58**, 267 (2007).
52. M. D. Malinsky, K. L. Kelly, G. C. Schatz, and R. P. Van Duyne, *J. Am. Chem. Soc.*, **123**, 1471 (2001).

53. Y. Sun, and Y. Xia, *Anal. Chem.*, **74**, 5297 (2002).
54. E. M. Larsson, J. Alegret, M. Kall, and D. S. Sutherland, *Nano Lett.*, **7**, 1256 (2007).
55. D. D. Evanoff Jr., R. L. Ryan, and G. Chumanov, *J. Phys. Chem. B*, **108**, 1522 (2004).
56. N. Nath, and A. Chilkoti, *Anal. Chem.*, **76**, 5370 (2004).
57. K. Sato, A. Hibara, M. Tokeshi, H. Hisamoto, and T. Kitamori, *Adv. Drug Delivery Rev.*, **55**, 379 (2003).
58. A. Manz, N. Graber, and H. M. Widmer, *Sens. Actuat. B*, **1**, 244 (1990).
59. S.-C. Wang, H.-P. Chen, C.-Y. Lee, and H.-C. Chang, *Biosens. Bioelectron.*, **22**, 563 (2006).
60. Y. Chuang, C.-Y. Lee, S.-H. Lu, S.-C. Wang, L.-K. Chau, and W.-H. Hsieh, *Anal. Chem.*, **82**, 1123 (2010).
61. P. E. Sheehan, and Whitman, *Nano Lett.*, **5**, 803 (2005).
62. P. R. Nair, and M. A. Alam, *Appl. Phys. Lett.*, **88**, 233120 (2006).
63. R. Blonder, E. Katz, Y. Cohen, N. Itzhak, A. Riklin, and I. Willner, *Anal. Chem.*, **68**, 3151 (1996).
64. G. Sakai, T. Sakai, T. Uda, N. Miura, and N. Yamazoe, *Sens. Actuat. B*, **24–25**, 134 (1995).
65. T.-J. Lin, K.-T. Huang, and C.-Y. Liu, *Biosens. Bioelectron.*, **22**, 513 (2006).
66. T.-J. Lin, and M.-F. Chung, *Sensors*, **8**, 582 (2008).
67. T.-J. Lin, and M.-F. Chung, *Biosens. Bioelectron.*, **24**, 1213 (2009).
68. K.-T. Huang, T.-J. Lin, and M.-H. His, *Biosens. Bioelectron.*, in press.
69. C.-Y. Chiang, M.-L. Hsieh, K.-W. Huang, L.-K. Chau,[1] C.-M. Chang, and S.-R. Lyu, *Biosens. Bioelectron.*, **26**, 1036 (2010).
70. K. E. Sapsford, J. Francis, S. Sun, Y. Kostov, and A. Rasooly, *Anal. Bioanal. Chem.*, **394**, 499 (2009).
71. A. Rasooly, *J. Food Protection*, **64**, 37 (2001).
72. J. Homola, J. Dostalek, S. Chen, A. Rasooly, S. Jiang, and S.S. Yee, *Int. J. Food Microbiol.*, **75**, 61 (2002).
73. J. L. N. Harteveld, M. S. Nieuwenhuizen, and E. R. J. Wils, *Biosens. Bioelectron.*, **12**, 661 (1997).
74. L.A. Tempelman, K.D. King, G.P. Anderson, and F.S. Ligler, *Anal. Biochem.*, **233**, 50 (1996).
75. G. Jeanty, and J. L. Marty, *Biosens. Bioelectron.*, **13**, 213 (1998).
76. T.-J. Lin, and C.-T. Lou, *J. Supercritical Fluids*, **41**, 317 (2007).

77. B. D. Gupta, H. Dodeja, and A. K. Tomar, *Opt. Quantum Electron.*, **28**, 1629 (1996).
78. V. V. R. Sai, T. Kundu, and S. Mukherji, *Biosens. Bioelectron.*, **24**, 2804 (2009).
79. C.-H. Chen, T.-C. Chao, W.-Y. Li, W.-C. Shen, C.-W. Cheng, J.-L. Tang, L.-K. Chau, and W.-T. Wu, *J. Laser Micro/Nanoeng.*, **5**, 1 (2010).
80. J.-L. Tang, S.-F. Cheng, W.-T. Hsu, T.-Y. Chiang, and L.-K. Chau, *Sens. Actuators B*, **119**, 105 (2006).
81. A. L. Weikel, S. D. Conkin, and J. N. Richardson, *Sens. Actuat. B*, **110**, 112 (2005).
82. J. N. Richardson, Z. Aguilar, N. Kaval, S. E. Andria, T. Shtoyko, C. J. Seliskar, and W. R. Heineman, *Electrochim. Acta*, **48**, 4291 (2003).
83. L. Yang, and S. S. Saavedra, *Anal. Chem.*, **67**, 1307 (1995).
84. S. S. Saavedra, and W. M. Reichert, *Anal. Chem.*, **62**, 2251 (1990).
85. S. B. Menders, and S. S. Saavedra, *Opt. Express*, **4**, 449 (1999).
86. M. D. Degrandpre, L. W. Burgess, P. L. White, and D. S. Goldman, *Anal. Chem.*, **62**, 2012 (1990).
87. O. S. Wolfbeis, *Trends Anal. Chem.*, **15**, 225 (1996).
88. S. Tao, and T. V. S. Sarma, *Opt. Express*, **31**, 1423 (2006).

Chapter 6

Fabrication of Biosensor Chips

Wei Te Wu,[a,*] Guo-Hua Feng,[b] and Wen Hsin Hsieh[b]

[a]*Department of Biomechatronics Engineering,*
National Pingtung University of Science and Technology,
1, Shuefu Road, Neipu, Pingtung 912, Taiwan, ROC
[b]*Department of Mechanical Engineering, National Chung Cheng University,*
168, University Road, Ming Hsiung, Chia Yi 621, Taiwan, ROC
[*]weite@mail.npust.edu.tw

This chapter introduces four production techniques based on polymer substrate as its core element for fabrication of biosensor chips, and also discusses the combined use of optical grating or fiber as an element to produce a sensor component. The four key technologies are photolithography, soft lithography, fabrication of diffraction gratings, and production of optical fiber windows.

6.1 Photolithography Process

Currently a variety of materials could be applied to the fabrication of biochips [1]. Among them, the PDMS-based biochip is most popular due to its easy preparation and low-cost merits. Typically, liquid PDMS is poured onto a designed mold, which is usually

From Bioimaging to Biosensors: Noble Metal Nanoparticles in Biodetection
Edited by Lai-Kwan Chau and Huan-Tsung Chang

ISBN 978-981-4267-24-3 (Hardcover), 978-981-4303-10-1 (eBook)
www.panstanford.com

made by glass, and then peeled off from the substrate after PDMS is solidified for subsequent biochip fabrication, e.g., serving as the chip cover. Besides that, some of silicon-based biochips/biodevices are popular due to their integration ability with CMOS circuitry [2, 3]. Researchers also directly work on glass slide as biochip substrate. For example, metal electrodes are deposited on glass slides for manipulating electrochemical reaction. However, the key components of the chips (e.g., flow channels or electrodes) need well-delineated patterns. Photolithography plays an important role to achieve these fabrication results. The purpose of this operation includes two aspects. Firstly, it is to create on the substrate surface a pattern whose dimensions are close to the design requirements as possible. Secondly, the multiple designed patterns correctly place on the wafer surface and the individual parts are in the correct positions relative to each other [4, 5]. Figure 6.1 shows the flow chart of the photolithography. To explain this technology in detail, four major process steps: (1) substrate cleaning, (2) photoresist selection and application, (3) mask fabrication and alignment, and (4) photoresist exposure and development are mentioned as following:

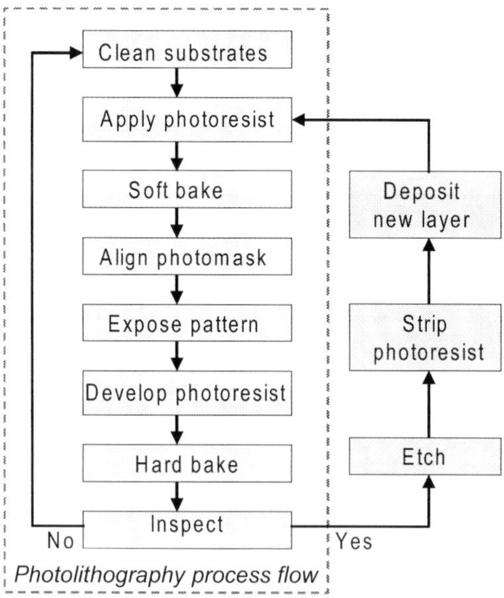

Figure 6.1 Photolithography process flowchart.

6.1.1 Substrate Cleaning

In this section we introduce how to process the substrate materials based on silicon and glass. Clean wafers are essential at all stages of the fabrication process. To clean silicon, four methods are commonly used and effective as below. Readers would try these methods according to their different needs and wafer conditions.

(a) Removes organic contaminants by acetone: Organic contaminants, usually produced in process steps of semiconductor fabrication such as photoresist residue and dry etched residue or exposed at organic molecule-contained environment for a long time, are required removal during the initial process. The simplest way is as follows: (i) immerse the whole wafer in acetone. Use a swab to wash the wafer surface or an ultrasonic bath would enhance the cleaning. (ii) Followed by processing the wafer with methanol and then rinse with water two to three times. (iii) Blow dry the wafer with N_2 gun or spin the wafer to use the centrifuge force drying the wafer.

(b) Oxygen plasma etching: Plasma cleaning is also a common way used to remove organic films and residues. Removing residues or photoresist from a substrate through gentle plasma cleaning is called descumming. Plasma is a cleaning agent and alternative to traditional wet chemical cleaning methods because it does not require using hazardous solvents. However, the cost of plasma etcher is much expensive than chemicals. If the equipment is available, the cleaning quality and uniformity can be well-controlled by properly adjusting the process parameters, such as oxygen pressure, plasma power, etc.

(c) Piranha clean (hot sulfuric acid / hydrogen peroxide mixture): Piranha is highly reactive. It attacks organic materials, such as photoresist or oil stain, strongly and effectively but need to use it carefully with full protective equipment. Usually when the above two methods are not workable, piranha cleaning could be a good try. The preparation of piranha is to mix 98% H_2SO_4 (sulfuric acid) and 30% H_2O_2 (hydrogen peroxide) in volume ratios of 2–4:1. Usually the samples are immersed in the piranha solution (Heat to 100°C) for 10–20 min and followed by water rinse for 15 min, and then blowing the processed samples dry with nitrogen gun.

(d) RCA clean: RCA clean is the industry standard for removing contaminants from silicon wafers. The RCA is called because Werner Kern developed the procedure in 1965 while working for RCA (Radio Corporation of America). The purpose of the RCA clean is to remove organic contaminants (such as dust particles, grease, or silica gel) from the wafer surface with a 5:1:1 H_2O:H_2O_2:NH_4OH solution; then remove any oxide layer that may have built up by using a diluted 20:1 H_2O:HF solution; and finally remove any ionic or heavy metal contaminants by using a solution of 6:1:1 H_2O:H_2O_2:HCl.

Regarding the glass substrate cleaning, hydrofluoride contained solution should not be used to avoid surface etching therefore roughen the substrate surface. Usually glass wafers (or slides) cleaning could be treated with soap solution first, and then cleaned by a solvent, and further processed by a mild acid clean. Water rinse and nitrogen blow dry are followed for each treatment. More detailed are described below.

(a) Soap clean: using soapy water to clean the glass substrate is simple and safe way. When the glass substrate is immersed in the soapy water, gently rubbing the surface to clean dirt and residues with lint-free wipe and cotton swab could be more effective. After finished, rinse the glass substrate with water and blow dry with nitrogen for further process if necessary.

(b) Solvent clean: similar to silicon cleaning, the main purpose of using solvent is to clean oils and organic residues on glass surfaces. Acetone is the most common solvent to be used. Note that, after the substrate cleaning with acetone, acetone leaves its own residues. Hence, a two-solvent method is often used — methanol rinse is followed to remove these residues. Then rinse the glass substrate in water and blow dry with nitrogen.

(c) Acid clean: If the glass substrate has metal residues or ionic contaminations, mild acid could be considered for cleaning. By using 30% HCl or 30% nitric acid solution, the metal ionic residues would be easily removed from the glass surface. The reaction time is usually several minutes, followed by water rinse and nitrogen blow dry.

6.1.2 Photoresist Selection and Application

Photoresists are the heart of the masking process. Their preparation, bake, exposure, and remove process needs to be well treated so that the designated pattern can be formed on the substrate. Basically, the photoresist is manufactured to respond to specific wavelengths of light and different exposing sources, as well as formulated with specific thermal flow characteristics to adhere to specific surfaces. Four major components included in the photoresist: light (energy) sensitive polymers, solvents, sensitizers, and additives. The light-sensitive polymers are functioned to change the structure of the photoresist from soluble to polymerized (or vice versa) after exposure. The solvents maintain the photoresist in liquid form and allow a thin photoresist layer to be applied to the wafer by spinning/spraying. The sensitizers act as the control of chemical reaction of photoresist while exposure. The additives are mixed with the photoresist to obtain various purposes, such as the dyes to absorb light rays in the photoresist.

Common photoresists are designed to respond to ultraviolet or laser sources. Some special photoresists react to X-ray or electron beams. Typically, two kinds of photoresists can be chosen for an application: positive (e.g., AE5214) or negative (e.g., SU-8) type, which is related to the contained light-sensitive polymers in photoresists. The basic positive photoresist polymer is the phenol-formaldehyde novolak resin. Before exposure, the polymer is insoluble. It converts to a soluble state in a special solvent (called development) after exposure. As for the negative photoresist, the exposure makes the polymer switched from unpolymerized structure to a cross-linked material which is etch-resistant (not soluble in developing solution).

To apply the photoresist on the wafers, adhesion promotion can be considered (e.g., HMDS) to get better adhesion, especially dealing with features less than 1 micron. Two methods are commonly used: spin coating and spray. Spin coating is a mature technique and the standard coating method for flat wafers in IC technology. Regularly, two spin speeds are used in one coating. The slow acceleration and spin speed is applied first, which allows the liquid photoresist to flow and spread the whole wafer. Then a fast spin speed causes the coating as uniform as possible. The viscosity of the resist solution and the spinning speed strongly affect the layer formed. Hence, the process optimization needs to focus on these two parameters. When the processed wafer is not flat, spray method could be a good choice to apply photoresist. The spray system uses a spray nozzle, which generates a distribution of droplets of micrometer size. During spray coating, rotating the wafer slowly could minimize the centrifugal force and allow photoresist coverage in all the angle of the cavities. To get the proper droplet size distribution of photoresist, a viscosity of less than 20 cSt is necessary.

Soft bake step is necessary after the photoresist coating. The purpose is to evaporate the solvent contained in the photoresist, which allows for better adhesion and avoid interfering with photosensitive components in the photoresist during exposure. Temperature and time are two major parameters for soft baking. Usually photoresist manufacturers will provide the required information and user could follow and fine-tuned for different applications. Convection ovens and hot plates are commonly used for this process.

6.1.3 Photomask Design/Fabrication and Alignment

Photomasks are high-precision plates containing microscopic images of specific patterns designed by users. It transfers the defined tiny feature-sized patterns onto the wafer. Commercial available substrate materials for making photomasks include quartz and soda lime glass due to their good optical transparent property and small thermal expansion coefficients. To block ultraviolet (UV) light the following materials are commonly coated on one-side of the mask plate: chrome, iron oxide, and emulsion. To fabricate a high resolution photomask is costly. The e-beam directly write the designed pattern on the specific photoresist which is coated on the block material, followed by development and etch process to remove unwanted block material. If the resolution is larger than 10 microns the transparency-type photomasks made by printing would be an alternative, especially for some microfluidics or biochip research areas.

When readers design the photomasks, two polarities of masks are needed to consider: light field (most regions are clear) and dark field (most regions are dark). Through different combination of light/dark field photomask and negative/positive photoresist, the intended patterns can be achieved in two ways. Figure 6.2 shows the use of clear field photomask and positive photoresist can obtain the same island patterns as the use of dark field photomask and negative photoresist. As for which selection is better for the final results, the accumulation of user experience could make a proper judgment.

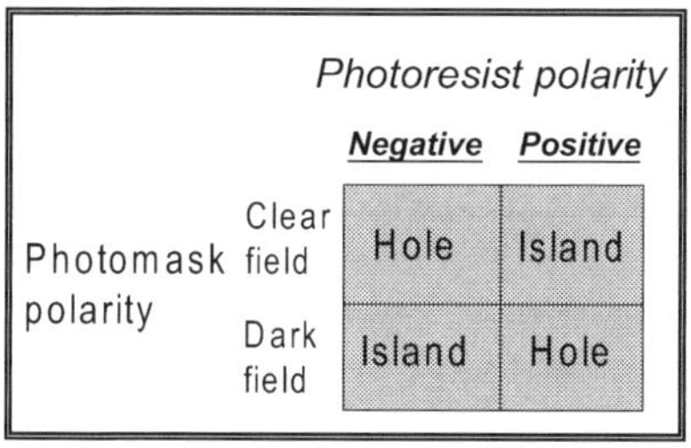

Figure 6.2 Photomask and photoresist polarity results.

An aligner system consists of two major parts: (1) movable mechanism to correctly position the patterns of the photomask on the wafer surface and (2) the exposure subsystem. Two major factors determine the quality of the aligner: resolution and registration capacities. The resolution is mainly a function of the wavelength of the exposing light. The exposing light with smaller or narrower wavelength possesses higher resolution ability due to the diffraction effect. Also, the short wavelength light reduces the scattering effect in the photoresist and from the wafer surface. The registration capacity is determined by how well the images are correctly placed to each other. This requires precise translation/rotation stages and associated mechanisms as well as the operators' experience of finding the best image matching position.

Three aligner types are commonly used: contact, proximity (or soft-contact), and projection. When the contact type aligner is operated, the photomask is positioned over the chunk, which the processed wafer is vacuumed onto. During alignment, the chunk is translated in XY plane, and rotated with an angle θ. Once the wafer and photomask are aligned properly, the chunk is pushed to contact the photomask and followed by exposure. Similar to contact aligner, the major difference of proximity type aligner is that a tiny gap existing between the wafer and photomask during exposure. Therefore, the contact type can make smaller pattern transfer to the wafer compared to the proximity type, but the wear degree of the photomask for the contact type is more severe compared to the soft-contact type. As for the projection type aligner, the major discrepancy from the above two types is the mask image projected onto photoresist by lenses and the projected image on wafer at 1:1 or 5:1 or 10:1 reduction. Hence, good lenses and optical system are must. Besides, due to its small projected region, step-by-step repeat projection onto a large wafer is needed. There is a trade-off between the speed and resolution.

6.1.4 Photoresist Exposure and Development

The photoresist sensitivity relates to the energy of specific wavelength provided by exposing source. Common positive and negative photoresists respond to UV light. Some are particularly designed to reactive to G, H, I lines, whose wavelengths are 365 nm, 405 nm, and 432 nm, respectively, because of current lithography systems use the high pressure Hg lamp which has high intensity in these lines. To enhance resolution, there are specific photoresists sensitive to deep ultraviolet (DUV) light spectrum which excited by excimer lasers.

The photoresist sensitivity is a parameter to measure the amount of energy required to initiate the basic chemical reaction. Users could usually find the information of specific photoresist from manufacturer's data sheet. The unit is often expressed as millijoules per square centimeter (mJ/cm^2) for a given thickness of coated photoresist. In practical operation, the intensity of light source will be tested first, and users can calculate the necessary time for exposure. Overexposure and underexposure could affect the fidelity of the designed patterns, especially when dealing with the micron-range features. Some process recipes will suggest the postexposure bake for a suitable temperature and bake time to reduce the standing wave effect.

After the wafer finishes the alignment and exposure steps, the designed pattern is transferred to the photoresist as exposed and unexposed regions. Development technique is to use the specific chemicals to dissolute the unpolymerized region (negative photoresist) or photosolublized part (positive photoresist) that an exact duplicate of patterns is formed on the photoresist.

The chemicals for developing photoresist associated with specific photoresists can be found from the data sheet provided by the photoresist manufacturers. Generally speaking, the factors affecting the developing results including the soft bake time and temperature; degree of exposure; developer concentration; the time, temperature, and method for development. Over or under development will cause problems such as poor dimension control or removal of excess photoresist intended for protection.

Development includes wet (e.g., immersion, spray, puddle) and dry (plasma) techniques. The most common and low-cost method is immersion. To process that, the developer solution is poured into a chemical resistant container, and then the wafer with patterned photoresist is immersed in the solution for a specific time, followed by rinsing with water. This could be a simple and effective way to develop the relative large patterns with feature size in the range of several microns. For small patterns, the surface tension of developing solution will prevent the chemicals from penetrating into small trenches. In practical operation, users should care the developer chemicals becoming diluted through multiple uses. Room temperature fluctuation can result in the changes in developing rate. Agitation is helpful in developing process to make soluble photoresist more uniform and allow the developer easily penetrates into small openings on patterned photoresist. The agitation can be achieved by mechanical stirring or activating ultrasonic waves in the developer.

Hard bake is usually treated after the developing step, and use the similar equipment and methods as soft bake. Nominal process temperature is from 130 to 200°C for 30 min in a convection oven. The purpose is to achieve good adhesion of the photoresist to the wafer surface. The heat makes the photoresist contained liquid evaporate and further polymerized, therefore improving its etch-resistant properties.

Finally, the development results are inspected to determine if the wafer is passed for further process, such as etching or deposition, otherwise, the rejected wafer will be striped the patterned photoresist and re-processed from the cleaning step again.

6.2 Soft Lithography

Sensor systems with micro-components created with micro-molding methods are now common due to the use of micro-injection molding and hot embossing technologies to produce large numbers of miniature fluid control components and systems. Micro-injection molding and hot embossing techniques are required when producing the mother mold, while the mother mold is manufactured using MEMS technique in the LIGA process. LIGA is a German acronym for Lithographie GaVanodormung Abformung, which in English translates to lithography, electroforming, and micro-molding. The process is significant for the production of deep-precision X-ray electrical deposition molds. The LIGA process is the combination of three technologies: deep lithography, micro-electroforming, and micro-molding. This process can be used to produce high-precision and high-aspect ratio structures. Since the standard LIGA process requires deep X-ray lithography, it can provide results accurate up to sub-micron level. However, due to the high production costs and complexity of the procedure, other technologies have been developed as alternatives, such as Deep UV (DUV) lithography, the excimer laser machine, or deep RIE/ICP. As a category, these LIGA-like processes have become more popular [6–7]. With the maturity of large-scale integrated circuit manufacturing technique, using UV light has become the most accessible alterative. Therefore, in the following description of biosensor chip manufacturing technique, UV LIGA will be used as the key light source. Following are the procedures used: (1) lithography: deep UV lithography; (2) electrodeposition: electroplating; (3) micro-molding: hot-embossing and micro-injection. By following these three production procedures to produce a micro-mold, a required large number of uniform biochips can be produced by injecting the mold with polymers at high temperature and pressure. This section introduces the chip fabrication and package techniques.

6.2.1 Lithography: Deep UV Lithography

The core concepts of DUV Lithography technique are described in the previous section. The biggest difference is the use of metal as the main substrate for the mother mold, particularly stainless steel because of its resistance to oxidization, acidity, and alkalis; good mechanical strength; and compatibility with existing plastic-molding technique. The general steps and procedures are as follows:

(a) Grind and polish the stainless steel plate to ensure that the plate is as smooth as possible.
(b) Degrease the surface of the plate by submerging the plate into in a 1:1 KOH and aqueous alkaline solution at room temperature using ultrasonic cleaning.

(c) Roughen the surface of the stainless steel, soaking it in a 2:8:90 solution of HF, HNO_3, and water. Wash at room temperature with ultrasonic cleaning.

(d) Implement the activation treatment on the surface of the stainless steel. Soak the stainless steel in a 10% sulfuric acid solution. Use ultrasonic cleaning to remove the surface oxide layer.

(e) Treat the stainless steel with nitrogen and dry with heat to remove moisture.

(f) Coat the stainless steel with suitable photo-resistant material. Refer to the previous section to select the correct positive/negative photo-resistance. If desired, the thickness of the photo-resistant material mold can be increased after completion.

(g) Soft bake the photo-resistant material. The purpose of the soft bake process (which has been described in the previous section) is to remove the solvent in the photo-resistant material, and is an important factor in controlling adhesion, exposure, and imaging parameters.

(h) If the photo-resistant stainless steel plated has been properly prepared, place the mask design on top and expose it with a 365 nm i-line light source, so the pattern of the mask will be transferred to the substrate. The exposure produces macromolecule polymerization (positive photo-resistance) and decomposition (negative photo-resistance) to achieve the transfer the mask pattern.

(i) Once the exposure is complete, the development process removes some unnecessary photo-resistant material. Negative photo-resistance will not wash away while positive photo-resistance development will be exposed as part of the wash, leaving behind the pattern that was not exposed.

(j) Finally, the hard bake procedure removes the remaining photo-resistant solvent and moisture. This condenses the photo-resistant resin bonding compounds and increase the photo-resistant heat stability and adhesion so the mask pattern can be protected.

Once the processing of the stainless steel substrate in complete, completing above steps lithography process results in the appearance of the lithography pattern, as shown in the Fig. 6.3. This process is followed by the electrodeposition process.

6.2.2 Electrodeposition: Electroplating

The electrodeposition manufacturing process can be divided into two categories: electroforming and electroplating, both of which operate according to the same principles, the biggest difference being that the electroforming process is independent of the substrate material, as shown in Fig. 6.4, whereas electroplating requires substrates with planned material, as shown in Fig 6.3. This section describes the electroplating technique following the lithography process. This technique forms micro-structures in the substrate and can greatly reduce the time required for molding and also increase the mechanical strength of the mother mold.

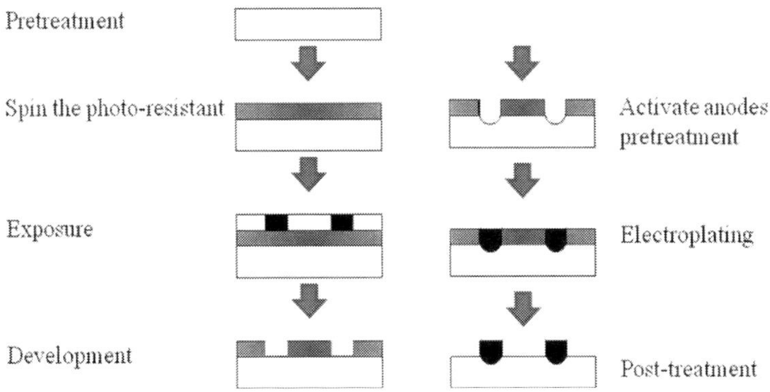

Figure 6.3 Soft lithography process flowchart (electroplating).

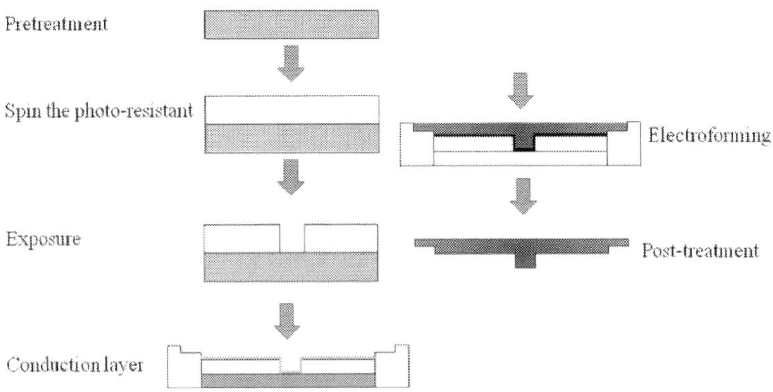

Figure 6.4 Soft lithography process flowchart (electroforming).

The basic theory of electrodeposition is to allow electric current conduction to move ions through the interior of the transmission. Upon contact with the electrode and solution, a reaction occurs between the electrode and the moving charge. At the anode, dissolution of the metal surface produces oxygen and oxidation (anodic oxidation), while on the cathode side; precipitation of metal produces a hydrogen reduction reaction (cathodic reduction). Basically, electroplating uses the appropriate potential energy from the electrical flow of current to produce electrochemical cathode precipitation and attract it to the material. Metal ions come from the electroplating solution or from the consumable anode; the electricity restores them and deposits them at the cathode. Electroplating is an electrochemical reaction, and Faraday's law of induction regulates the amount of plating. Electroplate the previously discussed photo-resistant processed side of a stainless steel substrate with nickel requires three steps: pre-treatment, plating, and post-treatment:

(a) Pre-treatment: With 20 ASD (A/dm^2) in a 10% sulfuric acid solution at room temperature activates anodes using a stainless steel plate that has been processed with lithography. The purpose of this procedure is for etching to increase the plating area at the bottom of the plate and to activate the oxidized layer materials.

(b) Plating: This requires a nickel-plating solution composed of the basic ingredients of a sulfuric acid bath (e.g., Ni_2SO_4), an ingredient to activate the soluble auxiliary anode and higher conductivity (e.g., Ni_2Cl_2, NH_4Cl), and an ingredient to prevent changes in buffer pH (e.g., boric acid). For low-cost plating, a low-stress sulfamate bath with high scalability, better sealing, and high concentration formulations has replaced most sulfuric acid baths. Coating structures and performance improvements, such as improved gloss and smoothness, are mainly achieved by using organic additives. Generally, nickel additives can be classified as brightener and wetting agents, structure modifiers, flattening agents, and carriers. A brightener enhances the reflective properties of metal coatings. For good performance, the roughness of metal reflective coatings must be considerably below the wavelength of incidental light. Therefore, adding a brightener is essential to reducing the size of sedimentary particles, and making the coating brighter. After a brightener is added to nickel plating, the cathode potential increases, which make the nickel harder to deposit, thus, requiring more energy. When gas is released from the electrodes, a wetting agent is often added to speed up the gas discharge. Adding a wetting agent reduces the surface tension between the gas and plating solution, thus allowing the gas bubble to grow larger. A structure modifier is used to improve the structure of metal coatings, and may change the lattice type and orientation. Coatings are also used to adjust stress. A flattening agent can reduce the rugged surface of the plated layer and smooth the coating surface. Many brighteners also have a leveling effect. Brightening and leveling agents can be combined under a wide range of current density for smoother coatings. The frequency and amount of fluid injections depends on the roughness of the substrate and the requirements for thickness, gloss, and smoothness. The ingredients in the bath should remain the consistent to maintain the coating quality. Nickel is the electroforming solution based on nickel sulfamate used to make the electroforming mold.

(c) Post-processing: To complete the formation of micro-structures, the coating layer usually has high electrical resistance, so galvanic grinding is done after the completion of excess coating removal. After grinding the photo-resistant layer, the plate is then placed in a heated alkali solution and then water to avoid shedding. After cleaning, moisture is removed with dry nitrogen, allowing the mother mold to set.

6.2.3 Micro Molding: Hot-Embossing and Micro-Injection

Micro-molding technique generally shapes polymer plastic materials with techniques including hot embossing, injection molding [8–9]. Using polymer plastic material as a biological sensor chip substrate provides five major advantages: (1) low-cost and high-scalability can increase market competitiveness; (2) transparency — compared to non-transparent silicon substrate, transparent plastic chips are useful for observing micro-flow channels in laboratory or clinical tests; (3) good biocompatibility; (4) they can be discarded after use and will not cause cross-contamination between samples; (5) better mechanical strength relative to high silicon and glass chips which are very brittle and are easily damaged during manufacturing or delivery. In contrast, plastic materials are more flexible and are less-easily damaged, and thus are easier to transport and store. The plastic polymer materials commonly used in the manufacturing of biosensor chips can be categorized into two types based on their thermal properties:

(1) Thermoplastic: the material is heated until it reaches glass transition temperature (T_g) and above to a deformable state. When the temperature drops, the material maintains the shape it took when it was heated. Common thermoplastic materials include polymethylmethacrylate (PMMA) and polycarbonate (PC).

(2) Thermosetting: This material is in liquid state before heating but, once heated, it is permanently shaped under pressure. Common thermosetting materials include polydimethylsiloxane (PDMS).

In the micro-forming technique, micro-compression molding can use either thermoplastic or thermosetting plastics with hot pressing. The main process involves putting a plastic granule or a sheet of plastic film on the mold, then using the heating rods or other heating devices to heat the mold. When the plastic material reaches the glass transition temperature (around 10~20°C), then the upper and lower templates are pressed together until the plastic material is pressed into shape prior to being packed, cooled, and stripped (as shown in Fig. 6.5). The micro-compression molding technique has major advantages in that the material's low flow rate makes it suitable for forming micro-structural elements over a large area.

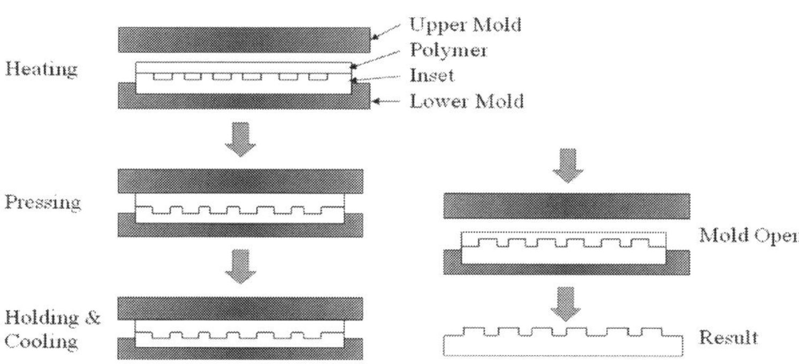

Figure 6.5 Hot-embossing flowchart.

Micro-injection molding makes extensive use of thermoplastics, but thermosetting plastics or ceramic materials are also used. The main process of injection molding requires putting plastic granules in a heating tube and heating them until they reach a liquid state. Then a nozzle is used for high-pressure, high-speed injection of the material, which passes through the sprue and runner to the mold to be completed under pressure in the cavity. After cooling, the molded object is released via the ejection system. The process includes filling, packing, cooling, and other steps (as shown in Fig. 6.6). The micro-injection molding technique provides the major advantage of being able to produce refined, complex shapes in small-sized finished products.

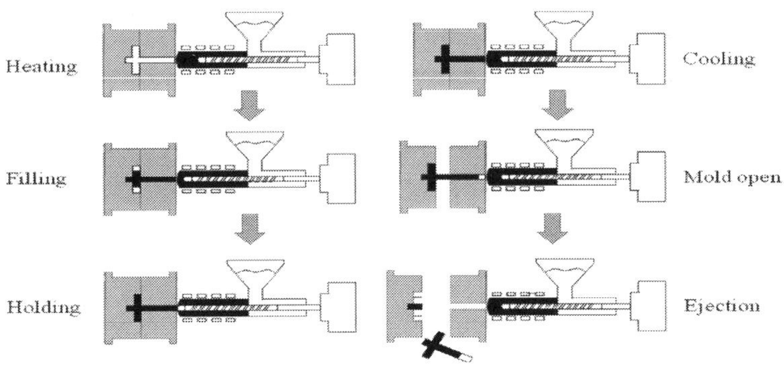

Figure 6.6 Micro-injection flowchart.

6.2.4 Bonding

The biosensor chip bonding technique is part of the manufacturing process, but it can affect the overall accuracy of the most critical aspect: a good and easy-to-operate interface. As such, the kind of interface between the plastic polymers to construct the biosensor chip by a bonding technique can be used as a basis for classification. It can be divided into two categories: attachable medium and non-attachable medium. Bonding methods for the attachable medium include the organic bonding medium, UV sensitive curable bonding medium, or double-sided tape style. The non-attachable medium uses fusion bonding for bonding. These bonding techniques can be characterized as follows.

Attachable medium mounting/bonding technique: Bond two plastic joints with organic dielectric [10] using appropriate pressure and heat. This approach cannot effectively ensure that the micro-flow around the joint is securely sealed. We often found infiltration from bonding medium of the microchannel, resulting in flow blockage. The characteristic of UV sensitive solidified bonding is that the medium will solidify after being exposed to UV light and bonding is complete. However, it still suffers from the infiltration problem mentioned above. The double-sided tape-bonding medium is used to put the bonding medium between two plastic chips. The flow movement of the bonding material between the two plastic chips is low, thus allowing the bonding tape to be adhered between the plastic chips, then heating to the appropriate temperature will complete the bonding. Although this method does not have the infiltration problem, it cannot assure that the sides are completely sealed. So, when the microchannel contacts with a solution, sometimes it may affect the operation of the biosensor chip.

Unattached bonding medium technique is a traditional high-temperature fusion bonding technique [11]. It uses a gradual heating process on the surfaces of two sides. When the thin surface outer layer has melted, the two chips are pressed together to form a seal, thus negating the infiltration problem. However, with the heating temperature close to glass transition temperature, it can greatly affect the size of the microstructure. This issue prompted the development of partial heating bonding technique [12]. The main concept of partial heating is to focus heating on a certain bonding area, such as the microchannel. Common heating sources are ultrasound and other high-energy lasers. These bonding techniques can prevent infiltration and can also solve the problem of imprecision from overall heating. However, this technique has two disadvantages: residual stress after bonding, expensive equipment, and inefficient process.

6.3 Fabrication of Diffraction Gratings

A diffraction grating is an optical component with a regular pattern whose elements are separated by a distance comparable to the wavelength of light under study. Due to its ability to disperse polychromatic light into its constituent monochromatic components, the diffraction grating has been widely used in astronomical, biological, chemical, metallurgical, and other analytical investigations. In bio-medical detection, diffraction gratings have been used as waveguide couplers and detectors [13–20]. In the following, common fabrication methods of diffraction gratings are discussed.

6.3.1 Diamond Ruling

Diamond ruling, using a carefully shaped diamond tool to mechanically rule the surfaces of grating substrates, produced the first diffraction gratings made for commercial use, and now-a-days continues to be widely used in producing various types of diffraction gratings. Due to the ability in controlling the shape of the diamond tool and thereby the shape of the ruled groves, diamond ruling enjoys a dominant position as the major method of fabricating blazed gratings. On the other hand, the linear motion of ruling machines makes this method be used mostly for producing diffraction gratings with straight groves. Figure 6.7 shows the SEM image of a planar blazed diffraction grating (grove density: 1200 groves/mm, blazed angle: 17.5°).

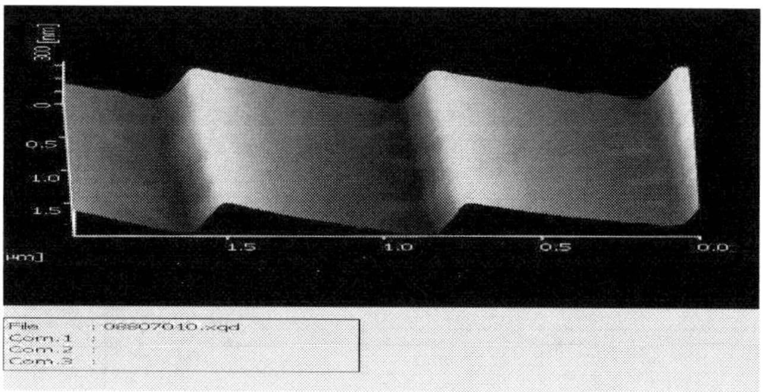

Figure 6.7 SEM image of a planar blazed diffraction grating.

6.3.2 Gray-Scale Lithography

In principle, gray-scale lithography adopts a gray-scale optical mask to modulate the intensity of the light through it and exposes a photoresist to different depths. After development, the photoresist will form a three-dimensional profile corresponding to the intensity pattern on the optical mask. The three-dimensional, developed photoresist will then in turn be used as the mask for anisotropic etching of the grating substrate. The fabrication processes are shown in Fig. 6.8. Due to the flexibility in the pattern design of the optical mask, gray-scale lithography can be adopted for the fabrication of diffraction gratings with complex geometries, such as two-dimensional, Fresnel, or blazed gratings.

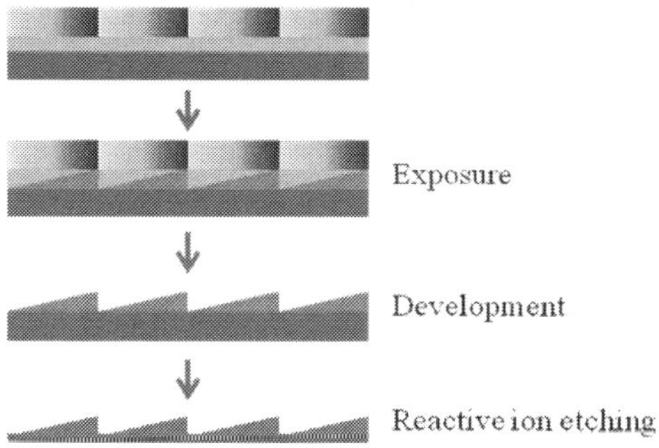

Figure 6.8 Fabrication processes of gray-scale lithography.

In 2003 Mouroulis *et al.* [21] adopted this method to produce blazed grating with grove spacing in the order of tens of microns. Figure 6.9 shows the planar Fresnel lens fabricated with gray-scale lithography on a silicon substrate [22]. The planar Fresnel lens consisted of 10 profiled gratings for X-ray diffraction, where each grating has a uniquely defined profile.

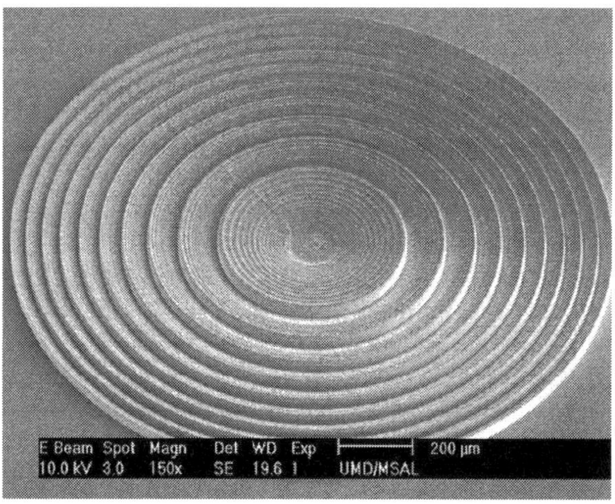

Figure 6.9 Planar Fresnel lens consisting of 10 profiled gratings for X-ray diffraction [22]. Each grating has a uniquely defined profile. The diameter of the lens is 1.6 mm.

6.3.3 Holographic Exposure

Holographic exposure uses the interference fringe pattern, consisting of a set of equally spaced bright and dark lines, of two intersected laser beans to expose the photoresist coated on a substrate. The exposed photoresist is then chemically developed to form a pattern of straight groves with a sinusoidal profile. The developed photoresist with a pattern of straight groves can be used as a master grating for replication, or as a mask for anisotropic etching of the substrate. Due to the fact that optical masks are not required in the fabrication processes, holographic exposure is also considered one of the maskless lithography techniques. It is suitable for fabricating gratings with high grove densities and large areas, and is widely used in the fabrication of commercial gratings and actively researched [23–28]. Holographic gratings, however, cannot be easily blazed because of their sinusoidal grove profile, and their efficiency is usually considerably less than a comparable ruled grating. Figure 6.10 shows the schematic diagram of the experimental facility

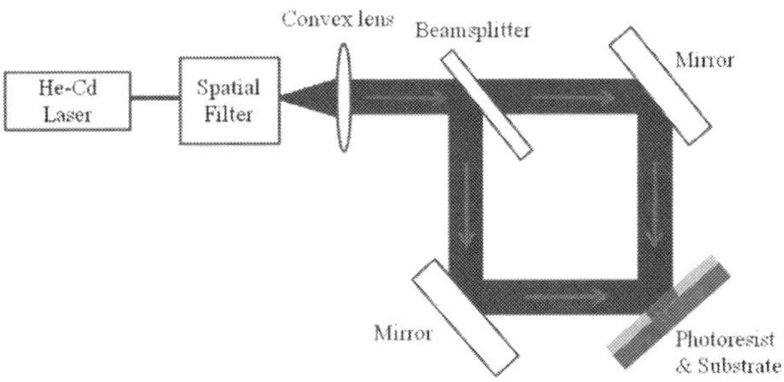

Figure 6.10 Schematic diagram of the experimental facility used for holographic exposure.

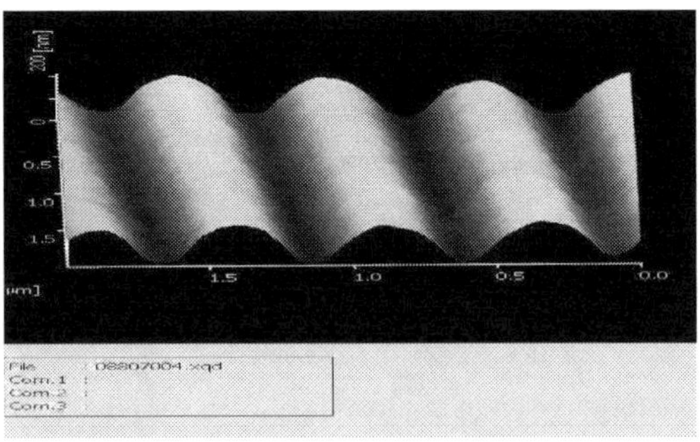

Figure 6.11 SEM image of a holographic grating with a grove density of 1800 groves/mm.

used for holographic exposure. Figure 6.11 is the SEM image of a holographic grating with a grove density of 1800 groves/mm.

6.3.4 Electron-Beam Direct Writing

Electron-beam direct writing is the method of scanning a beam of electrons in a patterned fashion across the surface of a substrate and selectively removing the exposed regions. The depth of the substrate removed by the electron beam depends on the energy and scanning velocity of the electron beam. As the diameter of the electron beam could be less than 5 nm, this method has a very high spatial resolution, far better than the diffraction limit of optical masks employed by other methods. This method, however, suffers from the long fabrication time, as it takes a long time to scan the electron beam across the entire substrate. Figures 6.12 and 6.13 show the photo of the ELIONIX ELS-7500 EX electron-beam direct writing system and the SEM image of a grating fabricated by this system, respectively.

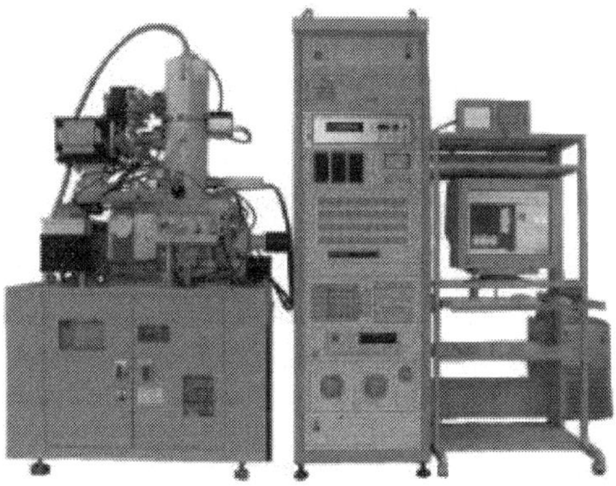

Figure 6.12 Photo of the ELIONIX ELS-7500 EX electron-beam direct writing system [29].

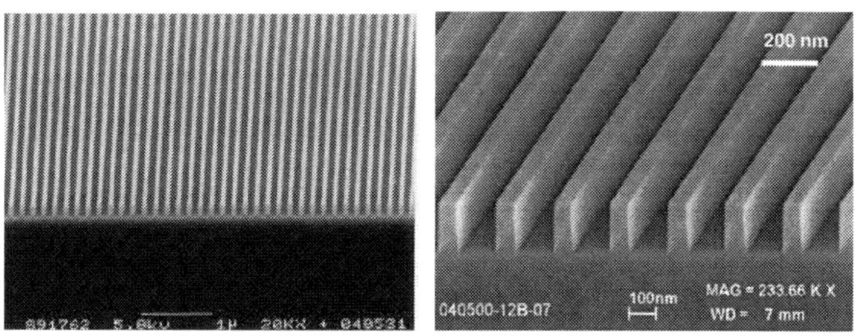

Figure 6.13 SEM image of silicon gratings [37].

6.3.5 Nanoimprint Lithography

Nanoimprint lithography was proposed by Chou *et al.* [30] in 1996 for the fabrication of nanometer scale patterns. Since then, this technique has been actively researched and extended to many applications [31–36]. In principle, it uses compression molding to create a thickness contrast pattern in a thin resist film carried on a substrate, followed by anisotropic etching to transfer the pattern through the entire resist thickness (shown in Fig. 6.14). The imprint resist is typically a monomer or polymer formulation that is cured by heat or UV light during the molding. To fabricate gratings, a master grating fabricated by a method discussed in the above sections is used as the mold during the imprinting to create replicates, which could be made of material different from the master grating, rapidly and cost effectively. In 2003 Yu *et al.* [37] adopted reactive ion etching to transfer a grating patter to a silicon substrate; the SEM image of the silicon gratings is shown in Fig. 6.13. On the other hand, anisotropic wet etching was used by Jiao *et al.* [38] to transfer the pattern to a gold film.

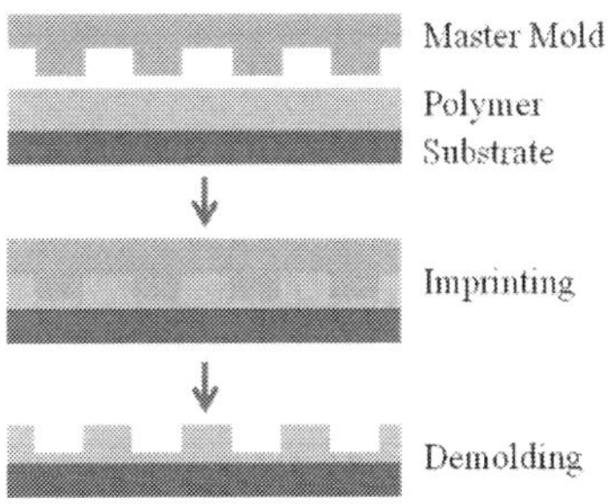

Figure 6.14 Process of nanoimprint lithography.

6.4 Manufacture of Optical Fiber Windows

Optical fiber can be used as a fiber optic sensor since light from a source can be guided via the optical waveguide to areas for testing physical or chemical characteristics, such as stress, strain, temperature, refractive index, molecular concentration, etc. Since these changes will result in changes to the optical characteristics, analysis of changes in optical characteristics can be used to find physical or chemical quantity changes in the tested area. The basic structure of the fiber is shown in Fig. 6.15. Optical fiber is essentially a cylindrical optical waveguide along its axis to radial, and can generally be divided by its refractive index into 3 layers: core, cladding, and the outside protection jacket. The core and cladding of the optical fiber transmit the basic elements of light. Fiber optic sensors are not affected by electromagnetic noise or magnetic interference. The impact of ionizing radiation can also be avoided though the use of radiation treatment making it suitable for demanding environments, such as nuclear power plants. Also, since the fiber optic sensors use the same fiber as both a sensor and signal transmission line, they can be placed in areas that traditional sensors with wires could not, such as small or not easily accessible locations. Fiber optic sensors use light as the transmission medium rather than current or voltage, so there is no risk of electric shock, making them suitable for medical measurements. Fiber optic materials do not corrode, and are thus suitable for deep-sea engineering and environments where there is risk of chemical corrosion. Glass fiber has a higher temperature resistance gauge than metal, and longer-term stability and fatigue resistance, making it suitable for long-term monitoring. Since optical fibers have been used in long distance optical fiber communications, fiber optic sensor technique is easily adapted to long-distance telemetry. In addition, the use of wavelength division multiplexing technique in optical communications also helped the same optical fibers with multi-point measurement, which has lead the fiber optic sensors being widely used in aerospace, medicine, chemistry, earth engineering, civil engineering, and other fields as well.

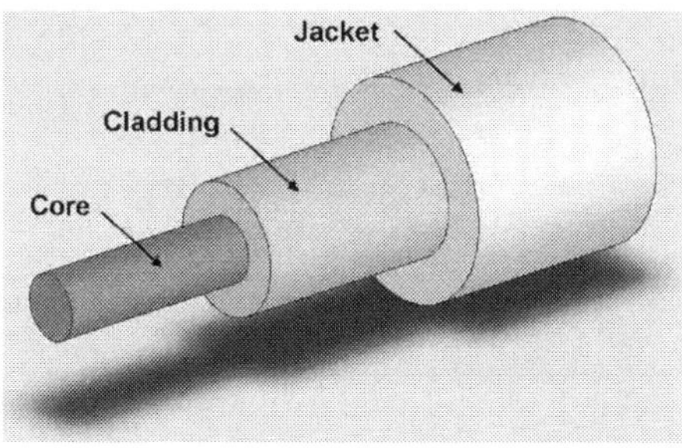

Figure 6.15 Structure of an optical fiber.

Fiber optic sensors rely on the measurement of physical (chemical) content, hence, finding a mechanism to modulate the physical quantity, and then measuring the results of the modulation indirectly by measuring the changes in the physical (chemical) content. For example, to measure physical qualities, such as the mechanical measurement of curvature, the bending of the fiber causes lost of light as it escapes from the fiber core. The more severe the bending, the more serious is the loss of light energy. In other words, light energy is modulated by the curvature, so if the optical fiber is affixed to a mechanical object, the curvature can be measured indirectly by measuring by the intensity of light through the optical fiber. As another example, a gas will absorb a specific wavelength of light, and this absorption increases as the concentration of the gas increases, with an appropriate light source guided by the fiber into a test area where the light temporarily leaves the fiber and is then is re-captured by the optical fiber at the other end, the concentration of the gas can be deduced by measuring the attenuation of the specific wavelength of light energy. A single mechanism for modulation can occur within the fiber, and may also occur in an external environment around the optical fiber. In addition, different modulation methods can be applied individually or in combination. Modulation mechanisms include (1) absorption modulation; (2) chromatic dispersion modulation; (3) scattering based modulation; (4) luminescence–fluorescence based modulation; (5) refractive index based modulation; (6) geometric effect based modulation; (7) interferometric and phase modulation; (8) wavelength modulation; and (9) Doppler's effect modulation.

Depending on sensor positioning, different modulation mechanisms can be categorized as three types: (1) extrinsic, (2) intrinsic, and between them (3) evanescent. With extrinsic sensing methods light is guided to the test area by optical fiber, temporarily leaves the fiber, is modulated by the external environment, and is then captured into the fiber and passed to the signal processor for analysis. The role of optical fiber is for signal transmission only, and is not involved in the sensing function. For intrinsic sensors, the light does not leave the optical fiber; modulation occurs from changes to the external environment or changes in the internal characteristics, which affect certain characteristics of the light (such as wavelength). Evanescent fiber optic sensors derive changes to the parameters tested in the external environment via the escape or loss of light during transmission. Though both this type and extrinsic sensors measure changes in light energy, the modulation mechanism for this type occurs in the optical fiber and energy is not allowed to escape the fiber to be recaptured. Therefore, this optical fiber not only acts as a signal transmission line, but also as a sensing component. To improve the sensitivity of optical fiber sensors for use in fiber optic biosensors, the fiber must be processed a second time by stripping a portion of cladding so the light-sensitive core layer can be in contact with the sample solution. The area where the cladding is removed is called an optical fiber window, as shown in Fig. 6.16. The fiber has a window gap structure and the depth of this gap can be controlled. A shallow depth would only require the removal of the jacket layer, while a deeper depth allows the fiber core to be exposed. This section describes three methods to fabricate optical fiber windows: etching, polishing, and high energy ultrashort pulse laser processing.

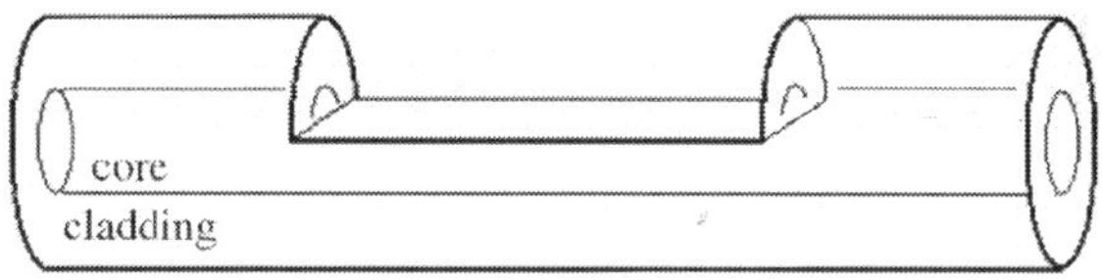

Figure 6.16 Schematic diagram of optical fiber window.

6.4.1 Etching Method

The core of glass fiber is fused silica. Fused silica is a noncrystalline (glass) form of silicon dioxide (quartz, sand). To generate good flat etching results, the BOE (Buffered Oxide Etch), rather than HF (Hydrofluoric Acid) is used to etch the optical fiber [39] because the BOE has lower etching rate. Besides, BOE etching is only effective for SiO_2, and the plastic coating covering on the D-shaped window optical fiber cannot be removed. Therefore, the etching length can be determined by controlling the length of the bare fiber, and the etching depth can be determined by controlling the etching time. However, the etching rate is dependent on the temperature and concentration of the BOE. Thus, the etching temperature must be controlled if accurate etching depth is required. For single mode optical fibers, an etching depth of at least 50 μm must be obtained to let the evanescent wave through. Before etching, part of plastic coating must be stripped, followed by BOE etching for a properly controlled etching time. The maximum etching time can be measured as the time when the core of the D-shaped window optical fiber is exposed to the air and finally all modes are cut off, thus allowing the maximum etching depth and maximum etching time to be determined. In other words, in a single mode optical fiber when the transmission light is cut off, the etching depth is 9 μm. Summarizing, the etching process consists of the following steps:

(a) Strip off coating
(b) BOE etching
(c) Cleaning with water and drying with nitrogen

6.4.2 Polishing Method

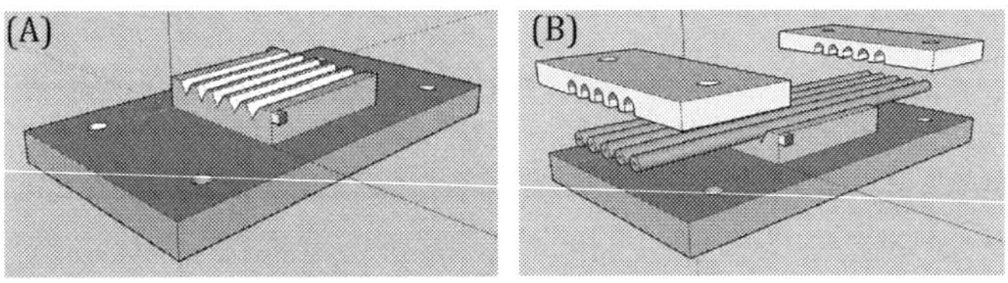

Figure 6.17 Polishing fixture diagrams: (A) V-shaped groove of the fixture, (B) location of optical fibers in the fixture.

Optical fiber windows can also be fabricated using polishing techniques. The fabrication technique requires an appropriate fixture (as shown in Fig. 6.17) to hold the fiber. The fixture has a groove, which is commonly V-shaped, and can be made of cut metal, or by crystal elements shaped by anisotropic etching. The polishing removal areas must be separated from the protected areas that are not to be processed. Once the fixture has been attached to the fiber and placed in the polishing machine, set the high precision polishing machine to use chemical mechanical polishing (CMP) to produce optical fiber windows. The polishing depth needs to be monitored in real-time through the optical line monitoring system. This system connects a fiber optic light source at one end, and at the other end of optical fiber sensors measure the intensity of the light. The overall schematic is shown in Fig. 6.18. The implementation steps are as follows [40]:

(a) Place fibers in grooves of a substrate
(b) Fix the fibers in grooves by bonding at least a portion of each fiber on the substrate

(c) Place the fibers and the substrate in a protection template to expose portions of the fibers to be polished while covering the remaining portions of the fibers
(d) Engage the protection template holding the fibers and the substrate to the wafer carrier of the CMP polisher
(e) Perform CMP polishing on the exposed portions of the fibers and the substrate

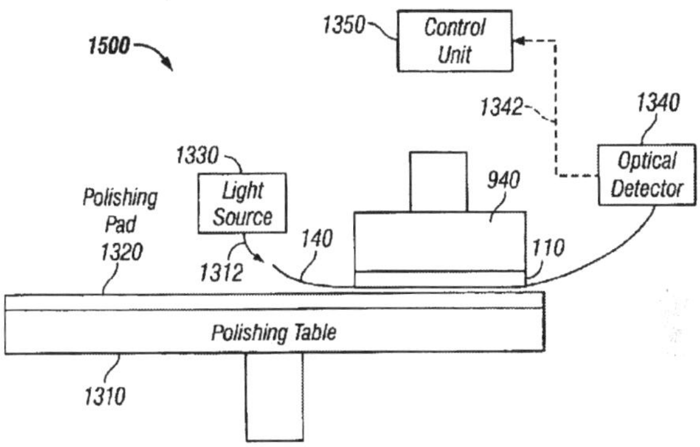

Figure 6.18 Schematic diagram of polishing system [40].

6.4.3 Ultrashort High-Energy Pulse Laser Processing Method

Lasers are highly directional, monochromatic, and have high coherence and energy density features. With the use of very small optical focusing systems they can produce power intensities of 108~1010 W/cm^2 or greater, and can be found in a wide range of applications. The advantage of laser processing is in its high power density, which allows it to process a wide range of materials, including industrial processing of materials and artifacts that cannot be handled by traditional methods, such as high-hardness materials and complex geometric structure works, for example, the three-dimensional internal processing within transparent materials. However, the fiber core of fused silica has a very high light transmission wavelength between 400 nm and 1500 nm [41]. In other words, light absorption by fused silica within this band is very low. High-energy laser pulses are needed to break this limit. The so-called ultra-short pulse laser has a very small pulse width with a heat transfer time in the tens to hundreds of picoseconds (picosecond, ps = 10^{-12} s). If this laser comes up short, the femtosecond laser has a pulse width of femtoseconds (femtosecond, fs = 10^{-15} s). Using a focused femtosecond laser, the pulse energy can be lowered to achieve a very high power density, with a high power output of 10 GW. When the laser pulse irradiates the processing surface, the instantaneous high power causes a high absorption of laser energy in the material, allowing it to be stripped as part of the processing mechanism [42]. The main processes on the material are femtosecond multiphoton absorption and multiphoton absorption material produced after avalanche ionization, so it can break through the fused silica material's light absorption properties in the 400~1500 nm wavelength. In addition, due to its very short laser pulse width, the material absorbs this energy so quickly that almost no heat is transferred, and the material in the processed area is almost entirely unaffected by heat. Unlike in continuous laser processing, the femtosecond laser pulse does not cause a plasma effect, resulting in high processing efficiency. In addition, unlike with traditional laser focusing spots, the femtosecond laser processing threshold value is clear and, if precise control is maintained of the femtosecond laser pulse power density, only a very small Gaussian beam centre area of energy is higher than the threshold value. The result is that, unlike with a traditional laser, the processing of the nonlinear absorption effect, optical diffraction limit, realization of submicron particles or nano-level of processing capacity, and the processing zone and the non-processing area boundaries can be accurately controlled and repeated.

Many researchers have used femtosecond lasers on multi-mode optical fibers to produce window fibers [43–45]. Optical fibers consist of three different layers. The outer jacket layer's material is mainly made of polymer. The other two layers are mainly made of fused silica. Therefore, the production of window fiber needs to set the laser's energy at different strengths, adjusting the energy level to where the outer layer of the polymer jacket layer is removed, then adjusted again when the fiber cladding layer and fiber core layer are off, processing to the set side, then using the defocused laser technique to heat the exposed core. This can improve the roughness on the surface that was created during processing. The femtosecond laser's high precision allows window fiber to form different shapes and arrangements, as shown in Fig. 6.19.

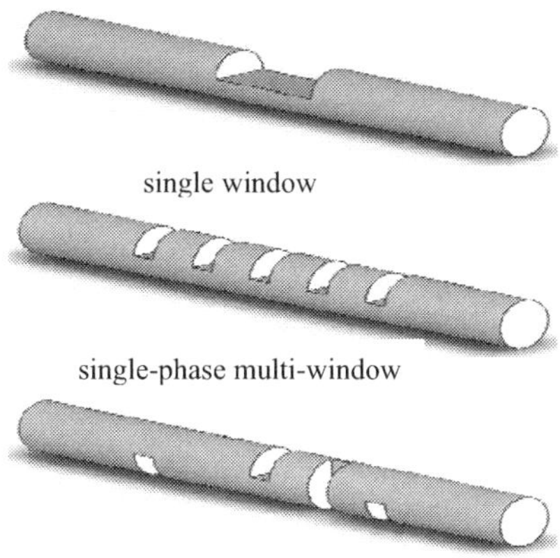

Figure 6.19 Schematic diagram of a variety of possible optical fiber windows.

6.5 Conclusions and Outlook

This chapter introduces four key technologies that are commonly used to fabricate biosensor chips: photolithography, soft lithography, fabrication of diffraction gratings, and production of optical fiber windows. Photolithography defines the microstructures in the biosensor chips through optical exposure technique. Soft lithography uses electrochemical processing technique to form metal molds in order to define the microstructures in biosensor chips. Grating or optical fiber window is often used in optical sensors. This chapter has overviewed the techniques to construct gratings and optical fiber windows. Since optical fiber after partial removal of cladding tends to be fragile and easily lose optical signals during transmission, this chapter has discussed how to re-process optical fiber to produce optical fiber windows, so the fiber not only transmits signals, and is not as fragile, but also functions as a sensor and as a component of the biosensor chip. Through the combined use of these four technologies, biosensor chips can be manufactured using polymer materials.

References

1. G. Shugar, and J. Ballinger, *Chemical Technicians' Ready Reference Handbook*, (McGraw-Hill: New York, 1996).

2. P. Van Zant, *Microchip Fabrication, 3rd edition* (McGraw-Hill: New York, 1996).
3. Gregory T. A. Kovacs, *Micromachined Transducers Sourcebook* (McGraw-Hill: New York, 1998).
4. N. P. Pham, T. L. M. Scholtes, R. Klerks, E. Boellaard, P. M. Sarro, and J. N. Burghartz, *Proc. Eurosensors* (2002).
5. Stephen A. Cambell, *The Science and Engineering of Microelectronic Fabrication* (Oxford University Press, 2nd edition, 2001).
6. E. W. Becker, W. Ehrfeld, P. Hagmann, A. Maner, and D. Munchmeyer, *Microelectron*, 35–56 (1986).
7. Y. Cheng, B. Y. Shew, C. Y. Lin, D. H. Wei, and M. K. Chyu, *J. Micromech. Microeng.*, 58–63 (1999).
8. L. Weber, W. Ehrfeld, H. Freimuth, Manfred Lacher, Heinz Lehr, and Bernhard Pech, *SPIE*, 156–167 (1996).
9. M. Heckele, W. Bacher, and K.D. Muller, *Microsyst. Technol.*, 122–124 (1998).
10. M. P. Martin, D. W. Matson, and W. D. Bennett, *Proc SPIE*, 172–176 (1998).
11. H. Mekaru, T. Yamada, S. Yan, and T. Hattori, *Springer-Verlag*, 682–688 (2004).
12. A Yussuf, and I Sbarski, *J. Micromesh. Microeng*, 1692–1699 (2005).
13. B. H. Schneider, E. L. Dickinson, M. D. Vach, J. V. Hoijer, and L. V. Howard, *Biosens. Bioelectron.*, 13–22 (2000).
14. M. Wiki, R. E. Kunz, G. Voirin, K. Tiefenthaler, and A. Bernard, *Biosens. Bioelectron.*, 1181–1185 (1998).
15. E. Brynda, M. Houska, A. Brandenburg, and A. Wikerstal, *Biosens. Bioelectron.*, 665–675 (2002).
16. F. F. Bier, F. Kleinjung, and F. W. Scheller, *Sens. Actuators, B*, 78–82 (1997).
17. V. A. Sychugov, A. V. Tishchenko, N. M. Lyndin, and O. Parriaux, *Sens. Actuators, B Chemical*, 360–364 (1997).
18. P. J. Skrdla, S. S. Saavedra, N. R. Armstrong, S. B. Mendes, and N. Peyghambarian, *Anal. Chem.*, 1332–1337 (1999).
19. T. O'Brien, L. H. Johnson, J. L. Aldrich, S. G. Allen, L. T. Liang, A. L. Plummer, S. J. Krak, and A. A. Boiarski, *Biosens. Bioelectron.*, 815–828 (2000).

20. J. Voros, R. Graf, G. L. Kenausis, A. Bruinink, J. Mayer, M. Textor, E. Wintermantel, and N. D. Spencer, *Biosens. Bioelectron.*, 423–429 (2000).

21. P. Mouroulis, F. Hartley, D. Wilson, V. White, A. Shori, S. Nguyen, M. Zhang, and M. Feldman, *Opt. Express*, 270–281 (2003).

22. B. Morgan, C. M. Waits, J. Krizmanic, and R. Ghodssi, *J. Microelectromech. Syst.*, 113–120 (2004).

23. F. Yu, P. Li, H. Shen, S. Mathur, C.-M. Lehr, U. Bakowsky, and F. Müklich, *Biomater.*, 2307–2312 (2005).

24. C. H. Chang, Y. Zhao, R. K. Heilmann, and M. L. Schattenburg, *Opt. Lett.*, 1572–1574 (2008).

25. N. D. Lai, Y. Di Huang, J. H. Lin, D. B. Do, and C. C. Hsu, *Opt. Express*, 3362–3369 (2009).

26. H. H. Solak, C. David, J. Gobrecht, L. Wang, and F. Cerrina, *Microelectron. Eng.*, 77–82 (2002).

27. H. J. Jiang, X. C. Yuan, Y. Zhou, Y. C. Chan, and Y. L. Lam, *Opt. Commun.*, 19–24 (2000).

28. H. H. Solak, C. David, J. Gobrecht, V. Golovkina, F. Cerrina, S. O. Kim, and P. F. Nealey, *Microelectron. Eng.*, 56–62 (2003).

29. ELIONIX. http://www.sts-elionix.com.

30. S. Y. Chou, P. R. Krauss, and P. J. Renstrom, *Science*, 85–87 (1996).

31. S. W. Ahn, K. D. Lee, J. S. Kim, S. H. Kim, S. H. Lee, J. D. Park, and P. W. Yoon, *Microelectron. Eng.*, 314–318 (2005).

32. H. Z. Liu, W. T. Jiang, Y. C. Ding, Y. P. Tang, B. H. Lu, H. B. Lan, Y. S. Shi, and L. Yin, *Microelectron. Eng.*, 4–9 (2009).

33. X. Y. Lei, L. Wu, P. Deshpande, Z. N. Yu, W. Wu, H. X. Ge, and S. Y. Chou, *Nanotechnology*, 786–790 (2003).

34. D. Y. Khang, H. Kang, T. Kim, and H. H. Lee, *Nano Lett.*, 633–637 (2004).

35. Z. N. Yu, and S. Y. Chou, *Nano Lett.*, 341–344 (2004).

36. S. Y. Chou, C. Keimel, and J. Gu, *Nature*, 835–837 (2002).

37. Z. Yu, L. Chen, W. Wu, H. Ge, and S. Y. Chou, *J. Vac. Sci. Technol.*, B, 2089–2092 (2003).

38. L. Jiao, H. Gao, G. Zhang, G. Xie, X. Zhou, Y. Zhang, Y. Zhang, B. Gao, G. Luo, Z. Wu, T. Zhu, J. Zhang, Z. Liu, S. Mu, H. Yang, and C. Gu, *Nanotechnology*, 2779–2784 (2005).

39. D. Markos, B. Ipson, K. Smith, S. Schultz, R. Selfridge, T. Monte, R. Dyott, and G. Miller, *Appl. Opt.*, 7121–7125 (2003).
40. V. Koinkar, T. Collins, J. Costa, and J. Levert, Vista, Patent No.: US 6,719,608 B1 (2004).
41. http://www.thorlabs.com.
42. R. R. Gattass, and E. Mazur, *Nat. Photonics*, 219–225 (2008).
43. C. H. Chen, T. C. Chao, W. Y. Li, W. C. Shen, C. W. Cheng, J. L. Tang, L. K. Chau, and W. T. Wu , *J. Laser Micr/Nanoeng.*, 1–5, (2010/2).
44. C. H. Chen, T. C. Chao, J. L. Tang, and W. T Wu, *Sensors*, 4794–4804 (2010/5).
45. C. H. Chen, T. C. Tsao, W. Y. Li, W. C. Shen, C. W. Cheng, J. L. Tang, C. P. Jen, L. K. Chau, and W. T. Wu, *Microsyst. Technol.*, 1207–1214 (2010/7).

Chapter 7

Microfluidics for Biosensor Chips

Shau-Chun Wang
Department of Chemistry and Biochemistry, National Chung Cheng University, 168 University Road, Ming-Hsiung, Chia-Yi 621, Taiwan
chescw@ccu.edu.tw

Microfluidic devices that integrate functional units to perform bioanalytical and diagnostic tests in chips have some unique advantages, such as reducing reagent and sample consumption, and avoiding contamination during sample transfer between analysis procedures. This chapter reviews biosensing techniques that utilize noble metal nanoparticles to develop various spectroscopic methods, including label-free scattering and fluorophore-tagged emission methods. Unlike bulk materials such as mirror-like metallic films, nanoparticles of noble metals, such as gold (Au) and silver (Ag), absorb and scatter the incident light to appear colors, known as localized surface plasmon resonance (LSPR) and also known as particle plasmon resonance (PPR). The resonance frequency of the collective oscillating electrons is dependent on the dielectric properties of the nanoparticles and their surrounding medium. In other words, the binding events of immobilized probes on the particle surfaces will change the scattering frequency sensitively. Also the surface

From Bioimaging to Biosensors: Noble Metal Nanoparticles in Biodetection
Edited by Lai-Kwan Chau and Huan-Tsung Chang

ISBN 978-981-4267-24-3 (Hardcover), 978-981-4303-10-1 (eBook)
www.panstanford.com

plasmon induced by the incident light can enhance inelastic Raman scattering of molecules absorbed on noble metal nanoparticles. In addition to act as a substrate to immobilize fluorescence labeled molecules, noble metal nanoparticles work as fluorescence quenchers or emission enhancement media. When using strong interactions between surface electrons and fluorophore dipoles, noble metal nanoparticles can assist Förster resonance energy transfer (FRET) and surface plasmon-coupled emission (SPCE) fluorescence detection. Noble metal nanoparticles also have strong light absorbance properties to convert absorbed light to thermal energies, causing detectable refraction index change of surrounding medium to facilitate thermal lens detections. These strong light absorbance properties make noble metal nanoparticles suitable candidates as the sample dispersion matrix to desorb molecules into gas phase and ionize using laser irradiation. The molecules, even proteins, ionized via this photonics mechanism, matrix-assisted laser desorption ionization (MALDI), usually remain intact in gas phase. Mass analyzers are able to determine the structures of these large ions. This chapter also reviews applying microfluidics devices to implement the light absorbance properties of noble metal nanoparticles to develop biosensing methods.

7.1 Introduction

The bioanalytical applications of microchip technologies have attracted considerable attention in the past two decades. In addition to microarray-based biochips,[1] lab-on-a-chip devices utilizing microchip electrophoresis and other types of microfluidic technologies have also proved their feasibility for use in combinatorial chemistry, genomics, and proteomics. These applications are essential to drug discovery and other biomedical research fields.[2,3] Having collaborated with the microfluidics company Caliper Technologies Corp., Agilent Technologies launched its first commercialized lab-on-a-chip biochemical equipment system, the Agilent 2100 Bioanalyzer in 1999. In the following years, several lab-on-a-chip products appeared on the market.[4] The substrates used to fabricate microfluidic chips are typically silicon-based materials or polymeric plastics. Various fabrication processes have been developed to make microfluidic chips, including chemical etching, plastics modeling, template imprinting, and laser ablation. Various detection technologies, such as optical spectroscopy, mass spectrometry, and electrochemical methods have been successfully integrated with microfluidic chips.

In addition to briefly reviewing microchip fabrication processes, this chapter discusses detection technologies that employ noble metal nanoparticles in microfluidic chips. These technologies include PPR spectroscopy, including hybrid instrumentation of PPR with mass spectrometry, fluorescence spectroscopy, and other detection techniques, such as surface-enhanced Raman scattering and thermal lens detections.

7.2 Fabrication of Microfluidic Devices

Most of the fabrication technologies discussed in this section have been reviewed in Chapter 6. Therefore, this section only outlines the major substrate materials used to make microfluidic chips, and briefly describes their fabrication procedures.[5]

Table 7.1 illustrates the substrate materials and fabrication technologies discussed in this chapter. Since fused silica capillary has been the most popular conduit for capillary electrophoresis (CE), SiO_2-based materials such as glass and quartz have been also used to fabricate microchip CE devices. Wet chemical etching processes with highly erosive reagents such as hydrofluoric acid can be used to create microchannels on these materials.[6] Before chemical etching with strong acidic and alkaline reagents, such as hydrofluoric acid and concentrated potassium hydroxide, glass or quartz substrate chips are coated with a layer of photoresist material. Covered with this mask, the chip is then exposed to UV light, which etches along the mask edges to create microchannels. The photoresist layer is further developed after UV light exposure. Etching reagents are then poured on the photoresist layer to erode the light exposed areas and the substrate underneath the areas to complete microchannel fabrication in approximately 30 min. The etching time depends on reagent concentrations. An alternative technique is to use Al_2O_3 powder blasting to craft a microchannel measuring 100 microns in depth and width; this process takes only minutes.[7] However, the channel roughness of using blasting technique is usually less than ideal, about 1 micron.

Table 7.1 Typical substrate materials and technologies to fabricate microfluidic chips

	SiO_2-based materials (glass; quartz)	Thermoplastics* (PMMA; PC; COC)	Elastomers** (PDMS)
Chemical etching	×		
Powder blasting	×		
Template embossing		×	
Ablation		×	
Injection molding		×	
Micro-milling		×	
Mold casting			×

*PMMA, polymethylmethacrylate; PC, polycarbonate; COC, cycloolefin copolymer.
**PDMS, polydimethylsiloxane.

After microchannel fabrication, the fabricated chip surface is treated with acidic reagents to slightly melt in a furnace and then bonded with another chip under pressure. This other chip is drilled with inlet and electrode holes prior to the fusion bonding step.

Polymeric substrates, including thermoplastics and elastomers, can also be used to fabricate microfluidic devices.[8] Polymeric substrates and related fabrication tools are less expensive than glass materials and their tools. In addition, the physical and chemical properties of polymeric substrates are easier to control. As a result, polymeric chips make it easier to realize complex conduit layouts.

Common thermoplastic materials used to make microchannels include polymethylmethacrylate (PMMA), polycarbonate (PC), cycloolefin copolymer (COC), and co-polyester. Plastic fabrication techniques, such as template embossing and laser ablation, have been implemented to craft microchannels on these substrates. Structured master molds, which are typically made of metallic alloys or silicon wafers, are pressed against plastic chips in an oven at a temperature a little higher than the melting point of the plastic for a few minutes to imprint channels. Ablation marker lasers using various types of light sources have also been employed to directly write microchannels on thermoplastic substrates.[9] These light sources include carbon dioxide lasers, solid state lasers, and argon-ion lasers. Higher-energy light sources, such as femto-second lasers, X-rays, or synchrotron radiation, have also been used to ablate microchannels with high aspect ratios on plastic substrates.[10] Techniques such as injection molding and micro-milling have also been used to fabricate microchannels on thermoplastic chips.[11] After the microchannels have been patterned, the structured plastic chip and the cover chip are sealed using thermal bonding techniques. This step usually involves organic solvents, which enhance the fusion strength of plastics at the gap between the two chips.

Elastomers such as polydimethylsiloxane (PDMS) are commonly used to fabricate microfluidic devices.[12] A typical procedure is to first develop a silicon master molds with a positive surface relief pattern. Next, a PDMS precursor solution is poured into the mold to start polymerizing when cured at approximately 65°C. When the polymerization processes are accomplished, patterned PDMS substrates can be peeled from the mold. The resulting structured chip can be sealed with either a PDMS chip or a glass chip. When the cover chips are nearly perfectly flat, the sealing can be accomplished by merely pressing the structured chip against the cover. Otherwise, ozone plasma is used to activate the silane surface of the PDMS or glass chip prior to the chip bonding step, which fuses the two chips using water or methanol smeared on the plasma-activated surfaces.

7.3 Particle Plasmon Resonance Detection in Microfluidic Devices Using Noble Metal Nanoparticles

When incident light impinges into the thin film surface of bulk dielectric materials such as noble metals, and is reflected, partial light absorption occurs. This is due to the interactions between the evanescent wave field of incoming light (penetrating the film) and the dielectrics, which only occur at certain angle ranges of incident light resulting in reflectance minima. The wave vector component parallel to the free electron dipole of the dielectric surface is almost absorbed. As a result, the reflectance intensity decreases dramatically. This phenomenon is known as surface plasmon resonance (SPR).[13] The electric permittivity of a dielectric film can be altered by immobilized molecules on the reverse side; therefore, the angle of reflectance minima is shifted when the planted probes are docked with detected molecules. Several commercial spectroscopic biosensors reviewed in recent research have utilized this label-free sensing scheme.[14] Commercial SPR detection equipment such as Biacore systems (GE Healthcare) have become popular tools for studying biomolecular interactions.

Although the thin film of bulk noble metals such as gold (Au) or silver (Ag) is mirror-like and shines at all wavelength ranges, the nanoparticles of these metals are colored to scatter or absorb light at specific wavelength ranges. This phenomenon is known as PPR, referring to the plasmon excitation phenomenon occurring on nanometer-sized metallic structures. The absorbed incident light induces the oscillation of conduction electrons confined in the metallic nano-scale substrates to scatter. When the electrons collectively oscillate at the resonance wavelength of incoming light, the scattering intensifies to the degree that the nanoparticles appear colored. The scattering wavelength is dependent on the permittivity of nanoparticles and their surrounding medium. Similar to the principles of developing SPR biosensing methods, the dielectric properties of nanoparticles are tailored when immobilized probes on the surface recognize targets to dock. The shifting of PPR scattering or absorbance bands can be observed to confirm the binding event. Chapters 3 and 4, respectively, illustrate colorimetric and spectroscopic biosensing assays and slide-based biosensors with PPR detection methods using functionalized noble metal nanoparticles.

7.3.1 Microfluidic Devices to Facilitate PPR Detection

These functionalized nanoparticles can be filled into microchannels or coated on channel walls to develop miniaturized assays. Dark-field microscopy is suitable for observing the color changes of these nanoparticles due to binding events in the micro-channel.[15] Gold nanoparticles of 80 nm diameter implanted with biotinylated antibodies are purged into PDMS (poly(dimethylsiloxane)) or PMMA (poly(methyl methacrylate)) microchannels to monitor the bindings of antigens such as *Helicobacter pylori* and *Escherichia coli* at the detection limit of 10 ng, which is comparable to the limit provided by dot blot assays.

Colorimetric assays can also be performed by measuring the light transmission through the coating layer of functionalized nanoparticles on substrate slides of transparent materials such as quartz. The slides can be integrated with microfluidic chips for the purpose of precise liquid delivery.[16,17] Gold nanoparticles are synthesized in a solution and immobilized on the quartz slide. One self-assembled thiol-based monolayer covers the nanoparticles to functionalize with antigen probes such as biotin molecules. A light-emitting diode (LED) light source irradiates through the slide to interrogate the changes of dielectric properties due to the binding of antibodies with the immobilized antigens. This type of biosensing chip has demonstrated a 270 ng/mL detection limit using anti-biotins samples, which is comparable with the limit using a Biacore SPR sensing chip.

Nanosphere lithography has been used to craft nanoparticle arrays on membrane substrates, in which Ag nanoparticles are orderly arranged. Cytochrome P450 enzymes, which prevent the nanoparticles from their inherent aggregation properties, are stabilized on the particle surface to study drug binding mechanisms via monitoring the shifts of the PPR spectrum.[18]

When these functionalized nanoparticles are coated on optical waveguide substrates, such as planner waveguides or optical fibers, the attenuated intensity of guided light due to PPR interactions with the nanoparticles can be used to determine specific sensing events on the particles. Chapter 5 discusses PPR biosensing applications using waveguide-based devices. Due to miniaturizing waveguide devices requiring less effort, developing microfluidic chips using waveguide-based PPR sensing is more straightforward than developing SPR chips.

For instance, one segment of plastic buffer wrapping optical fiber can be removed to coat Au nanoparticles on the cladding layer. An LED or laser light coupled into the fiber propagates along the fiber via internal reflection. As described in the previous section, the light attenuation due to reflection along the fiber is sensitive to the permittivity change of coated nanoparticles. When recognition probes are implanted on the particles coated on the fiber suspended in one flow cell, the intensity attenuation or PPR scattering wavelength shift can report the binding events of targets in sample solutions. Various assays using fiber optic-PPR (FO-PPR) systems have been developed to detect anti-DNP and anti-nuclear antibodies.[19,20] The size of FO-PPR flow cells can be reduced to a sub-mm scale to become microfluidic devices saving the consumption of reagents and samples and shortening PPR signal response time due to smaller diffusion distance from the fiber surface.

7.3.2 Microfluidic Mixer to Improve PPR Detection

Microfluidic-assisted PPR assays described in Section 3.1 employ devices of immobilized noble metal particles on substrates. Although the dimension of a micro-channel in delivering sample solutions is only hundreds of microns, large targets must still expend considerable diffusion time to contact with the immobilized probes on the nanoparticles to accomplish binding.

Reynolds number scaling with both fluid speed and container dimension is only 10 or smaller in the sub-millimeter flow channel when the fluid speed is approximately 1 mm/sec. Under this small Reynolds number, fluids in microchannels are irrotational and difficult for creating any turbulence in mixing solutes.

Non-linear electro-osmotic flows have been used to generate micro-vortices in microfluidic devices.[21,22] Non-linear electro-osmosis can occur at the charged surface of conducting substrates. Due to the conducting properties, external electric field lines can penetrate the substrate surface. Solution ions in the bulk are driven to migrate along the electric field lines. However, the electrical double layer (Debye layer) on the charged surface is ion-selective to prevent the co-ions of the surface charge from reaching the surface. The co-linearity between electric filed lines and ion migration paths is no longer valid to break down the irrotationality of the fluid. Additionally the depletion of co-ions at the regime near the substrate surface creates one extended electrical double layer, one or two orders of magnitude thicker than the original layer. When the counter ions accumulated in the extended layer are driven to migrate by the external field, these ions drag surrounding fluid to generate electro-osmotic flow (EOF) of which the speed is 10–100 times faster than typical EOF generated at the charge surface of an insulated substrate (such as a fused silica capillary wall). Ion migration speed and Debye layer thickness are both proportional to the external field strength; therefore, the EOF speed ascends quadratically with the field strength. High speed (~1 cm/sec) micro-vortices are observed near the surface of conducting ion-exchange resin under even moderate DC field 100 V/cm. When these resin granules move back and forth, the localized micro-vortices travel throughout the mixing cell to advect solutes chaotically, which accomplish mixing efficiently (100 times faster than diffusion mixing). Although the metal electrode is conducting, a high frequency AC field (~100 kHz) must be used to avoid polarization and allow the counter ion accumulation by diffusion to create an electrical double layer, because ion polarization at the electrode surface can completely screen the field line. The utility of a high frequency AC field across the print electrodes has demonstrated efficient mixing in microfluidic devices.[23]

Non-linear electro-osmosis can occur not only on the surface with permanent charges but also at the dielectric structure corner tips, accumulating induced charges by the external field. Similar to the mixing device using print electrodes, a high frequency AC field is required to sustain the electrical double layer in generating EOF.[24] The field application electrodes can be placed outside the mixing cell channel to avoid contamination due to chemical reactions on the electrode. Several relief-like strip structures with the thickness of 30 microns are fabricated on the FO-PPR sensing channel. When an external AC field (100 kHz, 50 V/cm) is applied, intense micro-vortices are generated at the corners of each strip.[25] The external field heating slightly raises the solution temperature to circulate the bulk flow via convection. When the circulation flow couples with the micro-vortices, efficient mixing is accomplished via chaotic solute advection to reduce the PPR sensing response time of streptavidin docking 10-fold shorter. The sensing of a virus extracted from orchid leaves is accelerated three times in this PPR sensing cell using induced ac EOF mixing.

In addition, slender structures fabricated in microchannels have been used to split a fluid into several narrow streams, traveling along paths of different lengths prior to merging together.[26] Such passive splitting and merging processes can drive solutes to mix via chaotic advection actions. Tilted grooves patterned on the bottom of microchannel, inducing secondary flows when fluid passes through the channel, are able to accomplish similar mixing processes. Alternatively, these grooves can be crafted with femto-second laser ablation on the cladding layer of optical fibers suspended in the flow cell to facilitate PPR detection.[27]

7.4 Integration of Biosensing Systems Using Noble Metal Nanoparticles with Mass Spectrometer

Like other bio-sensing systems using micro-columns, such as micro-liquid chromatography and CE,[28,29] the most straightforward means to establish hybrid microfluidic devices with a mass spectrometer is to use an electrospray ionization interface. Typically when coated with conducting materials such as metal deposit, a high voltage is applied to the end of a microcolumn or microchannel to create a strong electric field across the channel end and the ground electrode to induce charges at the liquid meniscus surface. Figure 7.1 shows that in this strong field, induced charges on the meniscus surface are pulled outward to become a conical tip, known as a Taylor cone. The accumulated charges of ionic solutes at the cone tip result in liquid instability, ejecting a small stream out of the microchannel. Because this sprayed micro-jet is highly charged, it further disintegrates into tiny aerosols. The sub-micron ionic solutes in these droplets finally pop out to become gas phase ions, completing the electrospray ionization process. These ionized gas phase species are then directed into a mass analyzer to determine their chemical structures. For instance, microfluidic digestion chips containing trypsin-immobilized Au nanoparticles have been hybrid with one micro-capillary to separate the fragmented proteins, which are determined with mass spectrometry via electrospray ionization.[30]

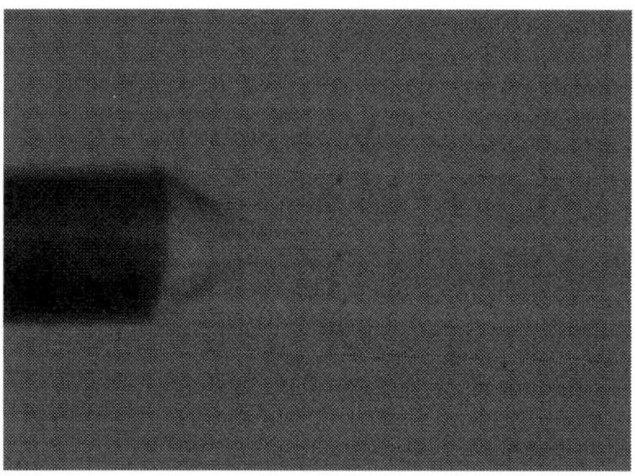

Figure 7.1 Image of Taylor cone formed at the tip of a hypodermic needle (0.21 mm O.D.) with a high voltage 3 kV. The sprayed liquid is 10 mM ammonium acetate solution (pH 8).

Besides, the core and ligand monolayer compositions of Au nanoparticles have been measured using electrospray mass spectrometry by tagging ionization functionalities, such as methoxy penta(ethylene glycol) thiolate groups.[31] Researchers have used similar methods to quantify the surface coverage of conjugate probes on functionalized Au nanoparticles. Having been modified with thiol-derivatized single-stranded DNA, Au nanoparticles are ionized to determine the coating thickness with electrospray-differential mobility analysis to estimate the surface coverage of DNA.[32]

Alternatively, having been dried on the plate, biomolecules docked with functionalized noble metal nanoparticles are able to desorb into gas phase by absorbing UV laser illumination to vaporize. These molecules are ionized via the matrix assisted laser desorption ionization (MALDI) processes.[33] One mass spectrometer is also able to analyze biomolecules ionized via the MALDI process.

Typically prior to MALDI processes, samples are dispersed in light-absorbing matrix such as sinapinic acid, which has very strong UV absorption. Next when illuminated by UV laser, the matrix is overheated to the point that it vaporizes and sometimes directly ionizes. During matrix evaporation, analytes dispersed in the matrix are desorbed into the gas phase in vacuum, and subsequently undergo three types of reactions: proton transfer, electron transfer, and cation transfer reaction. In the following reactions, m and A represent matrix and analyte molecules, respectively.

Proton transfer reaction:

$$mH^+ + A \rightarrow m + AH^+ \text{ and } (m\text{-}H)^- + A \rightarrow m + (A\text{-}H)^-$$

In this reaction, protonated matrix transfers H^+ to analyte, or deprotonated matrix extracts H^+ from analyte.

Electron transfer reaction:

$$m^+ + A \rightarrow m + A^+ \text{ and } m^- + A \rightarrow m + A^-$$

In the above, cationic matrix extracts an electron from analyte or anionic matrix transfers an electron to analyte.

Cation transfer reaction:

$$mNa^+ + A \rightarrow m + ANa^+$$

In this reaction, the cationic sodium — matrix complex transfer sodium ion to analyte for instance.

When molecules are homogeneously dispersed in a light sorbent matrix, the illuminated spot is instantaneously overheated upon irradiation. The analytes, matrix molecules, and other additives such as salts or acids at the heated point are therefore also vaporized. Charged additives of small ions such as protons or alkaline metal ions then attach on the moieties of high electronegativity to generate pseudo-molecule ions.

Since noble metal nanoparticles have strong light absorbance, docked molecules on the nanoparticle surfaces can desorb into gas phase when the particles are illuminated. For instance, absorbed peptides on the self-assembled monolayer of Au nanoparticles can be imaged with mass spectrometer via ionizing these peptide with precise laser focusing to spatially control desorption spots.[34]

7.5 Fluorescence Spectroscopic Detection in Microfluidic Devices Using Noble Metal Nanoparticles

Like other types of nanoparticles, noble metal nanoparticles have been used as supporting substrates to immobilize molecular probes and fluorophores. This facilitates biosensing with fluorescence detection in microfluidic chips. Various fluorescence detection schemes employing the interactions between fluorophore and noble metal particles have been developed. Examples include using gold nanoparticles as quenching acceptors for FRET detection and using silver nanoparticles for surface plasmon coupled fluorescence detection. In addition, molecular beacons can be immobilized on noble metal nanoparticles to determine metal species.

7.5.1 Applying Gold Nanoparticles as Quenching Acceptors to Förster Resonance Energy Transfer (FRET) Detections

Förster resonance energy transfer is a non-radiative process of dissipating the energy of electrons populated in the excited state.[35] This energy transfer process occurs when the transition dipoles of one pair of fluorophores, the donor and acceptor, have strong interactions. When the transition dipole of the donor fluorophore is excited enough to pump electrons from the ground state to an excited state, some of the extra energy of stimulated electrons on the donor fluorophore, presumably to emit fluorescence, is transferred to excite the transition dipole of an acceptor fluorophore. Finally, the detected fluorescence emission comes partially from the acceptor fluorophore. Alternatively, extra energies are absorbed by the acceptor, resulting in the disappearance of fluorescence emission. Figure 7.2 shows the mechanism of the FRET process.

The resonance frequencies of donor and acceptor transition dipoles must overlap to a certain degree to ensure the efficient transfer of the energy of the excited donor dipole. In the dimensions of noble metal nanoparticles (ca. 10 nm), the energy gap between the ground and the first excited electronic states of free electrons on the surface of nanoparticles often fits the wavelength range of visible light. In other words, the resonance frequencies of noble metal nanoparticles can match the emission frequencies of various donor fluorophores in the visible light range.

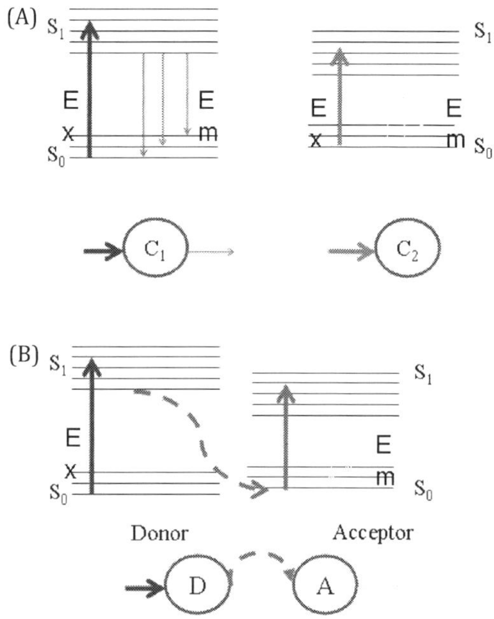

Figure 7.2 The mechanism of Förster resonance energy transfer process. (A) Two compounds, C_1 and C_2, are far away. They need light of specific wavelength for excitation (blue and green thick arrows), after relaxation, emission lights will appear (green and yellow thin arrows). (B) When C_1 and C_2 are close enough in a distance about 10 nm or less, they form a donor–acceptor pair. By exciting the donor, FRET occurs (grey dashed arrow). Acceptor receives the energy, then be excited (grey arrow), after relaxation, the emission light of the donor–acceptor pair comes mostly from the acceptor (yellow arrows). See also Color Insert.

This interaction between two transition dipoles becomes significant only when two dipoles are relatively close, typically 10 nm or less. Since the interaction between the induced dipole and induced dipole is inversely proportional to the sixth power of spacing distance between the two dipoles, this interaction is highly sensitive to distance. This energy transfer process must also proceed faster than the spontaneous emission of excited electrons (~10^{-9} s). As a result, resonance energy transfer fluorescence or quenching typically only occurs between two static fluorophores close to each other. The mean free paths of freely moving dyes in dilute solutions are usually too long to maintain close contact throughout the lifetime of spontaneous emission. In principle, when a fluorophore-tagged analyte docks with the recognition probe planted on noble metal nanoparticles, this excited fluorophore is able to dissipate its energy to the nanoparticles via FRET to quench its fluorescence.

When a tagged donor fluorophore on a single-strand DNA probe is initially absorbed on the noble metal surface, the hybridization of this probe with the complementary strand allows the absorbed fluorophore to jut away from the surface. Therefore, although the donor fluorescence is initially quenched, this dissipated emission is able to resume when DNA hybridization is complete. Chen and colleagues implemented this idea in developing a microfluidic biosensing device to detect the polymerase chain reaction (PCR) product of the dengue virus.[36] In their study, gold nanoparticles forming a self-assembled monolayer were deposited on the microchannel wall. Targeting dengue DNA probes tagged with Cy3 fluorescence dyes were immobilized in the monolayer via a thiol group at the end of probe. The DNA probe, whose dye-tagged end was bound to the nanoparticle surface, formed an arch conformation. The fluorescence of tagged dye was quenched to disappear at this conformation. When the PCR products of the dengue virus were added to hybridize DNA probes, the conformation of targeting DNA probes changed. The probes stretch outward and restore fluorescence. Prior to this hybridization step, the enterovirus PCR products were mixed in sample as a negative control.

7.5.2 Using Silver Nanoparticles in Surface Plasmon Coupled Fluorescence Detection

When the fluorophores spatially immobilize away from the surface of metallic nanoparticles, non-radiative quenching due to resonance energy transfer decreases dramatically. At a distance of hundreds of nanometers, fluorophore emission can couple with surface plasmon of metallic nanoparticles to occasionally, sometimes to enhance emission intensity. This mechanism is called SPCE.[37]

Chapter 1 described the principles of LSPR in detail. Briefly, this phenomenon refers to the plasmon excitation phenomenon occurring on nanometer-sized metallic structures. The absorbed incident light induces the oscillation of conduction electrons confined in the metallic nano-scale substrates to scatter. When the electrons collectively oscillate at the resonance wavelength of incoming light, the scattering becomes so intense that the nanoparticles appear colored. Similarly, the emission of an excited fluorophore tagged on a dielectric film can also excite surface plasmon to create a radiative beam. Since the coupling of surface plasmon with incident light is angle dependent, emission caused by this plasmon excitation should be directional too. In addition, since evanescent wave field typically propagates 200–500 nm forward through a dielectric film, SPCE is limited to closely-tagged fluorophores on the surface of nanoparticles.

For instance, in a model immunoassay using anti-rabbit antibody probes tagged with fluorescence labels, the probes bind to rabbit immunoglobin on a surface coated with silver nanoparticles. The surface plasmon on the silver significantly enhances fluorescence.[38] Large particles with intense scattering, such as plastic beads or red blood cells, only slightly attenuate the intensity of coupled fluorescence. However, hemoglobin and smaller molecules strongly absorbed on the surface diminish the intensity of fluorescence. In a microchannel immunoassay, the lateral-flow configuration required to separate blood cells prior to detection is no longer necessary when SPCE detection is employed.

Since the sizes of nanoparticles are much larger than usual solutes, the slow diffusion makes rapid detections employing SPCE methods in microchannel, where fluid mixing is problematic due to small Reynolds number limitation (Section 7.3.2). Liquid–liquid mixing in discrete droplets can be accomplished using microfluidic networks.[39,40] Reagent and sample solutions are filled into a funnel microchannel via different inlets, in which each stream migrates along laminar flow lines without any mixing. The outlet of funnel channel connects through a tiny hole with the other channel filled with oil flows immiscible with the solutions. When the solution streams come out to merge into the oil flow, the streams wrap with each other to become discrete droplets. The downstream of oil flow channel is serpent-like, in which the droplets go through the cycles of stretching, folding, and re-orientation. Such baker's transformation action chaotically mixes the solutes in each droplet. A liquid–liquid droplet microfluidic mixer has been used to rapidly mix fluorophore molecules with silver nanoparticles to enhance near-infrared fluorescence.[41] This microfluidic platform can fine tune the salt concentration, colloid concentration, and mixing efficiency to avoid nanoparticle aggregations.

7.5.3 Immobilizing a Catalytic DNA Molecular Beacon on Au Nanoparticle to Detect Pb(II) Species

The strong absorption of thiol groups on gold surfaces makes it easier to tag enzymes on gold nanoparticles when enzyme molecules are modified with a –SH group for immobilized enzymatic assays. Sweedler and colleagues immobilized one thiol derivative of a Pb(II)-specific DNAzyme fluorescent sensor on gold nanoparticles.[42] In their method, a self-assembled monolayer of thiolated DNAzyme first forms when enzyme strands are strongly absorbed on gold nanoparticles. This immobilized DNAzyme monolayer is then hybridized with complementary fluorophore-containing substrate solutes. As soon as they react with Pb(II), the substrate strands are cleaved to liberate a fluorescent fragment that indicates the existence of lead ions. The linear relationship between fluorescence intensity and Pb(II) concentration spans four decades (1 nM to 10 μM). The detection limit of this immobilized assay is 1 nM, which is a full order of magnitude lower than that of the previous solution-based method. The immobilized DNAzyme is able to regenerate after cleavage to allow multiple sensing cycles. This immobilized enzymatic assay can be applied to a stand-alone portable device when the enzyme immobilized nanoparticles are reserved in the nanopore cavities of a microfluidic–nanofluidic hybrid multilayer device.

7.6 Other Detection Techniques in Microfluidic Devices Using Noble Metal Nanoparticles

7.6.1 Microfluidic Devices to Facilitate Surface-Enhanced Raman Scattering Detections

When an incident light beam interacts with a polarizable molecule, the induced molecular dipoles oscillate with the light frequency and scatter. This scattering, known as Rayleigh scattering, is elastic and emits light of the same frequency as that of the incident light. The molecular polarizability is changeable when the molecule bonds vibrate. The scattering is no longer elastic. This inelastic scattering can occur to contain shifted peaks different from the Rayleigh scattering wavelength, including Stokes shift and anti-Stokes shift, of which the wavelengths are longer or shorter than the Rayleigh scattering peak, respectively. Raman scattering, of which the spectrum peaks are determined by the vibration frequencies of probed molecular bonds, is a highly specific tool for elucidating molecular structures.

When fluorophore molecules are absorbed on plasmonic nanoparticles of noble metals such as Au or Ag or within the proximity of a few nano-meters near the particle surface, Raman scattering light intensity can be enhanced by a factor of 10^6 to 10^8 for an assembly of molecules. This scattering enhancement effect known as surface-enhanced Raman scattering (SERS) is due to the LSPR occurring on the particle surface that focuses the incident light energy and amplifies the density of states at shifted scattering frequencies.

Bead-based assays to complementarily hybrid with oligonucleotide sequences of PCR products in a microfluidic device are bound with Raman active probe dye Rhodamine to label. The microsphere beads are retained with a micro-filter and heated to wash out Raman dyes. The released dyes are mixed with one stream of Ag nanoparticle solution in the same chip to enhance Raman scattering detections. Similarly, adenine-absorbed Au nanoparticles can be pinched by the step junction of the microchannel–nanochannel that captures the particles with target molecules into optically enhanced SERS active aggregates by employing capillary force.[43] The adenine detection limit of 10 pM has been achieved. Deuterated isotopomers have been used as an internal standard to correct quantitative results when SERS detections have been used to detect nicotine and pyridine in microfluidic mixers.[44]

7.6.2 Microfluidic Devices to Facilitate Thermal Lens Detections

Gold nanoparticles have strong light absorption properties to create a temperature gradient under intense light irradiation in solution. This temperature gradient results in the refraction index change of surrounding liquid known as the thermal lens effect, which can be probed with the other wavelength. The resulting refraction index change can focus or de-focus the probed light beam co-axially as aligned with the irradiation heating beam using the same microscope objective.

Individual gold nanoparticles absorb a continuous light at 532 nm under one microscope objective to station simultaneously. The light-absorbing nanoparticles release heat to change the refraction index around them. Probing light at 670 nm is directed via the same objective to interrogate the refraction index variability.[45] Alternatively, gold nanoparticles pass through the detection area of a microchannel to be probed under a thermal lens microscope.[46,47] Detection has been found to be more efficient in a narrow channel (~1 micron in width) than in the channel of 100 microns.

7.7 Conclusion

When incident light directly interacts with free electrons on the surfaces of noble nanoparticles, the scattering wavelength and intensity dependence of reflectivity is determined by particle surface dielectrics. This phenomenon can be used for PPR spectroscopic detections because the scattering indicates the specific docking of immobilized probes, such as antigens, with targeted bio-molecules (for example, antibodies).

Noble metal nanoparticles for PPR detection can be designed as colorimetric assays or coated on a stripped optical fiber to monitor the intensity attenuation of propagating light along the fiber. Either colorimetric PPR or FO-PPR can be conducted in microchannels. However, due to slow diffusivity of detected bio-molecules, developing micro-mixing units are required to accelerate detection response. In addition, electrospray ionization can occur at the microchannel outlet to determine the desorbed bio-molecules with mass spectrometry via applying high voltage at the channel tip. Alternatively, using the strong light absorbance of noble nanoparticles, upon laser irradiation the docked molecules are desorbed and ionize to determine with mass spectrometry via MALDI processes.

Noble metal nanoparticles, which have a strong affinity for thiol groups, can immobilize a variety of bio-molecular probes, including proteins and nucleic acids. These functionalized particles are suitable carriers for enzymatic and DNA hybridization assays. In addition, when fluorophores are tagged on the functional moieties, the strong interactions between the nanoparticle surface electrons and fluorophore dipoles can facilitate ultra-sensitive fluorescence detection methods such as FRET and SPCE. Functionalized nanoparticles can be coated on the microchannel surfaces or filled into running solutions to be employed with microfluidic devices. Similarly, micro-mixing is helpful for improving slow diffusivity problems of targeted molecules.

Other types of assays using noble metal nanoparticles such as SERS and thermal lens based methods have also been reported to perform in microchannels.

Acknowledgment

This work was supported by the National Science Council, Taiwan.

References

1. P. Fortina, D. Graves, C. Stoeckert, Jr., S. McKenzie, and S. Surrey, in *Biochip Technology*, Eds. J. Cheng and L. J. Kricka, (Harwood Academic Publishers, Philadelphia, 2001), p. 185.
2. P. S. Dittrich, K. Tachikawa, and A. Manz, *Anal. Chem.*, **78**, 3887 (2006).
3. J. West, J. Becker, M. Tombrink, and A. Manz, *Anal. Chem.*, **80**, 4403 (2008).
4. M. J. Felton, *Anal. Chem.*, **75**, 505A (2003).
5. M. J. Madou, Fundamentals of Microfabrication: The Science of. Miniaturization, (Taylor & Francis, New York, 2002).
6. S. C. Jacobson, R. Hergenroder, L. B. Koutny, R. J. Warmack, and J. M. Ramsey, *Anal. Chem.*, **66**, 1107 (1994).
7. D. Solignac, A. Sayah, S. Constantin, R. Freitag, and M. A. M. Gijs, *Sensors Actuators*, **92**, 388 (2001).
8. T. D. Boone, Z. H. Fan, H. H. Hooper, A. J. Ricco, H. Tan, and S. J. Williams, *Anal. Chem.*, 78A (2002).
9. C. G. Khan Malek, *Anal. Bioanal. Chem.*, **385**, 1351 (2006).
10. C. G. Khan Malek, *Anal. Bioanal. Chem.*, **385**, 1362 (2006).
11. H. Becker, and C. Gärtner, *Electrophoresis*, **21**, 12 (2000).
12. J. C. McDonald, and G. M. Whitesides, *Acc. Chem. Res.*, **35**, 491 (2002).

13. R. B. M. Schasfoort, and A. J. Tudos Eds., *Handbook of Surface Plasmon Resonance* (RSC Publishing, Cambridge, 2008).
14. R. L. Rich, and D. G. Myszka, *J. Mol. Recognit.*, **21**, 355 (2008).
15. F. Y. H. Lin, M. Sabri, J. Alirezaie, D. Q. Li, and P. M. Sherman, *Clin. Diagn. Lab. Immunol.*, **12**, 418 (2005).
16. C. J. Huang, K. Bonroy, G. Reekmans, K. Verstreken, L. Lagae, and G. Borghs, *Microelectron. Eng.*, **86**, 2437 (2009).
17. C. J. Huang, K. Bonroy, G. Reekmans, W. Laureyn, K. Verhaegen, I. De Vlaminck, L. Lagae, and G. Borghs, *Biomed. Microdevices*, **11**, 893 (2009).
18. A. Das, J. Zhao, G. C. Schatz, S. G. Sligar, and R. P. Van Duyne, *Anal. Chem.*, **81**, 3754 (2009).
19. J.-L. Tang, S.-F. Cheng, W.-T. Hsu, T.-Y. Chiang, and L.-K. Chau, *Sensor. Actuat. B-Chem.*, **119**, 105 (2006).
20. N.-S. Lai, C.-C. Wang, H.-L. Chiang, and L.-K. Chau, *Anal. Bioanal. Chem.*, **388**, 901 (2007).
21. S.-C. Wang, Y.-W. Lai, Y. Ben, and H.-C. Chang, *Ind. Eng. Chem. Res.*, **43**, 2902 (2004).
22. S.-C. Wang, H.-P. Chen, Y.-W. Lai, L.-K. Chau, Y.-C. Chuang, and Y.-J. Chen, *Biomicrofluidics*, **1**, 034104 (2007).
23. D. Lastochkin, R. Zhou, P. Wang, Y. Ben, and H.-C. Chang, *J. Appl. Phys.*, **96**, 1730 (2004).
24. S.-C. Wang, H.-P. Chen, C.-Y. Lee, C.-C. Yu, and H.-C. Chang, *Biosens. Bioelectron.*, **22**, 563 (2006).
25. Y. Chuang, C.-Y. Lee, S.-H. Lu, S.-C. Wang, and L.-K. Chau, *Anal. Chem.*, **82**, 1123 (2010).
26. A. D. Stroock, S. K. W. Dertinger, A. Ajdari, I. Mezi, H. A. Stone, and G. M. Whitesides, *Science*, **295**, 647 (2002).
27. C.-T. Huang, C.-P. Jen, T.-C. Chao, W.-T. Wu, W.-Y. Li, and L.-K., Chau, *Sensors*, **9**, 6456 (2009).
28. S. A. Shamsi, *Electrophoresis*, **23**, 4036 (2002).
29. J. B. Fenn, M. Mann, C. K. Meng, S. F. Wong, and C. M. Whitehouse, *Science*, **246**, 64 (1989).
30. Y. Liu, Y. Xue, J. Ji, X. Chen, J. Kong, P. Y. Yang, H. H. Girault, and B. H. Liu, *Mol. Cell Proteomics*, **6**, 1428 (2007).
31. J. B. Tracy, G. Kalyuzhny, M. C. Crowe, R. Balasubramanian, J.-P. Choi, and R. W. Murray, *J. Am. Chem. Soc.*, **129**, 6706 (2007).

32. L. F. Pease, D.-H. Tsai, R. A. Zangmeister, M. R. Zachariah, and M. J. Tarlov, *J. Phys. Chem. C*, **111**, 17155 (2007).
33. F. Hillenkamp, M. Karas, R. C. Beavis, and B. T. Chait, *Anal. Chem.*, **63**, 1193A (1991).
34. Y. P. Kim, E. Oh, M. Y. Hong, D. Lee, M. K. Han, H. K. Shon, D.W. Moon, H. S. Kim, and T. G. Lee, *Anal. Chem.*, **78**, 1913 (2006).
35. J. R. Lakowicz, *Principles of Fluorescence Spectroscopy* (Springer, Singapore, 2006).
36. Y. T. Li, H. S. Liu, H. P. Lin, and S. H. Chen, *Electrophoresis*, **26**, 4743 (2005).
37. J. R. Lakowicz, *Anal Biochem.*, **324**, 153 (2004).
38. M. Evgenia, G., Ignacy, B. Anne, C. Nils, and G. Zygmunt, *Anal. Bioanal. Chem.*, **388**, 1127 (2007).
39. R. F. Ismagilov, A. D. Stroock, P. J. A. Kenis, G. Whitesides, and H. A. Stone, *Appl. Phys. Lett.*, **76**, 2376 (2000).
40. H. Song, and J. D. Tice, R. F. Ismagilov, *Angew. Chem.*, **115**, 792 (2003).
41. M. D. Furtaw, D. Lin, L. Wu, and J. P. Anderson, *Plasmonics*, **4**, 273 (2009).
42. C. B. Swearingen, D. P. Wernette, D. M. Cropek, Y. Lu, J. V. Sweedler, and P. W. Bohn, *Anal. Chem.*, **77**, 442 (2005).
43. M. Wang, N. Jing, I. H. Chou, G. L. Cote, and J. Kameoka, *Lab Chip*, **7**, 630 (2007).
44. A. Marz, K. R. Ackermann, D. Malsch, T. Bocklitz, T. Henkel, and J. Popp, *J. Biophotonics*, **2**, 232 (2009).
45. K. Mawatari, M. Tokeshi, and T. Kitamori, *Anal. Sci.*, **22**, 781 (2006).
46. N. Seta, K. Mawatari, and T. Kitamori, *Anal. Sci.*, **25**, 275 (2009).
47. P. S. Petrou, S. E. Kakabakos, and K. Misiakos, *Int. J. Nanotechnol.*, **6**, 4 (2009).

Chapter 8

Biodetection Based on Resonance Light Scattering of Noble Metal Nanoparticles

Tai-Chia Chiu and Cho-Chun Hu
Department of Applied Science, National Taitung University, 684, Section 1, Chunghua Road, Taitung 95002, Taiwan
tcchiu@nttu.edu.tw, cchu@nttu.edu.tw

Gold nanoparticles (Au NPs) and silver nanoparticles (Ag NPs) are two of the most efficient light scattering materials, and are extensively utilized in resonance light scattering (RLS) techniques. RLS techniques using these NPs are sensitive and selective for the analysis of biological and environmental samples. Although Au NPs are not as efficient as Ag NPs in RLS, their stability, ease in preparation and conjugation make them more popular. Because RLS signals are proportional to aggregate size, most RLS techniques are developed from measuring the RLS signal based on the aggregation of Au or Ag NPs, induced by the analytes. To develop highly sensitive RLS techniques, several important parameters such as the nature, size, and shape of NPs, as well as the intensity and frequency of the light source must be well controlled. Due to significant progress in nanoscience, it is expected that more efficient RLS probes will soon be developed for the detection of trace biomolecules and cell imaging.

From Bioimaging to Biosensors: Noble Metal Nanoparticles in Biodetection
Edited by Lai-Kwan Chau and Huan-Tsung Chang

ISBN 978-981-4267-24-3 (Hardcover), 978-981-4303-10-1 (eBook)
www.panstanford.com

8.1 Introduction

Light scattering causes many interesting phenomena in the universe. For example, the blue color of the sky is caused by the scattering of sunlight from the molecules and particles in the atmosphere.[1] Scattered light is emitted in all directions except the direction in which incident light beams is propagated, and scattered light is strongly related to the inhomogeneity of the medium.[2] Depending on the size of the photon-interacted particles (d) and the wavelength of incident light beams (λ), light scattering can be classified into Mie ($d >> \lambda$), Tyndall ($d \approx \lambda$), and Rayleigh scattering ($d \leq 0.05\lambda$).[2] Despite the wavelength difference between the incident and the scattered beams, light scattering can also be divided into elastic scattering, inelastic scattering, and quasi-elastic scattering.[3] Rayleigh scattering is elastic, while both Raman and Brillouin scattering are inelastic. Quasi-elastic scattering (dynamic light scattering) results from the Brownian movement of the scatters.[3]

Nanoparticles (NPs) of different sizes have unique optical and electric properties, and can thus become promising RLS probes. It is known that the RLS intensity is proportional to the sixth power of the radius of the nanoparticles, and is inversely proportional to the fourth power of the wavelength of incident light.[4,5] In addition, the RLS intensity is proportional to the light intensity. Thus, NP size, as well as the incident light's wavelength and intensity play important roles in determining the RLS signals.

Both Au and Ag NPs have visible absorption and capability for enhancing RLS signals. In addition to Au and Ag NPs, other NPs such as AgCl, PbS, HgS, Ag_2S, Fe_3O_4, CdTe, and C_{60} also provide enhanced RLS signals.[6–12] Due to its high sensitivity, RLS is a useful technique for determining the concentrations of analytes of interest.[13,14] RLS techniques, in conjunction with commercial spectrofluorometers, have been utilized in observing the formation of aggregated chromophores in complex systems.[15–17] Moreover, RLS techniques have proven themselves to be important and powerful tools for the quantification of nucleic acids, proteins, metallic ions, drugs (in artificial and real samples), and for characterization of the aggregation and assembly of biological and chemical species.[18–22]

This chapter briefly describes the basic concepts of RLS. Au and Ag NPs are the two most popular NPs used in RLS techniques, and thus their RLS properties and use in RLS bioassays are discussed in more detail. The roles that the nature, size, and shape of Au and Ag NPs play in determining RLS signals are emphasized here. The advantages and limitations of RLS techniques for bioassays are discussed using several representative application examples. Finally, the developed RLS techniques are summarized and their future trend is highlighted.

8.2 Basic Theory of RLS

In general, two processes (absorption and scattering) occur when light passes through a solution of aggregates. If the solvent itself is nonabsorbing, then energy is removed from the incident light through absorption and scattering by the aggregates. The light scattering component is a consequence of differences in polarizability between the aggregates and the solvent. The incident electromagnetic wave induces an oscillating dipole in the assembly, which radiates light in all directions. To understand the polarizability of the aggregates, two terms, absorption cross section (C_{abs}) and scattering cross section (C_{scat}), are presented. The ratio of the rate of energy absorption from the incident beam to the intensity of the incident beam is called C_{abs}. The ratio of the rate of energy scattering out of the incident beam (in all directions) to the intensity of the incident beam is called C_{scat}. If the induced dipole can be considered ideal — which is usually a valid assumption if the size of the aggregate is small compared to the wavelength (λ_m) of the light in the solvent — both cross sections are related to the polarizability of the aggregates in the following simple formulae[16]

$$C_{\text{abs}} = k_{\text{m}} \alpha_{\text{i}} \tag{8.1}$$

$$C_{\text{scat}} = \frac{k_{\text{m}}^4}{6\pi} |\alpha|^2 = \frac{k_{\text{m}}^4}{6\pi} \left(\alpha_{\text{r}}^2 + \alpha_{\text{i}}^2 \right) \tag{8.2}$$

where k_m is the wave vector of light in the solvent, $k_m = 2\pi/\lambda_m$, and α_r and α_i are the real and imaginary parts of the polarizability of the aggregates. Absorption at a certain wavelength band by a solution of aggregates can be understood to be the result of a maximum in the imaginary part of the polarizability in that region of the spectrum. The absorbance (A) of a sample of thickness (L) is presented as[16]

$$A = 2.3^{-1} \left(\frac{N}{V} \right) C_{\text{abs}} L \tag{8.3}$$

where N/V is the number of aggregates per unit volume. The real and imaginary parts of α are related to each other so that when α_i is maximized in some wavelength range, α_r also behaves anomalously in this region; hence, $|\alpha|^2$ is at a maximum in the absorption band, which also results in increased scattering. Under normal conditions, this increased scattering is difficult or impossible to detect because of the increased absorption and the weakness of the enhanced scattering effect. However, when this effect is investigated for aggregates of chromophores, the enhanced RLS can be enormous. The absorption depends on the first power of the polarizability, which in turn depends linearly on the volume of the aggregate. Thus, a solution with a fixed concentration of the aggregating component exhibits no change in A as aggregation occurs because the product of N/V and α_i remains constant. However, the amount of scattering depends on the square of the volume of the aggregate, and thus it increases as a consequence of aggregation. RLS is therefore extremely sensitive to aggregates.

8.2.1 RLS of Plasmonic NPs

When a metallic NP is exposed to an electromagnetic wave, the electrons in the metal (plasmons) oscillate at the same frequency as the incident wave. Subsequently, the oscillating electrons radiate electromagnetic radiation with the same frequency as the oscillating electrons. This re-radiation of light at the same incident wavelength is often referred to as plasmon scatter.[23,24] If the colloid is illuminated with light (λ) that matches the principle plasmon absorption maxima (λ_p), the NPs can then both absorb and scatter light outside of their physical cross-sections. For wavelengths longer than λ_p, light is only influenced over the physical constraints of its cross-section. Because the nature, size, and shape of NPs are important parameters for λ_p, they also affect scattering properties. For example, $C_{scat} = 8 \times 10^{-12}$ cm^2 for a 30 nm diameter Ag NP at 380 nm, which is about 2000-fold larger than that of polystyrene NP of 30 nm.[23] One 60 nm Au NP has the same scattering intensity as 3×10^5 fluorescein molecules. When compared to four of the most commonly used metal NPs (Ag, Au, Cu, and Al), Ag shows the most efficient plasmon scatter, which is about 10-fold higher than Au and 20-fold higher than Cu and Al.[23] Although Au NPs are less efficient at scattering than Ag NPs, their use is also popular, mainly because they are stable and easy to prepare and conjugate.

The scattering of light by very small (subwavelength) sized particles is well described by Rayleigh's theory.[23,24] For incident light horizontally polarized and observed in the same plane, the intensity of light scattered (I_{scat}) in the direction θ by a homogeneous spherical particle with radius (a), which is much smaller than the wavelength (λ) of the incident beam, is given by the Rayleigh expression[23,24]

$$I_{scat} = \frac{16\pi^4 a^6 n_{med}^4 I_0}{r^2\lambda^4}\left|\frac{m^2-1}{m^2+2}\right|^2 \cos^2\theta \tag{8.4}$$

where I_0 is the incident intensity of monochromatic light, n_{med} is the refractive index surrounding the particle, m is the refractive index of the bulk particle material, and r is the distance between the particle and where the scattered light is detected. From Eq. (8.4), the scattered light in the horizontal plane is 100% polarized. The scattered light intensities are highest at the observation angles $\theta = 0°$ and 180°, zero at $\theta = 90°$ and 270°, and proportional to $\cos^2\theta$ at all other angles. This spatial or angular distribution of plasmon scatter is characteristic of an electric dipole emitter.[23,24] For light vertically polarized and perpendicular to the scattering plane, the intensity of scatter is given by the well-known form of the Rayleigh expression[23]

$$I_{scat} = \frac{16\pi^4 a^6 n_{med}^4 I_0}{r^2\lambda^4}\left|\frac{m^2-1}{m^2+2}\right|^2 \tag{8.5}$$

8.3 Applications of NP-Based RLS Techniques

NP-based RLS probes are simple and sensitive techniques that can be performed using a commercial spectrofluorometer. When compared to fluorescence, RLS techniques face less problems of photobleaching and quenching due to changes in temperature, pH, and ionic strength.[13] As a result of these advantages, NP-based RLS techniques have become practical for the quantification of a number of analytes, including drugs, carbohydrates, antibodies, nucleic acids, and proteins in artificial and real samples. In addition, NP-based RLS techniques have also proven to be useful for the characterization of aggregation and assembly of biological and chemical species.

8.3.1 Au NPs as RLS Probes

Au NPs have been studied extensively in recent years due to their interesting optical properties and bio-compatibility.[25] Au NPs display intense colors ranging from rose red to purple. This is due to intense surface plasmon absorption and scattering at different wavelengths, which is highly dependent upon the NP size and shape.[26] The localized surface plasmon resonance (LSPR) band is due to electron oscillations in the metallic particles, induced by the incident light field. Upon increasing the size of Au NPs, LSPR bands undergo red shifts. Because of the strong oscillations from incident light in the visible region, RLS signals of analytes on the surface of Au NPs can be enhanced with magnitudes greater than 100-fold.[27] As a result, Au NPs have been shown to be effective matrices for the quantitative detection of analytes by RLS.

8.3.1.1 Small analytes

Because of strong interactions of thiol compounds with Au NPs through Au-S bonding, Au NPs have shown great selectivity for thiol-containing compounds such as cysteine and glutathione (GSH).[28,29] The determination of thiol-containing pharmaceutical compounds like thiamazole by RLS has been demonstrated using 13 nm diameter Au NPs.[27] At pH 5.2, the RLS spectrum of Au NPs shows a maximum peak at 555 nm and the RLS intensity is enhanced by trace amounts of thiamazole. The binding of Au NPs to thiamazole results in ligand-induced aggregation of Au NPs and significantly enhances the RLS intensity. Figure 8.1 demonstrates the relationship between relative RLS intensity and the ratio of thiamazole/Au NPs at a constant thiamazole concentration. An Au NP solution at higher particle concentration is less prone to aggregation, which is possibly due to the lack of enough thiamazole molecules per particle to induce aggregation. In term of sensitivity, it is suggested to use low concentrations of Au NPs when the analyte concentration is low. The RLS approach provides a linear range from 2.36 nM to 1.05 μM for thiamazole, with a limit of detection (LOD) at signal-to-noise ratio 3 ($S/N = 3$) of 2.01 nM ($n = 11$, RSD = 1.86%). Similarly, a RLS spectroscopy has been successfully applied to investigation of the aggregation process of Au NPs (10 nm diameter) induced by captopril.[30] In an aqueous medium of pH 2.09, Au NPs and captopril form core-shell assemble of $[(Au)_{31000}]@[(Captopril)_{2200}]$. As a result, a strong RLS signal occurs in the resonance region of the Au NPs. The RLS intensities characterized at 553 nm is proportional to the concentration of captopril over the range of 0.1–1.7 mg/L with the detection limit (S/N = 3) of 32.0 μg/L. This approach is useful to determine captopril in pharmaceutical preparations with the recovery of 97.0–104.5% and RSD less than 2.4%.

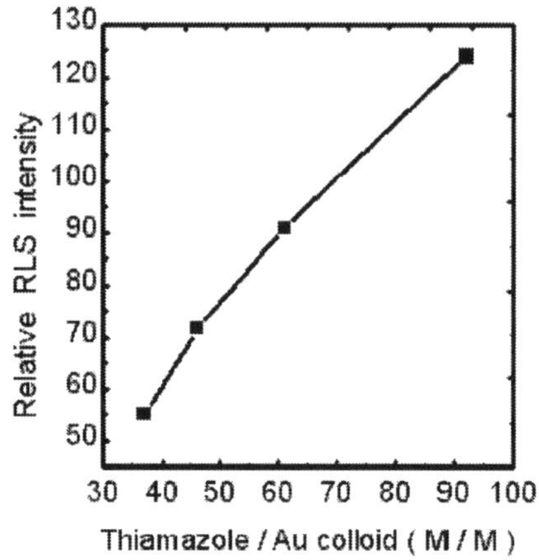

Figure 8.1 Relative RLS intensity as a function of thiamazole/13 nm diameter Au NPs (mol/L) ratio, with the same concentration of thiamazole (0.14 mM) and the Au NP concentration being 1.57, 2.36, 3.14, and 3.93 nM, respectively. Each sample was placed for 15 min before scanning and λ_{RLS} = 555 nm. Reprinted from Ref. 27 with permission.

RLS techniques are also popular for determination of small analytes in cells. One representative example is the determination and distribution of GSH within erythrocyte cells using Nile Red-absorbed 32 nm Au NPs.[31] When the Nile Red product is displaced by GSH on the Au NP surface, the fluorescence of the solution increases and the Au NPs aggregate, which results in increased RLS signals. Figure 8.2 displays the phase contrast, dark-field scattering, and fluorescence images of single erythrocytes. Representative scattering images of these three cells are presented in Fig. 8.2B, in which the bright spots illustrate the presence of Nile Red-absorbed 32 nm Au NPs within the cells. Figure 8.2C presents one representative fluorescence image (the upper cell in Fig. 8.2B), which indicates that the displacement and aggregation of Nile Red-absorbed 32 nm Au NPs induced by GSH occurs in a manner similar to the occurrence of those processes in free solution. The last two images clearly exhibit the localization of Nile Red-absorbed 32 nm Au NPs, showing that this dual detection system allows clear observation of GSH located in the central part in individual cells.

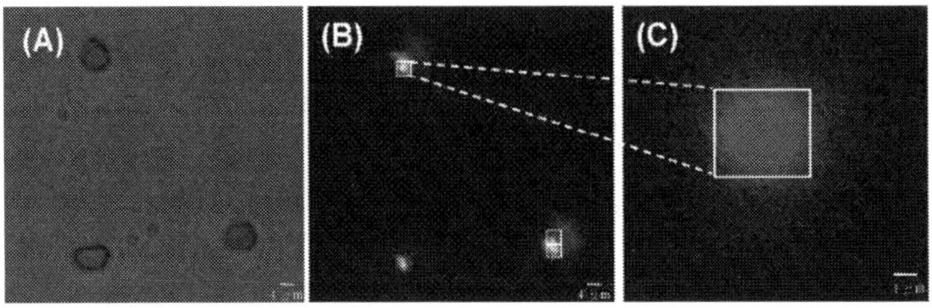

Figure 8.2 Comparison of the (A) phase contrast, (B) scattering, and (C) fluorescence images of erythrocytes incubated with 1 × Nile Red-absorbed 32 nm Au NPs for 12 h. The exposure times were (A) 0.25 s, (B) 0.5 s, and (D) 4 s, respectively. Light was collected using a 40 objective for the phase contrast and scattering measurements and a 100 objective for the fluorescence measurements. Reprinted from Ref. 31 with permission. See also Color Insert.

RLS spectroscopy can also be used to study the interactions between cysteine and Au NPs.[32] Through covalent interaction with the –SH group and the electrostatic binding with the $-NH_3^+$ group of cysteine, the self-assembling property of the Au NPs forms a network structure, which results in greatly enhanced RLS intensity. This RLS approach provides a linear range of cysteine concentrations, from 0.01 to 0.25 μg/mL, with an LOD of 2.0 ng/mL (16.5 nM). To minimize the interference of GSH, detection of cysteine by this RLS approach at pH 5.0 is proper. The RLS signals of GSH on Au reach a maximum at pH 3.2 and there is a sharp decrease in the RLS signal over the pH range 3.2–4.3. However, homocysteine interference cannot be prevented; homocysteine also induces an increased RLS signal at pH 5.0.

The RLS technique is also practical for the determination of glucose, based on the glucose-induced dissociation of aggregates of dextran (MW. 170 K) coated Au NPs with concanavalin A (Fig. 8.3).[33] Tetravalent protein concanavalin A is readily cross-linked with dextran-coated Au NPs (20 nm diameter), leading to a broadening and red shift in the LSPR band of Au NPs.[34] Addition of glucose that competitively binds to concanavalin A leads to aggregation of dextran-Au NPs with concanavalin A to a lesser extent. As a result, the RLS signals decrease, showing that the aggregations of Au NPs are indeed efficient at light scattering at a wavelength near the LSPR band of the Au NPs. By plotting the ratio of scattered light intensities at two different wavelengths, 560 and 680 nm, against glucose concentration, glucose concentrations can be readily determined from a few mM up to ~60 mM using a simple white light emitting diode and detection system. This simple and low-cost approach is ideal for monitoring physiological blood glucose where red scattering wavelengths (>600 nm) can be selected to eliminate the absorption of hemoglobin, water, and melanin.

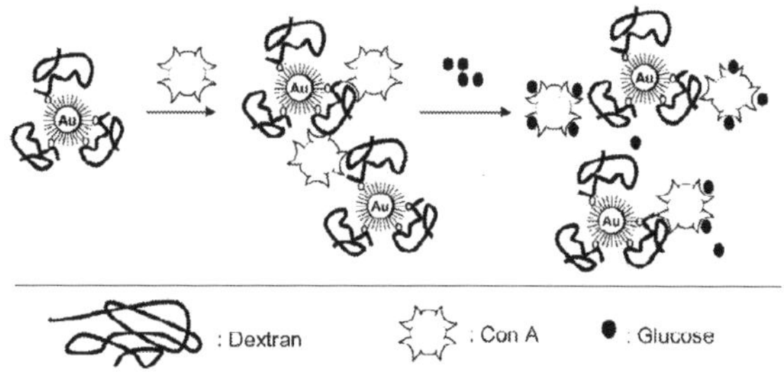

Figure 8.3 Glucose sensing scheme based on the dissociation of dextran-coated Au-NPs/concanavalin A aggregates and their respective light scattering properties. Reprinted from Ref. 33 with permission.

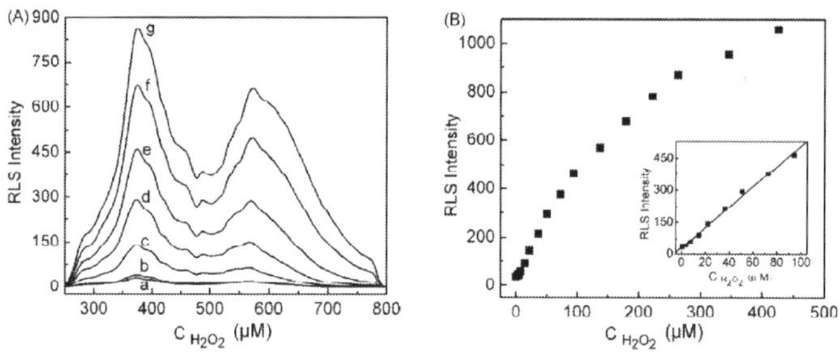

Figure 8.4 (A) RLS spectra of 3.0×10^{-10} M Au-NP seeds, upon growth in the presence of 2.4×10^{-4} M $HAuCl_4$ and 2.4×10^{-3} M CTAC in 0.01 M PBS (pH 7.0), with different concentrations of H_2O_2: (a) 0; (b) 2.5×10^{-6} M; (c) 2.2×10^{-5} M; (d) 5.0×10^{-6} M; (e) 9.4×10^{-5} M; (f) 1.8×10^{-4} M; and (g) 2.6×10^{-4} M. All spectra were recorded after a reaction time of 15 min. (B) The calibration curve corresponding to the RLS intensity at 375 nm vs. the concentration of H_2O_2 in the growth solution. The inset is the linear plots in the range of 5.0×10^{-7} M to 9.5×10^{-5} M. Reprinted from Ref. 35 with permission.

RLS techniques are useful for the determination of analytes based on the biocatalytic enlargement of Au NPs.[35] For example, H_2O_2, an important metabolite that is generated by many biocatalytic reactions can be determined by RLS (375 nm) because it effectively induces growth of the Au NP seeds. As the size of Au NPs increases, the RLS signal also intensifies (Fig. 8.4A). Thus, quantitative detection of H_2O_2 by RLS can be readily achieved (Fig. 8.4B). This RLS approach provides detection of glucose over a linear range of 1.0–110 μM, with an LOD of 0.68 μM.

Solutions containing Au NPs and rare-earth europium ions (Eu^{3+}) are interesting RLS systems because Au NPs can enhance the RLS signals of the metal ions.[36] In the absence of Au NPs, a solution containing Eu^{3+} has two RLS peaks at wavelengths of 400 and 780 nm, as shown in Fig. 8.5. When the solution contains Au NPs and Eu^{3+}, however, the two RLS peaks are both enhanced, mainly due to the energy transfer from the local field in Au NPs to Eu^{3+} ions. The RLS technique may also be utilized when investigating the interaction of 11-mercaptoundecanoic acid (MUA) capped Au NPs with Eu^{3+} ions and amino acids.[37]

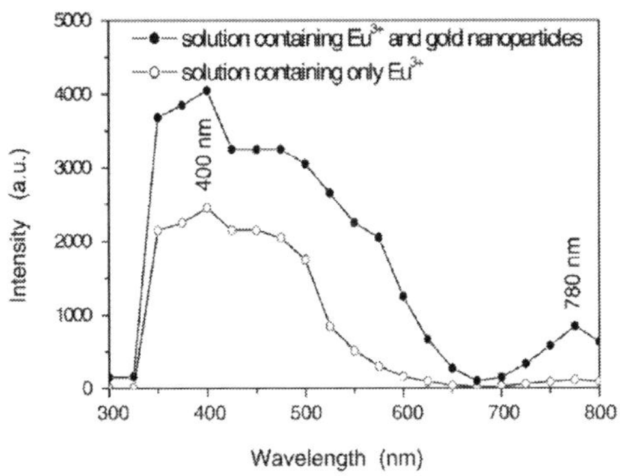

Figure 8.5 RLS spectra of solution containing only Eu^{3+} and solution containing both Au NPs and Eu^{3+}. Reprinted from Ref. 36 with permission.

Figure 8.6 conceptually illustrates how Eu binding events, in the presence of lysine, induce a change in the spacing and shape of the Au NPs. Aggregation of Au NPs, through the binding of Eu^{3+} to the carboxylate ions on the outer surface, results in the modification of most nanodots into nanorods. In the absence of Eu^{3+} ions, repulsive

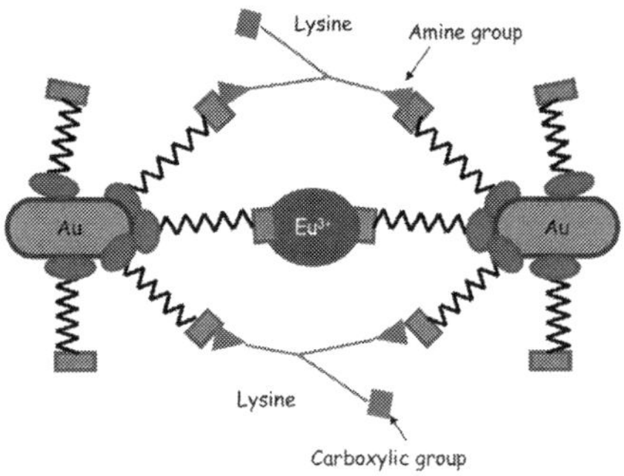

Figure 8.6 Schematic for the MUA-Au-NP resonance light scattering plasmon enhancement model. The RLS enhancement is achieved through cooperative binding with europium and lysine. Reprinted from Ref. 37 with permission.

forces among the negatively charged MUA-Au-NPs are strong enough to hinder the electrostatic attraction between the positively charged amino groups in lysine and the negatively charged MUA-Au-NPs. Because the RLS intensity of Eu^{3+} ion decreases upon increasing MUA-Au-NPs concentration, energy transfer from Eu^{3+} ions to MUA-Au-NPs occurs, significantly enhancing the efficiency of interplasmon coupling. In other words, Eu^{3+} ions act as sensitizers for the RLS emission (390 nm) of the Au NPs. Figure 8.7 displays

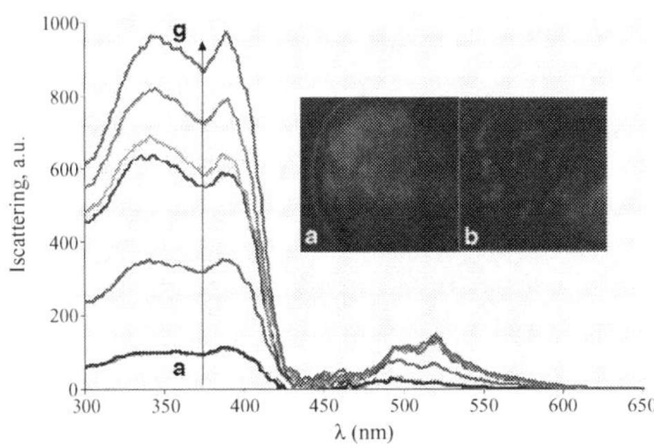

Figure 8.7 RLS spectra of: (a) MUA-Au-NPs; (b) MUA-Au-NPs-Lysine; (c) MUA-Au-NPs-Eu 1 × 10^{-3} M-Lysine; (d) MUA-Au-NPs–Eu 2.5 × 10^{-3} M-Lys; (e) MUA-Au-NPs-Eu 3.0 × 10^{-3} M-Lysine; (f) MUA-Au-NPs–Eu 5.0 × 10^{-3} M-Lysine; (g) MUA-Au-NPs-Eu 7.5 × 10^{-3} M-Lysine. Inset: Confocal fluorescence microscopy images of (a) agglomerated flocs of MUA-Au-NPs-Eu-Lysine and (b) isolated clusters of MUA-Au-NPs-Eu-Glutamine. [MUA-Au-NPs] = 5.3 × 10^{-12} M, [L-lysine] = 7.0 × 10^{-3} M, [Glutamine] = 7 × 10^{-3} M, pH = 6. Reprinted from Ref. 37 with permission. See also Color Insert.

the RLS signals and conformal fluorescence images of these various solutions, discussed above. The cooperative binding interactions of Eu^{3+} and lysine with Au NPs allow the discrimination of lysine from other amino acids. The RLS approach is therefore practical for the determination of lysine (130 ± 5 mg per 100 mL) in pharmaceutical syrups.

8.3.1.2 Proteins

Proteins can induce aggregation of Au NPs through changes in the surface charge density of Au NPs, or through specific interactions such as protein–protein, carbohydrate–lectin, and DNA–protein interactions.[38–43] For example, bovine serum albumin capped Au NPs form aggregates at around pH 4.5 because the protein does not possess a charge at its p*I* value. Another example is the platelet-derived growth factor induced aggregation of aptamer-capped Au NPs in 5 mM phosphate buffer (pH 7.4) containing 200 mM NaCl.[40]

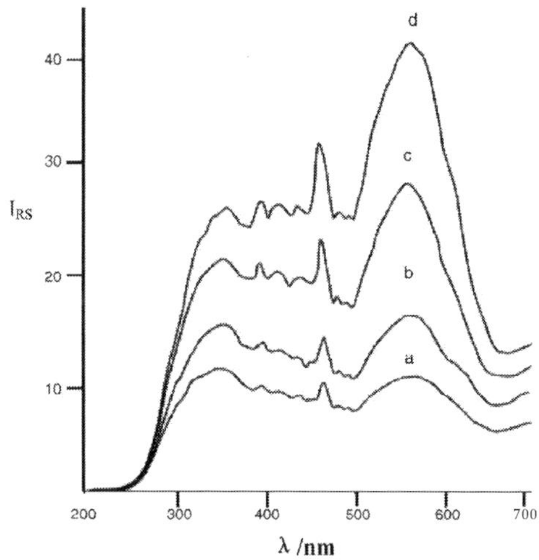

Figure 8.8 RLS spectrum of fibrinogen-gold-labeled goat anti-human fibrinogen system. (a) pH 6.2 PBS-23.2 g/mL gold-labeled goat anti-human fibrinogen-50 mg/mL PEG-4000; (b) pH 6.2 PBS-23.2 g/mL gold-labeled goat anti-human fibrinogen-50 mg/mL PEG-4000, 0.16 g/mL fibrinogen; (c) pH 6.2 PBS-23.2 g/mL gold-labeled goat anti-human fibrinogen-50 mg/mL PEG-4000, 0.54 g/mL fibrinogen; (d) pH 6.2 PBS-23.2 g/mL gold-labeled goat anti-human fibrinogen-50 mg/mL PEG-4000, 1.07 g/mL fibrinogen. Reprinted from Ref. 44 with permission.

RLS techniques using Au NPs bioconjugated with recognition molecules are useful for the determination of proteins, mainly because of analyte-induced increases in RLS signals of Au NPs. One representative example is the detection of fibrinogen using Au NPs (9.0 nm diameter) bioconjugated with goat anti-human fibrinogen (Fig. 8.8).[44] The gold-labeled anti-human fibrinogen has two characteristic RLS peaks at 340 nm and 560 nm (the peak at 470 nm is due to self-producing synchronous scattering). In 0.2 M Na_2HPO_4–NaH_2PO_4 buffer (pH 6.2) containing PEG-4000, the immune reaction between Au NPs bioconjugated with goat anti-human fibrinogen and fibrinogen takes place, leading to the release of goat anti-human fibrinogen from Au NP surfaces. As a result, Au NPs aggregate, leading to great enhancements in the RLS intensity at 560 nm. The value of I_{560nm} is proportional to the fibrinogen concentration over the range from 0.027 to 1.07 μg/mL. This approach provides an LOD of 1.14 ng/mL for fibrinogen, demonstrating great potential for the determination of fibrinogen in human plasma.

Immunoresonance scattering using Au NPs (8–10 nm diameter) as RLS probes is useful for the measurement of apolipoprotein AI (ApoAI) and apolipoprotein B (ApoB).[45] In order to further improve the intensity of RLS peaks at 560 nm, addition of PEG to the solution is essential. The analytes induce aggregation of apolipoprotein AI and apolipoprotein B antisera labeled Au NPs, leading to increased RLS signals, as shown in Fig. 8.9. Because of the correlation of RLS intensity with the size of the Au NPs, the intensity is greatly enhanced. The intensity is proportional to the concentration in the range of 8.33–333.3 ng/L for ApoAI and 1.97–197.2 ng/L for ApoB. The LODs are 2.04 and 0.96 μg/L for ApoAI and ApoB, respectively. This RLS approach is practical for the determination of the two analytes in human serum samples, with results being in good agreement with those obtained with an immunoturbidimetric method. Similarly, immunoresonance scattering using Au NPs (9.0 nm diameter) bioconjugated with goat anti-human prealbumin polyclonal antibody has proven useful for the analysis of trace prealbumin.[46] The immune reaction between the gold-labeled antibody and prealbumin takes place in a Na_2HPO_4–NaH_2PO_4 buffer (pH 7.6) in the presence of PEG-10000, leading to aggregation of Au NPs that have strong RLS signals at 580 nm. The approach provides a linear relationship between the RLS intensity and prealbumin concentration over the range from 16.67 to 666.67 ng/mL, with an LOD of 4.1 ng/mL. Homogeneous noncompetitive immunoassays by RLS, using a commercial spectrofluorometer, are practical for the determination of human immunoglobulin (IgG), based on analyte induced aggregation of goat-anti-human IgG-functionalized Au NPs.[47] Upon increasing IgG concentration over a dynamic range of 0.05–10 μg/mL, the RLS of bioconjugated Au NPs increases. The immunoassay can be accomplished in a homogeneous solution for the determination of human IgG in serum samples with one-step operation in under 10 min, and provides results that are consistent with those obtained by conducting an enzyme-linked immunosorbent assay. Detection of trace immunoglobulin M (IgM) using Au NPs (8 nm diameter) bioconjugated with goat antihuman immunoglobulin M (Au-GIgM) is also represented.[48] Aggregates form due to the interaction of Au-GIgG with IgM in KH_2PO_4–Na_2HPO_4 buffer (pH 4.9) containing PEG-6000, leading to an increased RLS intensity at 580 nm. The enhanced RLS intensity at 580 nm is proportional to the IgM concentration over the concentration range of 1.5–2000 ng/mL. The RLS approach is sensitive (LOD = 0.98 ng/mL) for IgM.

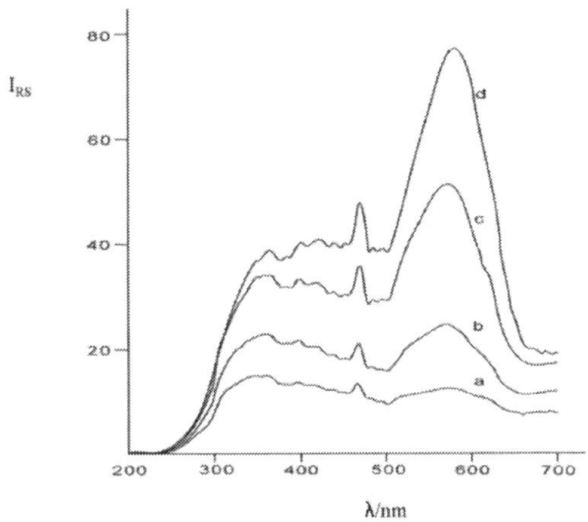

Figure 8.9 RLS spectra of gold-labeled goat anti-human ApoAI antiserum and ApoAI. Traces: (a) PB solution (pH 6.4) containing 23.18 mg/L goat anti-human ApoAI antiserum and 75 g/L PEG-6000; (b) PB solution (pH 6.4) containing 23.18 mg/L goat anti-human ApoAI antiserum, 0.033 mg/L ApoAI, and 75 g/L PEG-6000; (c) PB solution (pH 6.4) containing 23.18 mg/L goat anti-human ApoAI antiserum, 0.17 mg/L ApoAI, and 75 g/L PEG-6000; (d) PB solution (pH 6.4) containing 23.18 mg/L goat anti-human ApoAI antiserum, 0.33 mg/L ApoAI, and 75 g/L PEG-6000. Reprinted from Ref. 45 with permission.

Aptamer-conjugated Au NPs are selective and sensitive for detection of proteins and small analytes.[40–43] Through specific binding of the aptamers with the platelet-derived growth factor, MDA-MB-231 and Hs578T cancerous cells that over-express the platelet-derived growth factor, interact with aptamer-Au-NPs to greater extents than do H184B5F5/M10 normal cells.[49] Aggregation of the aptamer-Au NPs in the cytoplasm of the cancerous cells leads to the generation of a strong yellow scattered light upon photo-illumination; this phenomenon allows one to readily differentiate between the tested cancerous cells and normal cells using a laboratory-made dark field microscope.

8.3.1.3 DNA

Like proteins, DNA can induce aggregation of Au NPs bioconjugated with recognition molecules such as DNA and proteins. Aggregates of DNA functionalized Au NPs can be formed through cross-linking and non-cross-linking reactions. The latter refers to aggregation through van der Waal's forces. Factors that control the surface properties (e.g., charge density) of DNA-Au NPs, such as ionic strength and pH, are important. By carefully controlling ionic strength, colorimetric and fluorescence detections of Hg^{2+} and adenosine triphosphate using DNA-Au-NPs have been realized.[50–52] Cross-linking reactions through complimentary DNA hybridization are more common in the aggregation of DNA-Au NPs. Colorimetric sensors of DNA using DNA-Au NPs are useful for single-nucleotide polymorphisms study and disease diagnosis.[53–56] These successful colorimetric approaches indicate that RLS techniques using DNA-Au-NPs have potential for detection of DNA.

Figure 8.10 displays an application of 80 nm diameter Au NPs, bioconjugated with anti-biotin antibodies, for the detection of DNA hybridization on cDNA microarrays.[57] The arrays are composed of ~2000 human genes that were hybridized with colabeled (Cy3 and biotin) human lung cDNA probes at concentrations ranging from 8.3 ng/μL to 16.7 pg/μL. After hybridization, the arrays were treated with 80 nm diameter Au NPs, bioconjugated with anti-biotin antibodies and imaged in a white light CCD-based imaging system. For hybridizations with a probe concentration of 83.3 pg/μL, RLS detected ~1150 positive genes, while fluorescence detection only detected ~110 positive genes. RLS using DNA-Au-NPs is also practical for the detection of DNA in homogeneous solutions.[58] The assay relies on the observation of greatly enhanced RLS signals that originate from the aggregation of DNA-Au-NPs, induced by the target DNA. The reproducibility of this RLS assay is quite good (RSD 2.6%, n =11).

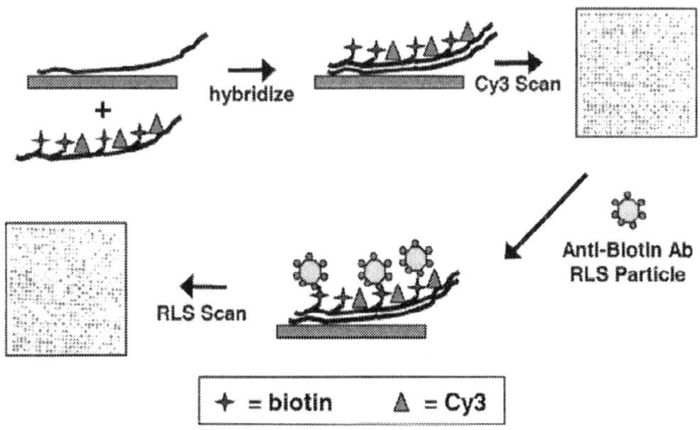

Figure 8.10 Outline of experimental protocol. cDNA probes generated by the colabeling of lung RNA with Cy3 and biotin are hybridized to an array. Following several wash steps to remove unbound probe, the array is scanned in a fluorescence scanner to capture the Cy3 fluorescence image. Treatment of the array with RLS NPs is accomplished by incubating the slides with anti-biotin antibody-coated 80 nm diameter Au NPs. The same array is then imaged in a CCD-based white light imaging system to generate the RLS image. Reprinted from Ref. 57 with permission.

In addition to DNA-Au-NPs, bare (non-bioconjugated) Au NPs also make useful RLS probes for the detection of DNA, based on non-cross-linking reactions. Recognition of a quadruplex DNA structure using unmodified Au NPs is realized using a simple, label-free, RLS approach, based on charge variations before and after DNA folding.[59]

The adsorption of uncoiled DNA on the surface of Au NPs prevents the NPs from aggregation in highly concentrated ionic media. Potassium ions induce the telomere DNA to change its conformation from an uncoiled to a quadruplex structure *via* intermolecular hydrogen bonding, leading to aggregation of the Au NPs and thus, increased RLS signals. A single point energy calculation shows that, when compared to the unfolded DNA, the quadruplex

DNA has greater surface negative charge density, symmetrical charge distribution, and well self-structural stabilization. As a result, adsorption of quadruplex DNA molecules on the surface of Au NPs is more difficult. Similar strategies can also be applied for DNA hybridization detection. Figure 8.11 displays a protocol of the detection of the human immunodeficiency virus type 1 by RLS using Au nanorods and a label-free probe DNA that recognizes the gene related to the virus.[60] These anisotropic nonspherical and positively charged Au nanorods show high stability against aggregation under high ionic strength conditions without requiring any additional stabilizing reagent. The addition of target DNA to a mixture of label-free probe DNA and nonmodified Au nanorods (in suspension) in high ionic-strength buffer, leads to a color change from red to light purple in less than 5 min and displays a strong RLS signal. The strong RLS signal is ascribed to the aggregation of Au nanorods, induced by forming double-stranded oligonucleotides, through the hybridization of target DNA with probe DNA. This approach allows detection of target DNA down to 0.1 pM and offers advantages of simplicity, sensitivity, specificity, and reliability for detection of the human immunodeficiency virus gene.

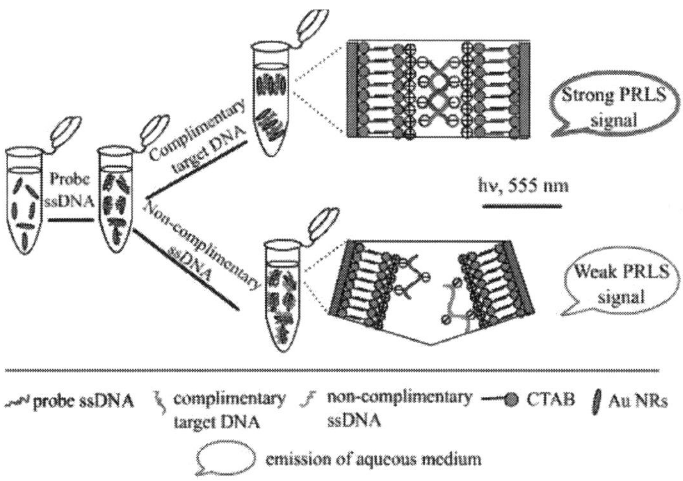

Figure 8.11 Schematic representation of the DNA hybridization detection with gold nanorods genosensing system. The different colors of gold nanorods represent the dispersed and aggregated states, respectively. Reprinted from Ref. 59 with permission. See also Color Insert.

8.3.2 Ag NPs as RLS Probes

Like Au NPs, Ag NPs are useful nanomaterials for many applications, mainly because of their interesting optical, electronic, and catalytic properties.[61–63] Ag NPs interact with photons more efficiently than any other type of NP of the same dimension, making them useful in a wide variety of optical applications.[61–63] The LSPR bands of spherical Ag NPs occur at around 410 nm, which are shorter that those of spherical Au NPs, which are around 520 nm. Based on the fact that RLS intensity is proportional to the fourth power of frequency, Ag NPs are more useful RLS probes than Au NPs. However, Ag NPs are not as stable as Au NPs. In addition, it is more difficult to prepare high-purity Ag NPs that have a narrow size distribution. In order to overcome this disadvantage, seeding methods have been suggested for the preparation of Au-Ag NPs.[64–66]

8.3.2.1 Small analytes

By taking advantage of the high reduction potential of Ag ions, analytes can be detected by RLS through the induced formation of Ag NPs. To determine the analytes that are capable of the reduction of Ag ions, Ag ions and the analytes are mixed to form Ag NPs. The RLS intensity of the formed Ag NPs is then measured. This method is useful for the determination of Sudan dyes in food products.[67] Sudan dyes including I, II, III, and IV posses nitrogen–nitrogen double bonds and phenol groups in their molecular structures, which are able to reduce Ag ions to form Ag NPs. The formation of Ag NPs induced by Sudan IV can be easily observed as light scattering when using a laser pointer and a light emitting diode to irradiate solutions (Fig. 8.12). Upon increasing Sudan IV concentration, the RLS intensity increases. Although the wavelength of the laser pointer (653 nm) is located at the far end of the RLS spectra, it is still a useful light source for generating these RLS signals because its output power (2.0 mW) is much higher than that of the light emitting diode (0.5 mW, 458 nm). Although color change from the red of Sudan to the brown of Ag NPs can be observed by the naked eye, its sensitivity is too poor (1.0 μM) for colorimetric detection to be practical. In order to improve the sensitivity, a commercial spectrofluorometer is effective to detect the enhanced RLS signals characterized at 452 nm. The RLS intensities are proportional to the dye concentrations over the range of 0.2–2.4 μM Sudan I, 0.1–2.4 μM Sudan II, 0.1–2.4 μM Sudan III, and

0.2–3.0 μM Sudan IV. The RLS approach provides LODs of 3.2, 3.0, 3.2, and 2.9 nM, for Sudan I, II, III, and IV, respectively, which are about 3000-fold more sensitive than with simple absorbance detection. A similar strategy has been employed to determine the concentration of ferulic acid, with an LOD of 15.2 nM.[68] Unlike reduction, oxidation of Ag NPs can be applied to detection of analytes that are capable of oxidizing Au NPs. As the size of the Ag NPs decreases, a decrease in RLS signal occurs, which is proportional to the analyte concentration. An example of this approach is the determination of chlorine dioxide in ammonia–ammonium nitrate solution (pH 9.1).[69] The RLS signal of Ag NPs at 470 nm decreases with increasing concentration of chlorine dioxide over the range of 1.1–185.0 ng/mL, with a correlation coefficient of 0.9995. This method is simple, rapid, sensitive (LOD 0.50 ng/mL), and cost-effective for the determination of chlorine dioxide in drinking water.

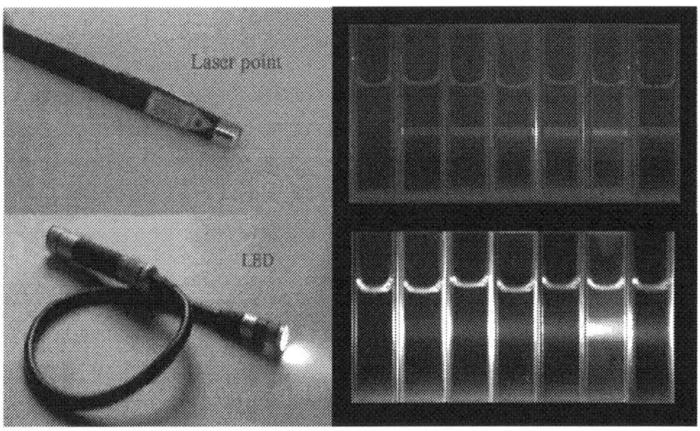

Figure 8.12 RLS signals based on visual detection of Sudan IV using a portable laser pointer (653 nm, 2.0 mW, up) and a light emitting diode (458 nm, 0.5 mW, down) as irradiated light sources. Concentrations: $AgNO_3$, 4.5×10^{-4} M; NaOH, 8.0×10^{-3} M; $NH_3{\cdot}H_2O$, 0.02%; Sudan IV (from left to right, mM), 0, 0.1, 0.2, 0.4, 0.6, 1.2, and a real sample of cayenne oil. Triton X-100, 0.012%. Reprinted from Ref. 67 with permission. See also Color Insert.

8.3.2.2 Biopolymers

Ag NPs are not as popular as Au NPs for the determination of biopolymers, mainly because they deteriorate through some types of reactions. For this reason, Ag NPs are usually used to improve detection sensitivity after selective capture of analytes of interest by using other functionalized nanomaterials such as DNA-Au NPs. Cetyltrimethylammonium bromide-capped Ag NPs as the RLS probe has been shown to be useful in the detection of DNA and RNA.[70] The interactions among Ag NPs, cetyltrimethylammonium bromide, and DNA through electrostatic attraction and/or chemical affinity occur, leading to aggregation of Ag NPs and thus, increases in RLS signals. Under optimum conditions (1.0 μg/mL Ag NPs, 8.0 μM cetyltrimethylammonium bromide, 5.0 mM Tris-HCl at pH 7.6), there are linear relationships between the quenching extent of RLS and the analytes over the concentrations ranges of 4.0×10^{-9} to 2.0×10^{-6} g/mL for fish sperm DNA, 7.0×10^{-9} to 1.8×10^{-6} g/mL for calf thymus DNA, and 6.0×10^{-9} to 1.0×10^{-6} g/mL for yeast RNA. This RLS method provides LODs of 2.7×10^{-10} g/mL, 4.8×10^{-10} g/mL, and 7.2×10^{-10} g/mL for fish sperm DNA, calf thymus DNA, and yeast RNA, respectively.

8.4 Conclusions and Outlook

The RLS signal of a scattered particle depends on its absorption feature, size, shape, concentration, and refractive index relative to the surrounding medium. In addition, the intensity and frequency of a light source are likewise important. Thus, control of these parameters is important for developing sensitive RLS techniques. Although Ag NPs are more efficient at light scattering than Au NPs, the latter have been used in most of the RLS techniques, mainly because of its stability and ease in preparation. It is thus possible to enhance RLS sensitivity by using more stable Ag-based nanomaterials such as Ag-Au NPs.

Having advantages of high sensitivity, rapidity, and simplicity, RLS techniques have been applied to the determinations of the concentrations of a number of analytes, including proteins, nucleic acids, pharmaceutical drugs, and carbohydrates in artificial and real samples. Successful examples have demonstrated the great potential of RLS techniques for diagnosis of disease, food quality control, cell imaging, and so on. Although RLS techniques are not as popular as colorimetric assays using Au NPs, they are more sensitive. Theoretically, most developed colorimetric assays using Au and Ag NPs can be readily applied to RLS techniques. Thus, it is expected that RLS techniques will soon gain popularity as the techniques become well recognized.

Acknowledgment

This work was supported by the National Science Council of Taiwan under contract numbers NSC 97-2113-M-143-001-MY2 and NSC 99-2113-M-143-001-MY2.

References

1. C. F. Bohren, D. R. Huffman, Eds., *Absorption and Scattering of Light by Small Particles* (Wiley, New York, 1998).
2. R. Pecora, Eds., *Dynamic Light Scattering* (Plenum Press, New York, 1985).
3. Q. Zuo, Eds., *Laser Light Scattering and its Application in Polymer Science* (Henan Science and Technology Press, Zhengzhou, 1994).
4. H. Liang, X. C. Shen, F. Li, Z. L. Jiang, *Chin. Chem. Lett.*, **11**, 251 (2000).
5. Z. L. Jiang, Z. W. Feng, X. C. Shen, *Chin. Chem. Lett.*, **12**, 551 (2001).
6. C.-Q. Zhu, D.-H. Li, Q. Z.-Zhu, H. Zheng, Q.-Y. Chen, H.-H. Yang, J.-G. Xu, Fresenius *J. Anal. Chem.*, **366**, 863 (2000).
7. L.-Y. Wang, L. Wang, H. Q. Chen, L. Li, L. Dong, T.-T. Xia, F. Z. Dong, Z. Q. Xu, *Anal. Chim. Acta*, **493**, 179 (2003).
8. L.-Y. Wang, L. Wang, L. Dong, Y.-L. Hu, T.-T. Xia, H.-Q. Chen, L. Li, C.-Q. Zhu, *Talanta*, **62**, 237 (2004).
9. H. Pan, X. Tao, C. Mao, J.-J. Zhu, F. Liang, *Talanta*, **71**, 276 (2007).
10. Y. Cheng, Z. Li, Y. Su, Y. Fan, *Talanta*, **71**, 1757 (2007).
11. J. Li, X.-W. He, Y.-L. Wu, W.-Y. Li, Y.-K. Zhang, *Anal. Sci.*, **23**, 331 (2007).
12. G.-C. Zhao, P. Zhang, X.-W. Wei, Z.-S. Yang, *Anal. Biochem.*, **334**, 297 (2004).
13. C. Z. Huang, Y. F. Li, *Anal. Chim. Acta*, **500**, 105 (2003).
14. K. Aslan, J. R. Lakowicz, C. D. Geddes, *Curr. Opin. Chem. Biol.*, **9**, 538 (2005).
15. R. F. Pansternack, C. Bustamante, P. J. Collings, A. Giannetto, E. J. Gibbs, *J. Am. Chem. Soc.*, **115**, 5393 (1993).
16. R. F. Pansternack, P. J. Collings, *Science*, **269**, 935 (1995).
17. P. J. Collings, E. J. Gibbs, T. E. Starr, O. Vafek, C. Yee, L. A. Pomerance, R. F. Pansternack, *J. Phys. Chem. B*, **103**, 8474 (1999).
18. W. Lu, P. Feng, Y. F. Li, C. Z. Huang, *Anal. Lett.*, **35**, 227 (2002).
19. W. Lu, C. Z. Huang, Y. F. Li, *Analyst*, **127**, 1392 (2002).

20. P. Feng, W. Q. Shu, C. Z. Huang, Y. F. Li, *Anal. Chem.*, **73**, 4307 (2001).
21. S. P. Liu, H. Q. Luo, N. B. Li, Z. F. Liu, W. X. Zheng, *Anal. Chem.*, **73**, 3907 (2001).
22. Y. K. Zhao, Q. E. Cao, Z. D. Hu, Q. H. Xu, *Anal. Chim. Acta*, **388**, 45 (1999).
23. J. Yguerabide, E. Yguerabide, *Anal. Biochem.*, **262**, 137 (1998).
24. J. Yguerabide, E. Yguerabide, *Anal. Biochem.*, **262**, 157 (1998).
25. M.-M. Daniel, D. Astruc, *Chem. Rev.*, **104**, 293 (2005).
26. C. L. Nehl, J. H. Hafner, *J. Mater. Chem.*, **18**, 2415 (2005).
27. X. Liu, H. Yuan, D. Pang, R. Cai, *Spectroc. Acta Pt. A-Molec. Biomolec. Spectr.*, **60**, 385 (2004).
28. S.-J. Chen, H.-T. Chang, *Anal. Chem.*, **76**, 3727 (2004).
29. Y.-F. Huang, H.-T. Chang, *Anal. Chem.*, **78**, 1485 (2006).
30. Z. D. Liu, C. Z. Huang, Y. F. Li, Y. F. Long, *Anal. Chim. Acta*, **577**, 244 (2006).
31. W.-L. Tseng, K.-H. Lee, H.-T. Chang, *Langmuir*, **21**, 10676 (2005).
32. Z. P. Li, X. R. Duan, C. H. Liu, B. A. Du, *Anal. Biochem.*, **351**, 18 (2006).
33. K. Aslan, J. R. Lakowicz, C. D. Geddes, *Anal. Chem.*, **77**, 2007 (2005).
34. K. Aslan, J. R. Lakowicz, C. D. Geddes, *Anal. Biochem.*, **330**, 145 (2004).
35. L. Shang, H. Chen, L. Deng, S. Dong, *Biosens. Bioelectron.*, **23**, 1180 (2008).
36. Z. Jian, Z. Xiang, *Spectroc. Acta Pt. A-Molec. Biomolec. Spectr.*, **61**, 3002 (2005).
37. A. C. Enriquez, I. A. R. Espejel, E. A. García, M. E. Díaz-García, *Anal. Bioanal. Chem.*, **391**, 807 (2008).
38. J.-M. Nam, C. S. Thaxton, C. A. Mirkin, *Science*, **301**, 1884 (2003).
39. J.-M. Nam, S. I. Stoeva, C. A. Mirkin, *J. Am. Chem. Soc.*, **126**, 5932 (2004).
40. C.-C. Huang, Y.-F. Huang, Z. Cao, W. Tan, H.-T. Chang, *Anal. Chem.*, **77**, 5735 (2005).
41. C.-C. Huang, S.-H. Chiu, Y.-F. Huang, H.-T. Chang, *Anal. Chem.*, **79**, 4798 (2007).
42. C.-C. Huang, C.-K. Chiang, Z.-H. Lin, K.-H. Lee, H.-T. Chang, *Anal. Chem.*, **80**, 1497 (2008).
43. C.-C. Huang, C.-T. Chen, Y.-C. Shiang, Z.-H. Lin, H.-T. Chang, *Anal. Chem.*, **81**, 875 (2009).
44. Z.-L. Jiang, S.-J. Sun, A.-H. Liang, C.-J. Liu, *Anal. Chim. Acta*, **571**, 200 (2006).

45. Z. Jiang, S. Sun, A. Liang, W. Huang, A. Qin, *Clin. Chem.*, **52**, 1389 (2006).

46. M. Hou, S. Sun, Z. Jiang, *Talanta*, **72**, 463 (2007).

47. B. Du, Z. Li, Y. Cheng, *Talanta*, **75**, 959 (2008).

48. Z. Jiang, L. Wei, M. Zou, A. Liang, M. Meng, *J. Biomol. Screen.*, **13**, 302 (2008).

49. Y.-F. Huang, Y.-W. Lin, Z.-H. Lin, H.-T. Chang, *J. Nanopart. Res.*, **11**, 775 (2009).

50. S.-J. Chen, Y.-F. Huang, C.-C. Huang, K.-H. Lee, Z.-H. Lin, H.-T. Chang, *Biosens. Bioelectron.*, **23**, 1749 (2008).

51. C.-W. Liu, Y.-T. Hsieh, C.-C. Huang, Z.-H. Lin, H.-T. Chang, *Chem. Commun.*, 2242 (2008).

52. C.-K. Chiang, C.-C. Huang, C.-W. Liu, H.-T. Chang, *Anal. Chem.*, **80**, 3716 (2008).

53. B. Dubertret, M. Calame, A. J. Libchaber, *Nat. Biotechnol.*, **19**, 365 (2001).

54. H. Li, L. J. Rothberg, *J. Am. Chem. Soc.*, **126**, 10958 (2004).

55. E. Tan, J. Wong, D. Nguyen, Y. Zhang, B. Erwin, L. K. Van Ness, S. M. Baker, D. J. Galas, A. Niemz, *Anal. Chem.*, **77**, 7984 (2005).

56. J. Li, X. Chu, Y. Liu, J.-H. Jiang, Z. He, Z. Zhang, G. Shen, R.-Q. Yu, *Nucleic Acids Res.*, **33**, e168 (2005).

57. P. Bao, A.G. Frutos, C. Greef, J. Lahiri, U. Muller,T. C. Peterson, L.Warden, X. Xie, *Anal. Chem.*, **74**, 1792 (2002).

58. B.-A. Du, Z.-P. Li, C.-H. Liu, *Angew. Chem. Int. Ed.*, **45**, 8022 (2006).

59. W. He, C. Z. Huang, Y. F. Li, J. P. Xie, R. G. Yang, P. F. Zhou, J. Wang, *Anal. Chem.*, **80**, 8424 (2008).

60. C. Z. Huang. Q. G. Liao, L. H. Gan, F. L. Guo, Y. F. Li, *Anal. Chim. Acta*, **604**, 165 (2007).

61. D. D. Evanoff Jr., G. Chumanov, *Chem. Phys. Chem.*, **6**, 1221 (2005).

62. B. Wiley, Y. Sun, Y. Xia, *Acc. Chem. Res.*, **40**, 1067 (2007).

63. V. K. Sharma, R. A. Yngard, Y. Lin, *Adv. Colloid Interface Sci.*, **145**, 83 (2009).

64. Y.-F. Huang, Y.-W. Lin, H.-T. Chang, *Nanotechnology*, **17**, 4885 (2006).

65. G. Compagnini, E. Messina, O. Puglisi, V. Nicolosi, *Appl. Surf. Sci.*, **254**, 1007 (2007).

66. J. F. Sánchez-Ramírez, U. Pal, L. Nolasco-Hernández, J. Mendoza-Álvarez, J. A. Pescador-Rojas, *J. Nanomater.*, 620412 (2008).

67. L. P. Wu, Y. F. Li, C. Z. Huang, Q. Zhang, *Anal. Chem.*, **78**, 5570 (2006).
68. H. Y. Wang, Y. F. Li, C. Z. Huang, *Talanta*, **72**, 1698 (2007).
69. C. Y. Kang, D. L. Xi, Y.-Y. Chen, Z. L. Jiang, *Talanta*, **74**, 867 (2008).
70. J. Zheng, X. Wu, M. Wang, D. Rana, W. Xua, J. Yang, *Talanta*, **74**, 526 (2008).

Chapter 9

Photoluminescence of Gold Nanoparticles and Their Applications to Sensing and Cell Imaging

Chih-Ching Huang* **and Yu-Shen Lin**

Institute of Bioscience and Biotechnology and Center of Excellence for Marine Bioenvironment and Biotechnology, National Taiwan Ocean University, 2, Beining Road, Keelung, 20224, Taiwan

*huanging@ntou.edu.tw

Metallic nanomaterials, which are among the most fascinating materials in modern science, exhibit unique optical, electronic, magnetic, and catalytic properties. Because of their photo-optical distinctiveness and biocompatibility, luminescent gold (Au) nanomaterials have become interesting components in bioassays. This chapter focuses on the preparation and bioapplications of polymer-stabilized Au nanoclusters (NCs), thiol-stabilized Au NCs, and luminescent Au nanoparticles (Au NPs, <2 nm). Varying the experimental conditions, such as the molar ratio of the capping agent to Au ions, allows the luminescence wavelengths of these systems to be tuned from the ultraviolet to the near-infrared. The luminescence quantum yields of Au NCs are several orders of magnitude higher than those of bulk Au and larger Au NPs. The biocompatibility of Au NCs and luminescent Au NPs has led to their application in the detection of antibodies, proteins, and metal ions, as well as in cell imaging.

From Bioimaging to Biosensors: Noble Metal Nanoparticles in Biodetection

Edited by Lai-Kwan Chau and Huan-Tsung Chang

ISBN 978-981-4267-24-3 (Hardcover), 978-981-4303-10-1 (eBook)

www.panstanford.com

9.1 Introduction

In their bulk forms, noble metals exhibit many interesting properties, including high conductivity, excellent chemical stability, and beautiful surface luster.[1] In the form of nanomaterials, however, these noble metals display features distinct from those found in the bulk. The chemical and physical properties of noble metal nanomaterials are highly dependent on their size, shapes, surface functionality, and the refractive indices of their surrounding media.[1–3] For example, small-diameter gold nanoparticles (Au NPs) exhibit greater catalytic activities than their larger congeners.[4] Likewise, spherical Au NPs feature only one absorption band (near 520 nm), whereas Au nanorods possess two: one at ca. 520 nm and the other one centered at a longer wavelength (600–1200 nm), depending on the aspect ratio (length/width).[5]

The study of few-atom metal nanoclusters (NCs), which bridge the divide between the properties of isolated atoms and those of NPs or even bulk metals, has attracted great interest because of their distinct optical and catalytic properties.[6–9] Nanoscale metals are roughly classified into three size domains: large NPs, small NPs, and NCs, according to their length scales (R) relative to the wavelength (λ) of the external electromagnetic field.[10,11] The optical responses of large metal NPs ($R > \lambda$) toward external electromagnetic fields depend on their sizes and their free-electron density. Mie theory can be used to describe the optical properties of large NPs.[10] When the particle size approaches the electron mean free path (e.g., 50 nm for Au or silver (Ag)), collective excitations of electrons become dominant, leading to plasmon resonance.[11] Mie theory also provides an adequate description if the size effects are suitably incorporated. Eventually, when the particle size becomes comparable with the third characteristic length — the Fermi wavelength of an electron (i.e., de Broglie's wavelength of an electron at the Fermi energy, or 0.5 nm for Au or Ag) — the optical, electronic, and chemical properties of metal NCs differ dramatically from those of the other two size regimes.[12,13] In the smallest size regime, metal NCs behave as molecule-like species, often displaying strong single-electron excitations with discrete states.[14–16] Among the primary topics of this chapter is a discussion of such highly polarizable, few-atom Au NCs.

Luminescence (photoluminescence, PL) of metals is normally extremely weak because of efficient nonradiative decay and the absence of an energy gap.[17–19] When the dimensions of a metal object decrease, quantum confinement effects become significant, resulting in many interesting physical and chemical properties, including luminescence.[6,20] Au NPs (<2 nm diameter) and Au NCs capped with ligands, including citrate, poly(amidoamine) (PAMAM) dendrimers, and thiolates, display luminescence at different wavelengths with significantly different quantum yields.[6,20] Au NCs capped with PAMAM or thiol compounds exhibit strong luminescence characteristics, but Au NPs capped with citrate do not. The luminescence energies of PAMAM-bound Au NCs vary strongly with respect to their size, from 3.2 eV for Au_5 to 1.4 eV for Au_{31}.[21] In contrast, for thiolate-protected Au NPs they vary more modestly with size; for example, the energy gaps of glutathione monolayer-protected Au NCs ranging in size from Au_{10} to Au_{39} lie in the range 1.4–1.7 eV.[22] Au_{13}, Au_{38}, and Au_{140} NCs capped with monolayers of various thiols [*N*,*N*,*N*-trimethyl(mercaptoundecyl)ammonium thiol, hexanethiol, tiopronin] possess energy gaps ranging from 1.1 to 1.3 eV, corresponding to near-infrared (NIR) emissions.[23] Variations in the luminescence intensities of the Au NPs and NCs are, on the other hand, more consistent with changes in their sizes; the emission intensities of both PAMAM- and thiolate-protected NCs increase upon decreasing their size.[21,22] Usually, Au NCs at the smallest sizes provide impressive quantum efficiencies (>10%).

In addition to Au NCs, alkanethiol (RSH)-capped Au NPs (<2.0 nm) — so-called luminescent Au NPs or Au nanodots — are interesting because they display PL with large Stokes shifts and long lifetimes.[24–27] The emissions of these luminescent Au NPs might arise from electronic transitions of Au(I) coupling to the ligand–metal charge transfer transition.[28–30] Unlike larger Au NPs, these small luminescent Au NPs do not feature surface plasmon absorption. Like Au NCs, the PL properties of these luminescent Au NPs are not directly related to their sizes.[24–27] Not surprisingly, contributions from surface characteristics become greater at diminished NP sizes because, as the size decreases, the surface-to-volume ratio increases and a larger fraction of the NP core atoms become involved in bonds to the core-capping ligands. The properties of these new types of luminescent Au NPs are also discussed in this chapter.

Luminescent Au NCs and Au NPs have great practicality in several fields, including sensing and cell imaging.[24,25,31–36] Because of their excellent physical and chemical properties, many methods for the preparation and characterization of luminescent Au NCs and NPs have been demonstrated during the past decade. In this chapter, we discuss the synthesis, optical properties, and applications of luminescent Au NCs and NPs. Herein, we categorize the preparation and optical properties of these luminescent Au NCs and NPs in three parts: polymer-stabilized Au NCs, thiol-stabilized Au NCs, and luminescent Au NPs. We then emphasize their analytical applications, notably in the detection of biomarkers, cells, and bacteria. Finally, the chapter concludes with a brief summary of the present and future directions of research in luminescent Au NCs or NPs.

9.2 Preparation and Optical Properties of Polymer-Stabilized Au NCs

Luminescent Au NCs are usually prepared in the presence of polymers that act as capping agents. To provide Au–Au interactions, OH- and NH_2-terminated PAMAM dendrimers are used to initiate and then stabilize the formation of few-atom NCs.[21] PAMAM dendrimers are near-spherical, highly branched macromolecules presenting symmetrically emanating dendrons of defined molecular weight and size. Water-soluble, monodisperse, blue-emitting (450 nm) Au_8 NCs that are stabilized by encapsulation in biocompatible PAMAM dendrimers exhibit a stable and high luminescence (fluorescence) with a quantum yield of 41%.[21] One general procedure for the synthesis of Au NCs is co-dissolving PAMAM and $HAuCl_4$ in distilled water and then reducing the Au^+ ions by slowly adding an equivalent amount of $NaBH_4$. Simultaneous formation of small luminescent Au NCs (i.e., PAMAM-encapsulated NCs) and large Au NPs is common when using this approach.[37] To produce stable luminescent Au NCs, it is necessary to stir the solutions at room temperature for at least 2 days to complete the reaction and aggregation processes. The solutions are subsequently subjected to purification through centrifugation to remove the large Au NPs, leaving clear, luminescent Au-NC solutions. The presence of the fluorescence signal is attributed to the Au NCs; the pure dendrimer does not fluoresce. Through slow reduction of gold salts (e.g., $AuCl_4^-$ or $AuBr_3$) with different concentrations of aqueous PAMAM solutions, the sizes of the luminescent Au NCs are readily controlled. Differently sized Au NCs exhibit discrete excitation and

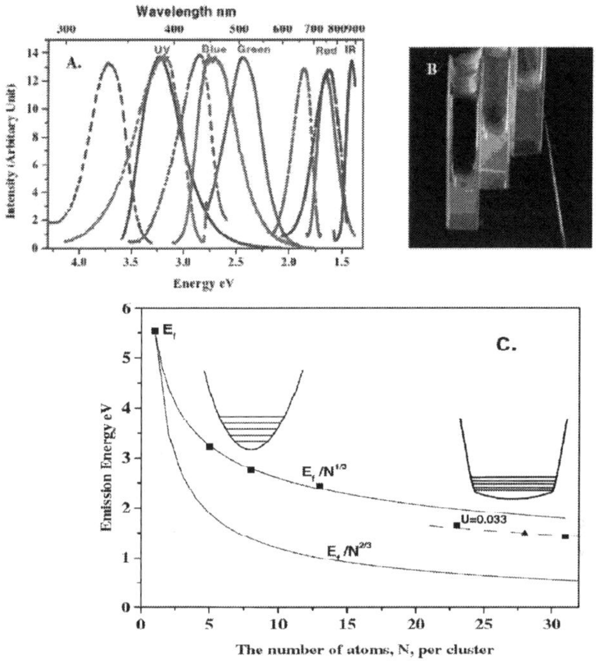

Figure 9.1 (A) Excitation (dashed) and emission (solid) spectra of various Au NCs. Emission from the longest wavelength-emitting sample was limited by the detector response. (B) Emissions from the three shortest wavelength-emitting Au NC solutions (from left to right) under long-wavelength UV lamp irradiation (366 nm). (C) Correlation of the number of atoms, *N*, per NC with emission energy. Reprinted with permission from Ref. 6. See also Color Insert.

emission signals that can range from the ultraviolet to the NIR region.[21] The discrete absorptions and emissions scale with the number of atoms, *N*, as $N^{1/3}$, precisely predicted by the spherical jellium model, but different from the $N^{2/3}$ scaling for semiconductor quantum dots (QDs), which do not exhibit the free-electron shell-filling degeneracies that are characteristic of metals.[38–40] The jellium approximation is the simplest model for describing the behavior of delocalized, free conduction electrons relative to the atomic NC core; it is also a basic model for explaining plasmon absorption in large NPs. Figure 9.1 presents a fluorescence image and discrete excitation and emission spectra of various dendrimer-encapsulated Au NCs in aqueous solutions. Varying the molar ratio of Au ions to

PAMAM from 1:1 to 1:15 allows both the excitation and emission energies of the observed fluorescent species to be tuned from the UV to the NIR. Interestingly, the PAMAM scaffold stabilizes Au NCs of various sizes and yields fluorescence quantum yields that are orders of magnitude higher than that of bulk Au. Mass spectrometric characterization revealed that the differently colored fluorescent Au NCs in Fig. 9.1 were Au_5 (UV), Au_{13} (green), Au_{23} (red), and Au_{31} (NIR), with each encapsulated within a PAMAM scaffold (i.e., Au NCs). The photophysical properties of these various water-soluble Au NCs indicate that they behave not only as quantum-confined but also as molecular and size-tunable fluorophores. Their high quantum yields are comparable with those of the best water-soluble emitters currently available, ranging from 70% for UV-emitting Au_5 to 10% for Au_{31} in the NIR. In contrast to the preparation of larger semiconductor NCs, complicated high-temperature syntheses with toxic precursors are not required when preparing dendrimer-encapsulated Au NCs.

Because Au NCs are too small to have the continuous density of states and plasmon absorptions characteristics that occur for larger Au NPs (>2 nm), the transition energy, rather than the plasmon-absorption width, should scale inversely with the NC radius.[38–40] The dependence of the emission energy on N in each Au NC may be fit quantitatively for the smallest NCs with no adjustable parameters when applying the simple scaling relation $E_{\text{Fermi}}/N^{1/3}$, where E_{Fermi} is the Fermi energy of bulk Au.[41–43] For a spherical NC, the radius (R) is equal to $r_s \times N^{1/3}$, where r_s is the Wigner–Seitz radius.[44,45] Identical to the electronic absorption for gas-phase alkali-metal NCs, the transition energy scaling with the inverse NC radius indicates that the electronic structure of Au NCs is determined solely by their free electron density and size. These observations suggest that the free electron shell-filling model corresponds exactly to the spherical jellium approximation.[21] Observation of this simple energy scaling ($E_{\text{Fermi}}/N^{1/3}$) for fluorescent Au NCs offers clear and direct experimental evidence for the discrete nature of the excited state in noble metal NCs, and of the evolution from discrete intraband transitions of the free electrons to the plasmon of large NPs in the condensed phase.[6] The jellium approximation accurately describes the size-dependent electronic structures and relative electronic transitions of small NCs.[6,21] These quantum-confined protoplasmonic transitions of the free conduction electrons suggest that the NCs are nearly spherical electronic structures with electrons bound by an approximately harmonic potential in three dimensions. Thus, the emission energies of smaller Au NCs (<Au_{20}) fit well to the energy scaling law $E_{\text{Fermi}}/N^{1/3}$ (Fig. 9.1C).[21] For Au NCs of larger sizes (Au_{23}–Au_{38}), however, small anharmonicities distort the potential well.[6,21]

A simple protocol, similar to that for the preparation of PAMAM-stabilized fluorescent Au NCs, can be used for the synthesis and purification of fluorescent pentaerythritol tetrakis(3-mercaptopropionate)-terminated poly(methacrylic acid) (PTMP-pMAA)-capped Au NCs that have an emission band at 700–750 nm.[46] The PTMP-pMAA ligand acts as a "multidentate" capping agent to control the growth of the Au NCs. By varying the polymer-to-Au molar ratio, the size of the NCs can be finely tuned, allowing observation of a transition from non-fluorescent to fluorescent NPs that have core diameters ranging from 1.1 to 1.7 nm. Using 4 mM PTMP-pMAA and 0.5 mM $HAuCl_4$ results in the preparation of the most highly fluorescent Au NCs, which have a particle size of 1.1 nm and a quantum efficiency of 3%.

Alternatively, highly fluorescent, water-soluble Au NCs can be prepared through ligand-induced etching processes.[47] First, a modified Brust–Schiffrin method is applied to prepare Au NPs (ca. 8 nm).[48] Tetraoctylammonium bromide is added to transfer $HAuCl_4$ from the aqueous phase to the toluene phase, where reduction of Au ions by $NaBH_4$ occurs under vigorous stirring. Subsequently, ligand exchange reactions using multivalent coordinating polymers, such as hyperbranched polyethyleneimine (PEI; M_n = 1800 g/mol), are performed to etch the thus-prepared Au NPs. As a result, fluorescent Au NCs having quantum yields between 10% and 20% are formed. The excitation and emission wavelength maxima are located at 421 and 505 nm, respectively. After a reaction with a strong reducing agent ($NaBH_4$), the excitation and emission peaks of the Au NCs shift to 353 and 445 nm, respectively. Electrospray ionization (ESI) mass spectrometry data revealed that the NCs comprised only eight Au atoms (Au_8). There are two possible chemical pathways that lead to the formation of atomic Au NCs. In one, Au_8 NCs are liberated in a single step during ligand exchange and are immediately protected by a multivalent, hyperbranched PEI ligand, which may also function to activate the Au atoms and to subtract Au_8 NCs from the NC surface. The formation of Au_8 NCs probably results from the extraordinary stability of this magic NC with closed electronic shells. In the other, Au(I) ions are possibly released from the Au NCs during the ligand exchange reaction, similar to that of triphenylphosphine-protected 1.5 nm Au NPs when using thiol compounds.[49] Also, it is known that Au(I) species tend to aggregate through strong aurophilic interactions, due to hybridization of the empty 6s/6p orbital and filled 5d orbital.[30] With its high density of binding groups, PEI can facilitate the formation of aggregates from Au(I) atoms.

9.3 Preparation and Optical Properties of Thiol-Stabilized Au NCs

$HAuCl_4$, $NaBH_4$, and thiols are commonly used for preparation of thiolate monolayer–protected Au NCs.[49] The as-prepared thiol-stabilized Au NCs possess molecule-like PL properties, with their emission wavelengths centered in the NIR region upon excitation in the visible region. Voltammetric data reveal that Au NCs capped with alkanethiolate and phosphine ligands possess redox-like and quantized double layer charging properties.[50–56] Table 9.1 summarizes the optical properties of the luminescent Au NCs, along with those of other ligand-protected Au NCs,[50–56] as well as assignments of the corresponding transitions for the PL bands of the Au NCs. One feature of these Au NCs is that their fluorescence emission wavelengths are all longer than 600 nm, making them useful for bioassays because sample matrix interference is usually low in this region. For example, tiopronin-coated NCs ($Au_{201}Tio_{85}$) feature a broad emission from 650 to 1250 nm and glutathione (GSH)-passivated Au_{28} NCs fluoresce over the range 840–1080 nm.[57–59] One disadvantageous property of these Au NCs is their low emission quantum efficiency (from 10^{-6} to 10^{-2}), which limits their practical use in assays.

There are several explanations for the PL properties of thiol-stabilized Au NCs. The interband transition (from d band electrons to the sp conduction band) and the relaxed radiative recombination across the energy gap between the highest and lowest occupied molecular orbitals (HOMO–LUMO gap) within the sp conduction band are responsible for luminescence.[50–59] For Au NCs that comprise a Au core of 28 atoms and a GSH layer of 16 molecules [i.e., $Au_{28}(SG)_{16}$], the two visible luminescence wavelengths correspond to an excitation of the d band electrons into the sp conduction band (interband transition) and to radiative recombination after being excited at 2.48 eV (500 nm) (Fig. 9.2A,B).[59] Because the visible luminescence is independent of the excitation wavelength between 3.10 and 2.07 eV (400 and 600 nm), the high energy luminescence band corresponds to the recombination of the excited electron from higher excited states in the sp band with the hole in the lower-lying d band (interband transition). The low energy luminescence band is assigned to the relaxed radiative recombination across the HOMO–LUMO gap at 1.3 eV within the sp conduction band (intraband transition) (Fig. 9.2B). To make it easier to understand the transitions for the luminescence bands, let us consider well-known transitions in luminescence: two luminescence bands corresponding to the two radiative transitions from the lowest excited singlet state (S_1, referred to as fluorescence) and the lowest excited triplet state (T_1, referred to as phosphorescence).[59] Accordingly, the two luminescence bands served for $Au_{28}(SG)_{16}$ can be assigned to the singlet (fluorescence) and triplet (phosphorescence) excited states of the molecule-type Au NC (Fig. 9.2C).

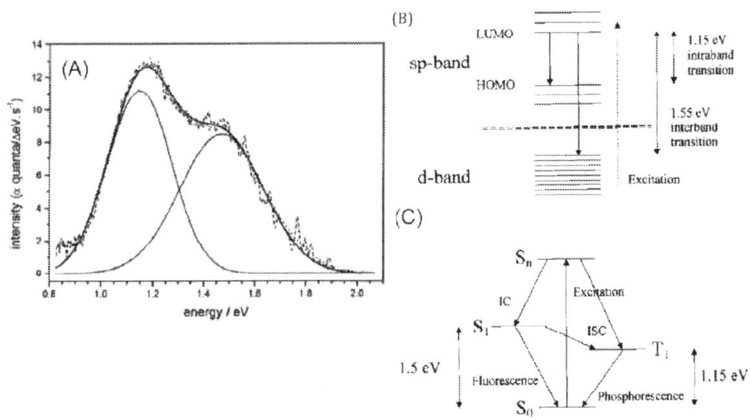

Figure 9.2 (A) Luminescence spectrum of $Au_{28}(SG)_{16}$ NCs in D_2O. (B) Solid state model for the origin of the two luminescence bands. (C) Molecular model for the origin of the two luminescence bands. Reprinted with permission from Ref. 59.

Table 9.1 Photoluminescence properties of Au MPCs

Core size (nm)	Ligand	$\lambda_{em}^{max\ a}$	Quantum yield	Assignment	Ref.
0.8 (Au_{12})	DMSA	630 (395)	1×10^{-6}	$T_1 \rightarrow S_0$	50
	DMSA–TOA	643 (404)	3×10^{-5}	$T_1 \rightarrow S_0$	
1.1 (Au_{38})	Mixed ligands: phenylethanethiolate and $PEG_{135}SH$	902 (680) 1025 (680)	1.2×10^{-2}	sp → sp (HOMO-LUMO)	51
Au_{13}	Mixed ligands: triphenylphosphine and dodecanethiol	~1000 (718)	1.3×10^{-3}	sp → sp (HOMO-LUMO)	52
1.1 (Au_{38})	Dodecanethiol	~1200 (1064)	—	sp → sp (HOMO-LUMO)	53
1.7 (Au_{147})	Dodecanethiol	~1200 (1064)	4.4×10^{-5}	sp → sp (HOMO-LUMO)	53
0.8	Dodecanethiol	840 (680)	$<3 \times 10^{-7}$	—	54
1.8 (Au_{201})	Tiopronin	770 (451)	$(3 \pm 1) \times 10^{-3}$	sp → d	55
0.9 (Au_{28})	Glutathione	830 (500) 1080 (514)	$(3.5 \pm 1.0) \times 10^{-3}$	sp → d or ($S_1 \rightarrow S_0$) sp → sp (HOMO-LUMO) or ($T_1 \rightarrow S_0$)	56

[a] Wavelengths of emission maxima. Numbers in parentheses represent excitation wavelengths (nm).

Key issues in the study of the optical properties of very small NPs are their size and shape effects and the contributions from surface characteristics. These issues are interrelated because the surface-to-volume ratio increases as the size decreases. To precisely assign the luminescence peaks that allow study of size dependence of the optical properties of NCs, solutions containing monodisperse NPs are essential. Luminescence becomes broad when the size distribution of the NPs is large. Polyacrylamide gel electrophoresis and ESI mass spectrometry are powerful tools for characterizing small Au NCs; for example, spectroscopic measurements of a fractionated series of Au_n NCs (n = 10–39) protected by GSH ligands [$Au_{10}(SG)_{10}$, $Au_{15}(SG)_{13}$, $Au_{18}(SG)_{14}$, $Au_{22}(SG)_{16}$, $Au_{22}(SG)_{17}$, $Au_{25}(SG)_{18}$,

$Au_{29}(SG)_{20}$, $Au_{33}(SG)_{22}$, $Au_{39}(SG)_{24}$] revealed that they are molecules in nature and that their optical and photophysical properties are highly dependent on the core sizes and the number of GSH ligands.[60] The optical band gaps of these GS-protected Au NCs and other Au NCs (Au_{140}, Au_{38}, Au_{11}) all increase upon decreasing their size. These blue shifts in emission maxima upon reducing the NCs' sizes are due to increased energy gaps between the quantized levels (interband or intraband transitions) ascribed to the smaller core sizes as well as to the higher coverage of thiolates or other capping molecules (e.g., phosphine).[60] The luminescence properties of the GS-protected Au NCs are quite different from those for the Au(I)–GS complexes. In contrast, many luminescent Au NCs, such as those listed in Table 9.1, do not exhibit a size-dependence of their optical band gaps.

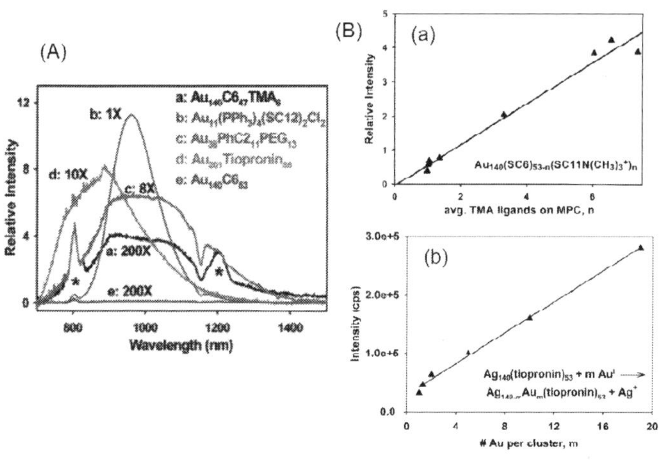

Figure 9.3 (A) Au MPCs with different core sizes and monolayers. C6, C12, PhC2, PEG, and PPh_3 represent hexanethiolate, dodecanethiolate, phenylethanethiol, poly(ethylene glycol) (MW 350) thiolate, and triphenylphosphine, respectively. Asterisks indicate artifacts from second- and third-order excitation peaks (800 and 1200 nm); the dip at 1165 nm is partly due to solvent/ligand absorption. (B) (a) Luminescence intensity (at 1000 nm) vs. number of TMA ligands exchanged onto $Au_{140}(C6)_{53}$ MPCs. (b) Luminescence at 690 nm of products of core metal galvanic exchange reactions of Ag tiopronin MPCs (average core diameter: 1.6 nm) with Au(I)[*p*-$SCH_2(C_6H_4)C(CH_3)_3$]. Reprinted with permission from Ref. 23. See also Color Insert.

Figure 9.3A reveals the visible–NIR luminescence of five different Au NCs (all <2 nm in diameter) that have Au core atoms (Au_{11}–Au_{201})

but feature monolayers of different thiols.[23] The core size-independence of the emission energy reflects the participation of localized core surface states that have a size-independent energy; this hypothesis is supported by ligand place exchanges and galvanic exchange of Ag core atoms with Au core atoms (Fig. 9.3B). Figure 9.3B(a) reveals that the luminescence intensity increases linearly (with a near-zero intercept) with the average number of polar *N,N,N*-trimethyl(mercaptoundecyl)ammonium (TMA) ligands exchanged onto $Au_{140}(C6)_{53}$ (nonpolar hexanethiolate-protected Au MPCs). Nuclear magnetic resonance (NMR) spectroscopy is a powerful tool for determining the ratio of TMA (3–4 ppm) and hexanethiolate (0.8–1.0 ppm) units in the mixed monolayer; UV absorbance and transmission electron microscopy (TEM) measurements are effective for confirming that no difference exists in the metal core size before and after the ligand place exchange reaction. The luminescence appears to be localized at specific surface sites occupied by the TMA ligands. A similar quantitative dependence (Fig. 9.3B(b)) can be found in core metal galvanic exchange reactions of tiopronin-coated Ag NCs with $Au(I)[p\text{-}SCH_2(C_6H_4)C(CH_3)_3]$, at various molar ratios.[61] During the reaction, the emission spectrum changes from that of Ag NCs (ca. 500 nm) to that of Au NCs. The final Au NC-like emission increases linearly upon increasing the reactant ratio of $Au(I)[p\text{-}SCH_2(C_6H_4)C(CH_3)_3]$ to Ag NCs, mainly because of increases in the number of Au atoms per NC core. Considering that one Au atom replaces one Ag surface atom, the fluorescence intensity reveals that the surface Au atoms act as discrete surface state emitters. This result parallels those from the ligand exchange experiment in Fig. 9.3B(a), suggesting that the NIR emission is an electronic surface state phenomenon. The emission intensities depend on the nature of both the NP core metal and the ligands attached to it. Similarly, the NIR luminescence of monolayer-protected Au_{38} and Au_{140} NCs is intensified after exchanging nonpolar ligands (phenylethanethiol) by more polar thiolate ligands, including alkanethiolates (ω-terminated with alcohol, acid, or quaternary ammonium groups) and thio-amino acids.[62] Remarkably, place exchanges of (i) the initial phenylethanethiolates on Au_{38} NCs with *p*-substituted thiophenolates or thio-amino acids and (ii) hexanethiolates on Au_{140} NCs with ω-quaternary ammonium-terminated undecylthiolates result in changes in the NIR luminescence intensities that increase linearly with respect to the number of exchanged polar ligands (Fig. 9.4).[62] The intensity increases are systematically larger for thiophenolate ligands that contain more electron-withdrawing groups. Analogous effects on intensities are also observed in the NIR emissions of Au_{140} NCs upon place exchange of alkanethiolates with thiolates having short connecting alkanethiolate chains to quaternary ammonium and ω-carboxylic acid termini.

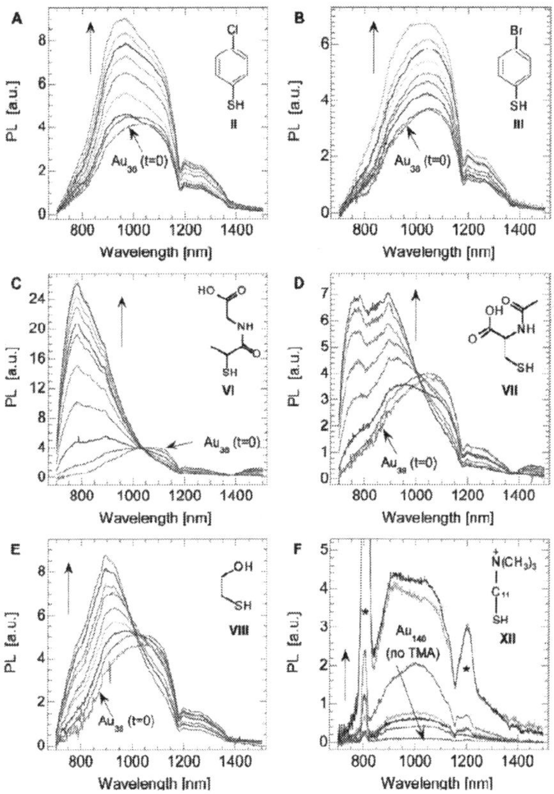

Figure 9.4 Luminescence spectra of $Au_{38}(SC2Ph)_{24}$ MPCs in THF (excited at 450 nm) during (*in situ*) ligand exchange with (A) 4-chlorothiophenol, (B) 4-bromothiophenol, (C) tiopronin, (D) *N*-acetyl-L-cysteine, and (E) 2-mercaptoethanol. Panel F presents luminescence spectra (excited at 400 nm) of $Au_{140}[S(CH_2)_5CH_3]_{53}$MPCs in CH_2Cl_2 for increasing lengths of time (bottom to top) of ligand exchange with TMA, following isolation and cleanup of the exchange product. Asterisks indicate artifacts from second- and third-order excitation leakage, due to wide slits; the sharp minimum at 1165 nm was due to background solvent/ligand absorption. Reprinted with permission from Ref. 62. See also Color Insert.

9.4 Preparation and Optical Properties of Luminescent Au NPs

Unlike large Au NPs (>2 nm), luminescent Au NPs capped with thiols exhibit luminescence. The luminescence of luminescent Au NPs is not simply dependent on the number of free electrons in the NCs, as is the situation for PAMAM-protected Au NCs.[6] Au(I)–thiol complexes are located on the surface of each small Au NP (<2 nm). Because Au(I)–thiol complexes exhibit luminescence,[29,30] the luminescence of luminescent Au NPs arises from both the complexes and the Au cores. In luminescent Au NPs, Au ions provide available states and hybridize with organic ligands to form charge transfer bands.[24–27] Luminescence is roughly attributed to metal–metal electronic transitions, coupled with strong ligand–metal/metal–metal unit charge transfer transitions.[28–30,62–64] These Au(I) complexes generally exhibit large Stokes-shifted luminescence with lifetimes in the microsecond regime.[62–64] Charge transfer between ligands and Au or Au–Au units is responsible for these large Stokes shifts and long-lifetime emissions. The emission center is usually assigned to metal–metal electronic transitions. In addition, at low temperature, the emission energy is inversely proportional to the Au–Au distance.[65] Moreover, lowering the temperature can result in a decrease in the Au(I)–Au(I) bond length, corresponding to a blue shift of the emission energy.[66]

A general strategy for synthesizing luminescent small Au NPs is using multidentate ligands featuring soft electron donor groups to coordinate with Au^{3+} ions.[67,68] With assistance of closed-shell interactions among Au(I) ions ($5d^{10}$) and bridging structures of the ligand groups, small luminescent Au(I) NCs can be prepared.[28–30,62–64] In these luminescent Au(I) NCs, closed-shell interactions drive the aggregation of Au atoms to form dimers and oligomers. The multidentate ligands are necessary to stabilize the Au(I) complexes/NCs because the bond energies of Au(I)–Au(I) bonds (20–50 kJ/mol) are much smaller than those (ca. 225 kJ/mol) of Au(0)–Au(0) bonds in fully reduced Au NPs or NCs.[68] The average Au(I)–Au(I) distance (2.7–3.4 Å) in such Au(I) NCs is also shorter than the sum (3.7 Å) of the two van der Waals radii of Au(I) ions, but it is longer than the average Au(0)–Au(0) distance (2.2–2.5 Å).[68]

GSH has been used to prepare larger (ca. 2 nm) GSH-encapsulated luminescent Au NPs.[27] These water-soluble, biocompatible, luminescent, large Au NPs were obtained through irradiation of a mixed aqueous solution of $HAuCl_4$ and GSH with room-light for 3 days. BRIGHT-yellow and red luminescence Au NPs having sizes of 2.2 ± 0.3 and 1.9 ± 0.3 nm are usually obtained from mixtures containing Au^{3+}-to-GSH molar ratios of 0.5 and 1.0, respectively. The absorption spectra of the luminescent Au NPs are distinct from those of fully reduced, ca. 2 nm Au NPs, which feature a weak, but distinguishable, plasmon absorption at ca. 520 nm. The luminescent Au NPs have no plasmon absorption, but feature a strong and broad absorption in the UV range (centered at 375 nm). The UV absorption likely arises from strong Au(I)–S charge transfer and/or Au(I)–Au(I) transitions. The strong emission bands of GSH-encapsulated luminescent Au NPs having diameters of 2.2 ± 0.3 and 1.9 ± 0.3 nm are centered at ca. 568 and 600 nm, respectively, with excitation wavelength maxima at ca. 398 nm and 265 nm, respectively. The strong UV excitation profiles and long lifetimes (ca. 5 μs) are reminiscent of the photophysical properties of the luminescent Au NPs at low temperature, suggesting that emission might result from analogous electronic transitions, such as interband transitions (dp–sp) mixed with ligand–metal charger transfer.

RS–Au NPs of various sizes luminesce at wavelengths within the range 501–613 nm, with quantum yields ranging from 0.0062 to 3.1%.[24] The luminescence wavelength of these RS–Au NPs can be controlled by varying the size of the alkanethiol. First, the non-luminescent Au NPs (ca. 2.9 nm) are prepared through reduction of $HAuCl_4 \cdot 3H_2O$ with tetrakis(hydroxymethyl)phosphonium chloride (THPC), which acts as both a reducing and capping agent. The Au NPs are self-assembled with alkanethiol ligands of various lengths (C_2–C_{11}) by introducing alkanethiol stock solutions into the as-prepared Au NPs. The positioning of these alkanethiol ligands on the surfaces of the as-prepared Au NPs results in fluorescent alkanethiol–Au NPs. TEM imaging revealed that the as-prepared alkanethiol–Au NPs are spherical and have smaller diameters than those of the original spherical particles. Presumably, this phenomenon is due to the formation of very strongly covalent, distinctly directional, Au–S bonds, and to the preference for dissociation into very small Au and Au–thiolate NCs (on the basis of fragmentation energies), as opposed to the breaking of the Au–S bonds and detaching the Au NCs from the thiolate radical.[69,70]

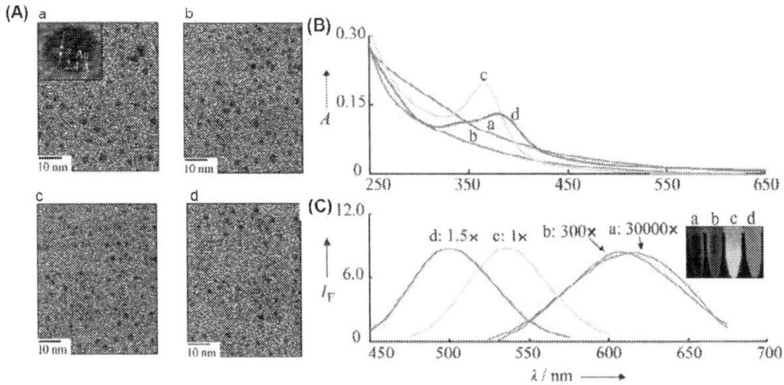

Figure 9.5 (A) TEM images, (B) UV–Vis absorbance spectra, and (C) normalized luminescence spectra of (a) Au NPs, (b) 2-ME–Au NPs, (c) 6-MH–Au NPs, and (d) 11-MU–Au NPs. Inset to (C): Photograph of the fluorescence of the various Au NPs upon excitation under a hand-held UV lamp (365 nm). The normalized luminescence intensities (I_F) are plotted in arbitrary units (a.u.); excitation wavelength: 365 nm. In (C), the concentration ratio of the Au NPs, 2-ME–Au NPs, 6-MH–Au NPs, and 11-MU–Au NPs was 3000:300:1:1.5. Reprinted with permission from Ref. 24. See also Color Insert.

Figure 9.5A displays TEM images of uncapped Au NPs and Au NPs capped with 2-mercaptoethanol (2-ME), 6-mercaptohexanol (6-MH), and 11-mercaptoundecanol (11-MU); these as-prepared alkanethiol-capped Au NPs, denoted as 2-ME–Au NPs, 6-MH–Au NPs, and 11-MU–Au NPs, respectively, have average diameters of 2.9 (±0.5), 2.3 (±0.3), 2.2 (±0.2), and 2.0 (±0.2) nm, respectively.[24] The smallest diameter, for the 11-MU–Au NPs, is due to greater degrees of breaking and detaching of larger-sized Au NCs and/or Au–thiol complexes. Figure 9.5B,C display the absorption and normalized luminescence spectra of the as-prepared Au NP, 2-ME–Au NP, 6-MH–Au NP, and 11-MU–Au NP solutions. The as-prepared Au NPs (2.9 nm) exhibit no apparent absorption band, revealing that the Au NPs prepared by THPC did not contain Au(I) atoms on the surface of each Au NP. Similarly, there is no apparent absorption band for the 2-ME–Au NPs. In contrast, the 6-MH– and 11-MU–Au NPs exhibit absorption band maxima at wavelengths (λ_{max}^{abs}) of 367 and 383 nm, respectively. The luminescence wavelength underwent a blue shift upon increasing the chain length of the thiol, primarily because of the decreased NP size and increased contribution of the alkanethiol-passivated surfaces, thereby decreasing the energy gap between the quantized levels as a result of a smaller core and a higher coverage of thiolate. As the particle size decreases, the surface-to-volume ratio increases and a larger fraction of the NP core atoms becomes involved in forming bonds with the core-capping ligands.

Based on the well-established spectral assignment for the Au(I)–thiolate complexes, the absorption of alkanethiol–Au NPs at 375 nm presumably originates from metal-centered and/or ligand–metal charge transfer (LMCT; S→Au) transitions.[28–30] In addition, the luminescent alkanethiol–Au NPs have large Stokes-shifted luminescence (1.03 eV) with long lifetimes (>250 ns) — typical characteristics of thiol–Au(I) complexes that display ligand–metal charge transfer and metal(I)–metal(I) interactions.[62–64] Thus, the luminescence of the alkanethiol–Au NPs presumably originates mainly from Au NP/polynuclear Au(I)–thiol (core/shell) complexes.[24–27] The presence of a shell of polynuclear Au(I)–thiol units suggests that the emission arises from a low-lying triplet state (phosphorescence), populated via intersystem crossing from the lowest singlet state.[62–64] The emission intensities of the luminescent RS–Au NPs are comparable with those of reported monolayer-protected Au NCs.[50–62] The emission peak of the RS–Au NPs (λ_{max}^{em} = 501–618 nm) is located at an energy higher than those of the $Au_{28}(GSH)_{16}$ NCs and the dodecanethiolate-protected Au_{38} NCs (<1.5 nm).[50–56] The blue shift in the emission maxima upon reducing the NC size results from the increase in the energy gaps between the quantized levels (interband or intraband transitions) ascribed to the smaller core sizes as well as the higher coverage of thiolates or other capping molecules (e.g., phosphine).[83] In contrast, the value of λ_{max}^{em} for the RS–Au NPs (ca. 2 nm) is inconsistent with those of the NCs, presumably due to the existence of the outermost layer of Au(I)–thiolate complexes.[24–27]

The luminescence properties of Au and Au/Ag NPs can be controlled by varying the molar ratios of THPC to Au ions (for Au NPs) and of Ag ions to Au ions (for Au/Ag alloy NPs).[26] Through variation of the initial molar ratio of THPC to $HAuCl_4$, Au NPs can be prepared having diameters ranging from 2.2 to 3.7 nm. Introduction of 11-mercaptoundecanoic acid (11-MUA) ligands onto the surfaces of the as-prepared Au NPs results in luminescent 11-MUA–Au

NPs. The as-prepared spherical 11-MUA–Au NPs of various sizes emit light at different wavelengths within the range 500–640 nm (Fig. 9.6A). Likewise, by controlling the molar ratio of Au and Ag ions, 11-MUA-protected Au/Ag NPs having similar sizes can be prepared; these NPs emit light at different wavelengths within the range 456–525 nm (Fig. 9.6B).

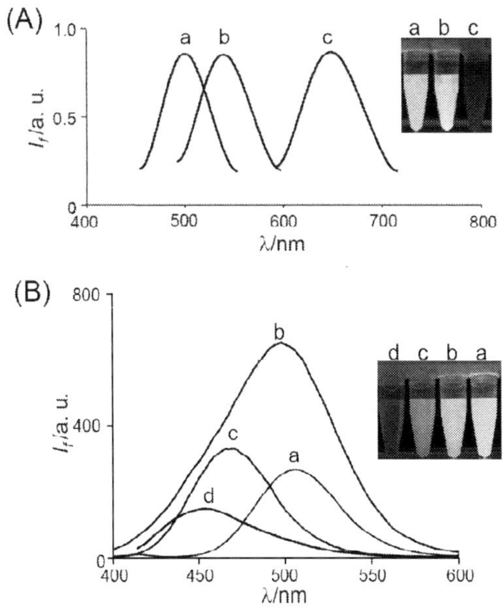

Figure 9.6 (A) Normalized luminescence spectra of 11-MUA–Au NPs prepared at THPC-to-$HAuCl_4$ concentration ratios of (a) 1.0, (b) 2.0, and (c) 3.5. (B) Luminescence spectra of 11-MUA–Au/Ag NPs prepared at $AgNO_3$-to-$HAuCl_4$ molar ratios of (a) 0, (b) 0.125, (c) 0.800, and (d) 2.000, respectively. Reprinted with permission from Ref. 26. See also Color Insert.

Similarly, water-soluble, biofunctional, luminescent mannose-capped Au NPs (Man–Au NPs) can be prepared through the reaction of 2.9 nm diameter Au NPs with 11-mercapto-3,6,9-trioxecyl-α-D-mannopyranoside (Man-RSH).[25] The luminescence intensity of these Man–Au NPs is highly dependent on the concentration of Man-RSH. The water-soluble Man–Au NPs having the highest quantum yield (9.4%) fluoresced ca. 260,000-fold more strongly than did the original Au NPs. The differently sized Man–Au NPs prepared using various Man-RSH concentrations (1–10 mM) all possess an absorption band at ca. 375 nm (Fig. 9.7A) and emitted luminescence at wavelengths centered in the region 525–550 nm (Fig. 9.7B). The corresponding TEM images (Fig. 9.7C) indicate that the Man–Au NPs prepared at Man-RSH concentrations of 0, 1, 2.5, 5, and 10 mM are well dispersed, having average diameters of 2.9 (±0.5), 2.1 (±0.2), 1.8 (±0.3), 1.7 (±0.2), and 1.5 (±0.1) nm, respectively. The decreasing size of these Au NPs upon increasing the concentration of Man-RSH results from significant fragmentation caused by strong Au–S interactions. No Au NPs were present in the solution when the concentration of Man-RSH was greater than 20 mM, revealing that the Au NPs had all dissociated into Au–thiolate complexes under these conditions. As a result, the as-prepared solution did not absorb light at 375 nm and did not luminesce (cf. spectra *f* in Fig. 9.7A,B).

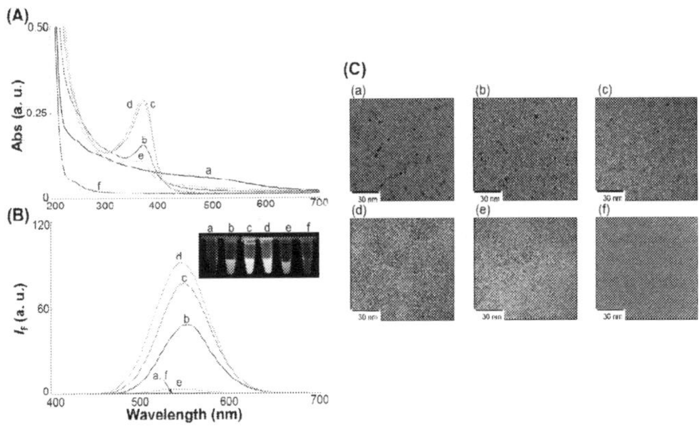

Figure 9.7 (A) UV–Vis absorption spectra, (B) luminescence spectra, and (C) TEM images of the 2.9 nm Au NP solutions after treatment with Man-RSH solutions having concentrations of (a) 0, (b) 1, (c) 2.5, (d) 5, (e) 10, and (f) 20 mM. Inset to (B): Photograph displaying the luminescence of the various Man–Au ND solutions upon excitation under a hand-held UV lamp (365 nm). Reprinted with permission from Ref. 25. See also Color Insert.

9.5 Applications

Luminescent, water-soluble Au NCs and Au NPs offer several features that make them attractive for use in bioassays, including large Stokes-shifted and long luminescence lifetimes, sizes comparable to those of biopolymers, and good water-solubility.

Unlike semiconductive QDs, they are more compatible with biological systems and are not prepared from toxic precursors under vigorous conditions. In addition, bioconjugation of Au NCs and luminescent Au NPs is quite simple when taking advantage of strong Au–S bonding.

Polymer-stabilized Au NCs are not popular for bioassays, mainly because of their low water-solubility and their difficult bioconjugation with recognition molecules. On the other hand, thiol-stabilized Au NCs have very low quantum yields, making them poor materials for developing sensitive nanosensors. Nevertheless, a few NCs have exhibited practical use in bioassays. Polyclonal, goat-derived anti-human IgG antibody-modified PAMAM–Au NCs have been used for the detection of human IgG antigen.[71] Coupling of goat-derived polyclonal anti-human IgG to the fluorescent PAMAM–Au NCs (λ_{em}^{max} = 450 nm) occurred through electrostatic interactions. Upon increasing the concentration of human IgG antigen, the luminescence intensity of the bioconjugated PAMAM–Au NCs decreased. Through interactions between the antigen and antibody in the form of a 2:1 complex, aggregation of the Au NCs occurred, leading to decreased luminescence intensity. The relationship between the luminescence intensity and the concentration of the human IgG was linear over the micromolar to nanomolar range. By conducting ligand exchange reactions, the PAMAM groups of the PAMAM–Au NCs can be exchanged by carboxylate-terminated *n*-alkanethiols, such as 11-MUA, allowing simple functionalization of the NCs with site-specific leading peptides, such as SV40 nuclear-localization signal (NLS).[72] To modify the surfaces of the 11-MUA-capped Au NCs with NLS for nuclear transport, 1-[(3-dimethylamino)propyl]-3-ethylcarbodiimide hydrochloride (EDC) is usually introduced to activate the carboxylic acid unit of 11-MUA prior to adding NLS. Figure 9.8 displays confocal microscopy images of the 11-MUA–Au NCs (without NLS) and the NLS–11-MUA–Au NCs inside HeLa cells. The one-color image features no luminescent signals (panel A) from the cells treated with the 11-MUA–Au NCs, implying that 11-MUA–Au NCs are not able to enter the cells efficiently, due, at least in part, to their negative surface charge. In contrast, intense blue PL (panels C and E) appears from the NLS–11-MUA–Au NCs, indicative of the internalization of the 11-MUA–Au NCs associated with NLS by HeLa cells. Counter-staining the cells with a specific membrane dye, wheat germ agglutinin conjugated Alexa 594 (WGA-Alexa 594), and a nuclear dye, SYTO 59, allowed observation of the intracellular and nuclear distributions of the NLS–11-MUA–Au NCs inside the cells. The two-color co-localization images (panels D and F) reveal that the blue luminescence from the NLS–11-MUA–Au NCs was distributed well within both the cytoplasm (panel D) and the nucleus (panel F); in contrast, the image of the cells treated with the 11-MUA–Au NCs (panel B) exhibits only the red fluorescence of WGA-Alexa 594. Therefore, the nuclear targeting of 11-MUA–Au NCs was possible because of the functionality of NLS, as revealed in panel F with the two-color co-localization images in the same confocal z-plane (blue: NLS–11-MUA–Au NCs; red: SYTO 59).

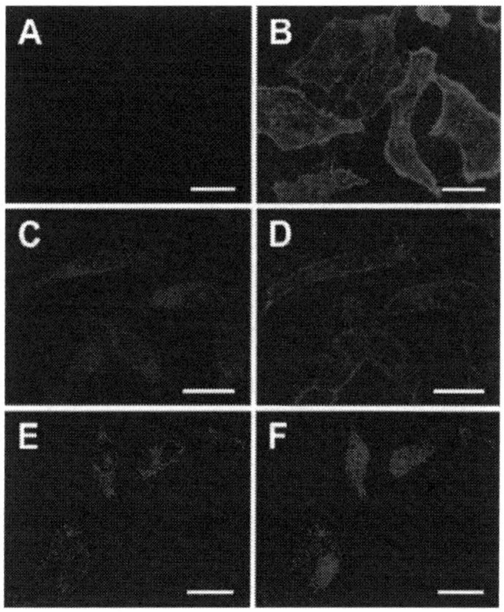

Figure 9.8 Confocal microscopy images of intracellular delivery of the Au NCs. HeLa cells were treated with 11-MUA–Au NCs (A, B) and NLS–11-MUA–Au NCs (E, F) for 1.5 h. The left panels present one-color images; the right panels present two-color co-localization images of the HeLa cells incubated with NLS–11-MUA–Au NCs and counterstained with a specific membrane dye (WGA-Alexa 594) and a nuclear dye (SYTO 59). Scale bar: 25 μm. Reprinted with permission from Ref. 72. See also Color Insert.

Water-soluble, fluorescent, thiol-capped Au NPs can also be selective and sensitive probe for the detection of various analytes of interest, such as heavy metal ion pollutants, which exert adverse effects on the environment and on human health. 11-MUA–Au

NPs are readily employed for the sensing of Hg^{2+} ions, based on luminescence quenching through Hg^{2+}-induced aggregation.[24] The interactions between 11-MUA–Au NPs and Hg^{2+} ions occur through Hg^{2+}-carboxylate bonding or Hg^{2+}–Au^{+} metallophilic interaction. In the presence of 2,6-pyridinedicarboxylic acid (PDCA), the 11-MUA–Au NPs bind to Hg^{2+}, leading to a decrease in fluorescence (Fig. 9.9). In the absence of PDCA, interference from Pb^{2+} and Cd^{2+} ions is strong. Such interference is minimized by adding 1.0 mM PDCA to the solution, mainly due to its strong interaction with Hg^{2+}.[73] This approach provides high sensitivity (limit of detection (LOD) = 5.0 nM) and selectivity (at least 10-fold against Pb^{2+} and Cd^{2+}). This LOD is lower than the maximum level (2.0 ppb) of mercury permitted in drinking water by the United States Environmental Protection Agency (EPA). This approach provides a sensitivity that is two orders of magnitude lower than those reported for heavy metal ion sensors based on chelation/aggregation-mediated colorimetry and for Au NP systems based on modulation of fluorescence quenching. Furthermore, this Au NP-based nanosensor can be applied to analyses of Hg^{2+} in environmental samples. For example, the concentration of Hg^{2+} in a pond water sample determined using this 11-MUA–Au NP sensor was 3.49 ppb, in good agreement with the value (3.20 ppb) determined using inductively coupled plasma mass spectrometry (ICP–MS).

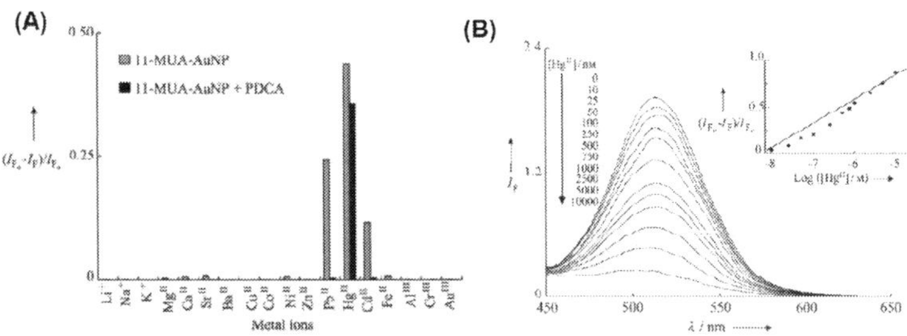

Figure 9.9 (A) Fluorescence ratios $[(I_{Fo} - I_F)/I_{Fo}]$ at 520 nm for the 11-MUA–Au NPs (10 nM) measured in the absence and presence of PDCA (1.0 mM) after the addition of 500 nM metal ions in 5 mM sodium tetraborate solutions at pH 9.2. (B) Fluorescence response of the 11-MUA–Au NPs upon the addition of Hg^{2+} ions (0, 10, 25, 50, 100, 250, 500, 750, 1000, 2500, 5000, and 10,000 nM). Inset: Plot of fluorescence ratios $[(I_{Fo} - I_F)/I_{Fo}]$ of 11-MUA–Au NPs at 520 nm versus log$[Hg^{2+}]$. [Reprinted with permission from Ref. 24].

Using two differently sized Au NPs, acting separately as donor and acceptor, homogeneous PL quenching assays have been developed for the analysis of proteins.[31] The introduction of a breast cancer marker protein, platelet-derived growth factor AA (PDGF AA), to a solution of 11-MUA-protected, 2.0 nm luminescent Au NPs provided PDGF AA–Au NPs as donors. Thiol-derived PDGF binding DNA aptamers (Apt) and 13 nm spherical Au NPs were used for the preparation of Apt–Au NP acceptors. Aptamers are DNA or RNA sequences recognizing specific target analytes; they are isolated from random-sequence DNA or RNA libraries through *in vitro* selection or systematic evolution of ligands by exponential enrichment (SELEX).[74–76] Relative to antibodies, aptamers possess certain advantageous features, including relatively simple and inexpensive syntheses through automation, tolerance to internal labeling, and long storage times without altering or losing their biological properties. The aptamer selected for PDGF has the sequence CAGGCTACGGCACGTAGAGCATCACCATGATCCTG; it exhibits strong binding affinity toward PDGF ($K_d \sim$ nM).[77] The consensus secondary structure motif of the PDGF aptamer is a three-way helix junction with a conserved single-stranded loop at the branch point; the helix junction domain represents the core of the structural motif required for high-affinity binding.[77]

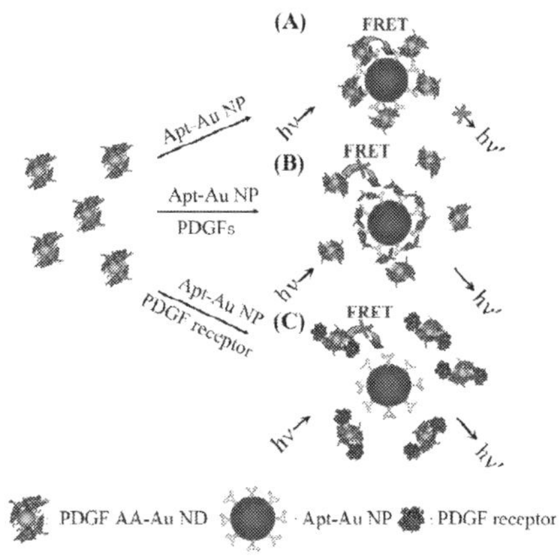

Figure 9.10 Schematic representation of PFGF and PDGF-receptor nanosensors that operate based on modulation of the photoluminescence quenching between PDGF AA–Au NPs and Apt–Au NPs. h – Planck's constant; ν – frequency of light. Reprinted with permission from Ref. 31. See also Color Insert.

In the assay, the PDGF AA–Au NPs and Apt–Au NPs were mixed in the absence and presence of PDGF. When mixed, the two differently sized Au NPs in the luminescent PDGF AA–Au NPs and Apt–Au NPs come into close contact, leading to luminescence quenching through electron and/or energy transfer. As a result, the luminescence of the PDGF AA–Au NPs at 520 nm decreases (Fig. 9.10A). This PDGF AA–Au NP/Apt–Au NP-based molecular light switching system allows the analysis of PDGFs as well as PDGF α-receptor in separate homogeneous solutions (Fig. 9.10B,C). In the presence of PDGFs, the interaction between the Apt–Au NPs and the PDGF AA–Au NPs weaken as a result of competitive reactions between the PDGFs and the Apt–Au NPs.

Similarly, the interactions between the Apt–Au NPs and the PDGF AA–Au NPs weaken as a result of competitive reactions between PDGF α-receptor and the PDGF AA–Au NPs. The LODs for PDGF AA and PDGF α-receptor were 80 pM and 0.25 nM, respectively. When using the Apt–Au NPs as selectors for (i) the enrichment of PDGF AA and (ii) the removal of matrices possessing intense background fluorescence from cell media and urine samples, the LOD for PDGF AA decreased to 10 pM. This Apt–Au NP-assisted PDGF-AA enrichment process provided greater sensitivity than those obtained using other signal aptamers.

Biofunctional Man–Au NPs are capable of sensing concanavalin A (Con A) through multivalent interactions.[25] Con A is a member of the lectin family; it binds selectively to α-mannopyranosyl and α-glucopyranosyl residues.[78,79] Con A exists predominantly as a tetramer of four identical subunits (each ca. 26,000 Da) at neutral and alkaline pH.[78,79] Man–Au ND–Con A aggregates can be formed through specific interactions between the carbohydrate units and the multivalent lectins. To minimize precipitation and collisions, which can cause fluorescence quenching, mixtures of Man–Au NPs and various concentrations of Con A were incubated for 60 min and then centrifuged prior to luminescence measurement. The recorded luminescence intensity of the supernatant is inversely proportional to the concentration of Con A. This approach provides an LOD of 75 pM for Con A, with remarkable selectivity over other proteins (e.g., bovine serum albumin, β-lactalbumin, carbonic anhydrase, conalbumin, myoglobin) and lectins (e.g., DBA from *Dolichos biflorus*; WGA from *Triticum vulgari*; PSA from *Pisum sativum*).[25] The biofunctional Man–Au NPs are also sensitive for the detection of *Escherichia coli* (*E. coli*). Type 1 fimbriae present on the surface of Enterobacteriaceae, such as *E. coli*, are responsible for their mannose- and mannoside-binding activities. Thus, incubation of *E. coli* with the biofunctional Man–Au NPs yielded brightly fluorescent cell NCs. The relationship between the luminescence signal and the *E. coli* concentration is linear over the range from 1.00 × 10^6 to 5.00 × 10^7 cells/mL (R^2 = 0.96), with the LOD of *E. coli* being 7.20 × 10^5 cells/mL (Fig. 9.11). In contrast to standard methods for pathogen detection, which require up to 2 days for analysis, the use of these luminescent carbohydrate-functionalized Au NDs allows the presence of *E. coli* to be detected within as little as 3 h.

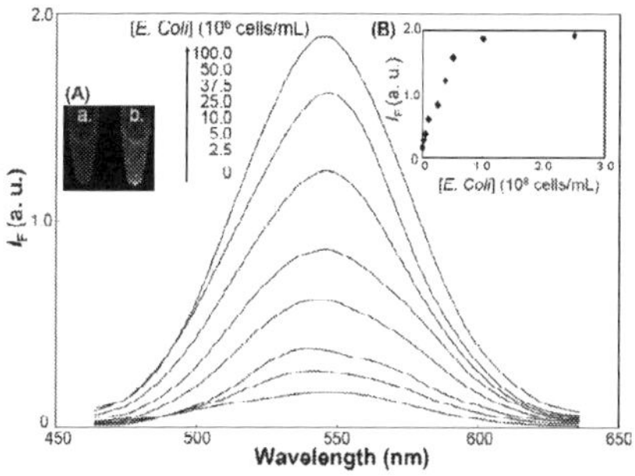

Figure 9.11 Luminescence spectra of Man–Au NPs (25 nM) used as probes for the detection of *E. coli* (from 2.50 × 10^6 to 1.00 × 10^8 cells/mL). Inset (A): Visualization of Man–Au NPs (25 nM) in the (a) absence and (b) presence of *E. coli* (2.50 × 10^8 cells/mL) upon excitation (365 nm) under a hand-held UV lamp. Inset (B): Plot of luminescence intensity (545 nm) versus *E. coli* concentration. Reprinted with permission from Ref. 25.

9.6 Conclusion

Research on luminescent Au NCs and luminescent Au NPs is attracting increasing interest. Great progress has been made in understanding the fundamental size- and surface-dependence of the optical properties of these Au nanomaterials, as well as in developing sensitive and selective sensors from them. Nevertheless, much work remains to be done to better understand and manipulate their properties. For example, the luminescence properties of luminescent Au NPs are different from those of Au NCs, but remain poorly understood. A quantitative explanation for the observed luminescence is missing; it should be investigated. In addition, surface modification and crystallinity, which affect the optical properties of such luminescent Au nanomaterials, are also important issues that require further study.

Many reports have suggested that these luminescent Au nanomaterials are promising tools for sensing and intracellular imaging. Their quantum yields are, however, low when compared with those of the more popular bioconjugated QDs. In addition, they are not as photostable as QDs, limiting their use in cell imaging. Thus, great efforts must be exerted to improve the photostability and quantum yields of Au nanomaterials, possibly by coating Au NCs and luminescent Au NPs with biopolymers, polymers, or SiO_2. In addition, the preparation of metal nanocomposites, such as fluorescent Au/Ag species, might extend their use in bioassays.

Acknowledgments

Our studies reported herein were supported by the National Science Council of Taiwan under contract 99-2113-M-019-001-MY2. We thank those authors who provided preprints or unpublished material for use in this article, and Huan-Tsung Chang for valuable comments on the early drafts.

References

1. P. K. Jain, X. Huang, I. H. El-Sayed, and M. A. El-Sayed, *Acc. Chem. Res.*, **41**, 1578 (2008).
2. P. C. Chen, S. C. Mwakwari, and A. K. Oyelere, *Nanotechnol. Sci. Appl.*, **1**, 45 (2008).
3. W. Zhao, M. A. Brook, and Y. Li, *Chem. Bio. Chem.*, **9**, 2363 (2008).
4. A. S. K. Hashmi, and M. Rudolph, *Chem. Soc. Rev.*, **37**, 1766 (2008).
5. M. Grzelczak, J. Pérez-Juste, P. Mulvaney, and L. M. Liz-Marzán, *Chem. Soc. Rev.*, **37**, 1783 (2008).
6. J. Zheng, C. Zheng, and R. M. Dickson, *Phys. Rev. Lett.*, **93**, 077402 (2004).
7. L. A. Peyser, A. E. Vinson, A. P. Bartko, and R. M Dickson, *Science*, **291**,103 (2001).

8. C. L. Cleveland, U. Landman, T. G. Schaaff, M. N. Shafigullin, P. W. Stephens, and R. L. Whetten, *Phys. Rev. Lett.*, **79**, 1873 (1997).
9. S. Fedrigo, W. Harbich, and J. Buttet, *J. Chem. Phys.*, **99**, 5712 (1993).
10. U. Kreibig, and M. Vollmer, in *Optical Properties of Metal Clusters* (Springer, Berlin, 1995).
11. N. W. Ashcroft, and N. D. Mermin, in *Solid State Physics* (Holt/Rinehart & Winston, New York, 1976).
12. R. Kubo, *J. Phys. Soc. Jpn.*, **17**, 975 (1962).
13. T. G. Schaaff, G. Knight, M. N. Shafigullin, R. F. Borkman, and R. L. Whetten, *J. Phys. Chem. B*, **102**, 10643 (1998).
14. W. T. Wallace, and R. L. Whetten, *J. Am. Chem. Soc.*, **124**, 7499 (2002).
15. C. T. Campbell, S. C. Parker, and D. E. Starr, *Science*, **298**, 811 (2002).
16. A. Sanchez, S. Abbet, U. Heiz, W.-D. Schneider, H. Häkkinen, R. N. Barnett, and U. Landman, *J. Phys. Chem. A*, **103**, 9573 (1999).
17. L. A. Peyser, T.-H. Lee, and R. M. Dickson, *J. Phys. Chem. B*, **106**, 7725 (2002).
18. I. Rabin, W. Schulze, G. Ertl, C. Felix, C. Sieber, W. Harbich, and J. Buttet, *Chem. Phys. Lett.*, **320**, 59 (2000).
19. W. Harbich, S. Fedrigo, J. Buttet, and D. M. Lindsay, *Z. Phys. D.*, **19**, 157 (1991).
20. L. Prodi, G. Battistini, L. S. Dolci, M. Montalti, and N. Zaccheroni, in *Frontiers in Surface Nanophotonics* (Springer Berlin, Heidelberg, 2007), V. 133.
21. J. Zheng, C. Zhang, and R. M. Dickson, *Phys. Rev. Lett.*, **93**, 077402 (2004).
22. Y. Negishi, K. Nobusada, and T. Tsukuda, *J. Am. Chem. Soc.*, **127**, 5261 (2005).
23. G. Wang, T. Huang, R. W. Murray, L. Menard, and R. G. Nuzzo, *J. Am. Chem. Soc.*, **127**, 812 (2005).
24. C.-C. Huang, Z. Yang, K.-H. Lee, and H.-T. Chang, *Angew. Chem. Int. Ed. Engl.*, **46**, 6824 (2007).
25. C.-C. Huang, C.-T. Chen, Y.-C. Shiang, Z.-H. Lin, and H.-T. Chang, *Anal. Chem.*, **81**, 875 (2009).
26. C.-C. Huang, H.-Y. Liao, Y.-C. Shiang, Z.-H. Lin, Z. Yang, and H.-T. Chang, *J. Mater. Chem.*, **19**, 755 (2009).
27. J. Zheng, *Fluorescent Noble Metal Nanoclusters*, PhD thesis, Georgia Institute of Technology, Atlanta (2005).

28. V. W.-W. Yam, and E. C.-C. Cheng, *Chem. Soc. Rev.*, **37**, 1806 (2008).
29. P. Pyykkö, *Inorg. Chim. Acta*, **358**, 4113 (2005).
30. P. Pyykkö, *Angew. Chem. Int. Ed. Engl.*, **43**, 4412 (2004).
31. C.-C. Huang, C.-K. Chiang, Z.-H. Lin, K.-H. Lee, and H.-T. Chang, *Anal. Chem.*, **80**, 1497 (2008).
32. S.-Y. Lin, N.-T. Chen, S.-P. Sum, L.-W. Lo, and C.-S. Yang, *Chem. Commun.*, 4762 (2008).
33. C.-A. J. Lin, T.-Y. Yang, C.-H. Lee, S. H. Huang, R. A. Sperling, M. Zanella, J. K. Li, J.-L. Shen, H.-H. Wang, H.-I. Yeh, W. J. Parak, and W. H. Chang, *ACS Nano*, **3**, 395 (2009).
34. L. Shang, and S. Dong, *J. Mater. Chem.*, **18**, 4636 (2008).
35. R. C. Triulzi, M. Micic, S. Giordani, M. Serry, W.-A. Chioue, and R. M. Leblanc, *Chem. Commun.*, 5068 (2006).
36. J. Yu, S. Choi, and R. M. Dickson, *Angew. Chem. Int. Ed.*, **47**, 1 (2008).
37. J. Zheng, J. T. Petty, and R. M. Dickson, *J. Am. Chem. Soc.*, **125**, 7780 (2003).
38. W. A. de Heer, *Rev. Mod. Phys.*, **65**, 611 (1993).
39. W. D. Knight, K. Clemenger, W. A. de Heer, W. A. Saunders, M. Y. Chou, and M. L. Cohen *Phys. Rev. Lett.*, **52**, 2141 (1984).
40. W. A. de Heer, K. Selby, V. V. Kresin, J. Masui, and M. Vollmer, *Phys. Rev. Lett.*, **59**, 1805 (1987).
41. W. A. Deheer, *Rev. Mod. Phys.*, **65**, 611 (1993).
42. K. Clemenger, *Phys. Rev. B*, **32**, 1359 (1985).
43. W. D. Knight, K. Clemenger, W. A. de Heer, W. A. Saunders, M. Y. Chou, and M. L. Cohen, *Phys. Rev. Lett.*, **52**, 2141 (1984).
44. T. Reiners, C. Ellert, M. Schmidt, and H. Haberland, *Phys. Rev. Lett.*, **74**, 1558 (1995).
45. W. A. de Heer, K. Selby, V. Kresin, J. Masui, M. Vollmer, A. Chatelain, and W. D. Knight *Phys. Rev. Lett.*, **59**, 1805 (1987).
46. N. Schaeffer, B. Tan, C. Dickinson, M. J. Rosseinsky, A. Laromaine, D. W. McComb, M. M. Stevens, Y. Wang, L. Petit, C. Barentin, D. G. Spiller, A. I. Cooper, and R. Lévy, *Chem. Commun.*, 3986 (2008).
47. H. Duan, and S. Nie, *J. Am. Chem. Soc.*, **129**, 2412 (2007).
48. M. Brust, M. Walker, D. Bethell, D. J. Schiffrin, and R. Whyman, *J. Chem. Soc. Chem. Commun.*, **801** (1994).
49. G. H. Woehrle, L. O. Brown, and J. E. Hutchison, *J. Am. Chem. Soc.*, **127**, 2172 (2005).

50. Y. Negishi, and T. Tsukuda, *Chem. Phys. Lett.*, **383**, 161 (2004).
51. D. Lee, R. L. Donkers, G. Wang, A. S. Harper, and R. W. Murray, *J. Am. Chem. Soc.*, **126**, 6193 (2004).
52. L. D. Menard, S.-P. Gao, H. Xu, R. D. Twesten, A. S. Harper, Y. Song, G. Wang, A. D. Douglas, J. C. Yang, A. I. Frenkel, R. G. Nuzzo, and R. W. Murray *J. Phys. Chem. B*, **110**, 12874 (2006).
53. T. P. Bigioni, R. L. Whetten, and Ö. Dag, *J. Phys. Chem. B*, **104**, 6983 (2000).
54. Y. Y. Yang, and S. W. Chen, *Nano Lett.*, **3**, 75 (2003).
55. T. Huang, and R.W. Murray, *J. Phys. Chem. B*, **105**, 12498 (2001).
56. S. Link, A. Beeby, S. FitzGerald, M. A. El-Sayed, T. G. Schaaff, and R. L. Whetten, *J. Phys. Chem. B*, **106**, 3410 (2002).
57. A. C. Templeton, S. Chen, S. M. Gross, and R. W. Murray, *Langmuir*, **15**, 66 (1999).
58. T. Huang and R. W. Murray, *J. Phys. Chem. B*, **105**, 1249 (2001).
59. S. Link, A. Beeby, S. FitzGerald, M. A. El-Sayed, T. G. Schaaff, and R. L. Whetten, *J. Phys. Chem. B*, **106**, 3410 (2002).
60. Y. Negishi, K. Nobusada, and T. Tsukuda, *J. Am. Chem. Soc.*, **127**, 5261 (2005).
61. T. Huang and R. W. Murray, *J. Phys. Chem. B*, **107**, 7434 (2003).
62. G. Wang, R. Guo, G. Kalyuzhny, J.-P. Choi, and R. W. Murray, *J. Phys. Chem. B*, **110**, 20282 (2006).
63. A. Vogler and H. Kunkely, *Coord. Chem. Rev.*, **219–221**, 489 (2001).
64. R. L. Whetten and R. C. Price, *Science*, **318**, 407 (2007).
65. J. M. Forward, D. Bohmann, J. P. Fackler, Jr., and R. J. Staples, *Inorg. Chem.*, **34**, 6330 (1995).
66. Z. Assefa, B. G. McBurnett, R. J. Staples, J. P. Fackler, B. Assmann, K. Angermaier, and H. Schmidbaur, *Inorg. Chem.*, **34**, 75 (1995).
67. H. Shan, Y. Yang, A. J. James, and P. R. Sharp, *Science*, **275**, 1460 (1997).
68. P. Pyykkö, *Chem. Rev.*, **97**, 597 (1997).
69. J. A. M. Sondag-Huethorst, C. Schonenberger, and L. G. J. Fokkink, *J. Phys. Chem.*, **98**, 6826 (1994).
70. M. Konôpka, R. Rousseau, I. Štich, and D. Marx, *J. Am. Chem. Soc.*, **126**, 12103 (2004).
71. R. C. Triulzi, M. Micic, S. Giordani, M. Serry, W.-A. Chioue, and R. M. Leblanc, *Chem. Commun.*, 5068 (2006).

72. S.-Y. Lin, N.-T. Chen, S.-P. Sum, L.-W. Lo, and C.-S. Yang, *Chem. Commun.*, 4762 (2008).
73. E. Norkus, I. Stalnionienë, and D. C. Crans, *Heteroat. Chem.*, **14**, 625 (2003).
74. G. F. Joyce, *Gene*, **82**, 83 (1989).
75. A. D. Ellington, and J. W. Szostak, *Nature*, **346**, 818 (1990).
76. C. Tuerk and L. Gold, *Science*, **249**, 505 (1990).
77. L. S. Green, D. Jellinek, R. Jenison, A. Östman, C.-H. Heldin, and N. Janjic, *Biochemistry*, **35**, 14413 (1996).
78. C. W. Cairo, J. E. Gestwicki, M. Kanai, and L. L. Kiessling, *J. Am. Chem. Soc.*, **124**, 1615 (2002).
79. D. F. Senear, and D. C. Teller, *Biochemistry*, **20**, 3076 (1981).

Chapter 10

Biodetection Based on Fluorescence Quenching and Surface-Enhanced Fluorescence Using Noble Metal Nanoparticles

Yang-Wei Lin[a], Chi-Wei Liu[b], and Huan-Tsung Chang[b,*]

[a]*Department of Chemistry, National Changhua University of Education, 1, Jin-De Road, Changhua City 500, Taiwan*

[b]*Department of Chemistry, National Taiwan University, 1, Section 4, Roosevelt Road, Taipei, Taiwan*

[*]changht@ntu.edu.tw

Fluorescence is popular in carbohydrate, protein, and DNA arrays; cell imaging; and single molecule detection because of its sensitivity. To achieve high sensitivity, fluorophores possessing high quantum yields are necessary. However, most analytes do not fluoresce strongly. In order to overcome this shortage, techniques based on fluorescence quenching and surface-enhanced fluorescence using novel metal materials have been applied. Fluorescence quenching and enhancements are both dependent on the distance of fluorophores from the metal surface; quenching usually occurs at a distance no greater than 50 Å while fluorescence enhancement commonly takes place at a distance between 70 and 100 Å. In addition to distance, the nature, size, and shape of metal materials are important parameters for fluorescence quenching and enhancement. With advanced nanotechnology, researchers have demonstrated techniques

From Bioimaging to Biosensors: Noble Metal Nanoparticles in Biodetection
Edited by Lai-Kwan Chau and Huan-Tsung Chang

ISBN 978-981-4267-24-3 (Hardcover), 978-981-4303-10-1 (eBook)
www.panstanford.com

entailing fluorescence quenching and enhancement using novel metal nanomaterials for the sensitive analysis of proteins, DNA, and small solutes.

10.1 Introduction

Noble metal nanoparticles (NPs) containing dye molecules have recently gained considerable interest in photonics, optoelectronics, and materials science because of their unique optical and electronic properties. For example, TiO_2-Au and ZnO NPs containing N_3 dye are useful materials in the fabrication of solar cells,[1,2] fullerene-functionalized Au NPs are effective in the fabrication of light-harvesting devices,[3,4] and Au NPs that are conjugated with 5-((2-(and-3)-S-(acetylmercapto)succinoyl)amion)- fluorescein and 5-[1,2]dithiolan-3-ylpentanoic acid and 1,6-bis((*N*-carbazol-3-yl)methyl)-2,4-hexadiyne ester are useful in the preparation of light emitting devices.[5,6]

Noble metal NPs are among the most polarizable inorganic templates capable of producing enhanced optical fields near their surfaces under visible electromagnetic radiation. When located in close proximity to a metallic NP, a dye undergoes strong changes in its electronic and optical properties likely as a result of a mixing of the molecule and metal electronic levels as well as an interaction of the molecule with the surface plasmon resonance. The changes are dependent on several parameters, including the size and species of the NPs, the distance between the fluorophores and the metal surface, the roughness of the metal surface, and the orientation of the fluorophore transition moment. Fluorescence quenching occurs in the case of the adsorption of a dye on a metal surface while a fluorescence enhancement occurs when the dye is located at distances between 70 and 100 Å from the metal surface. Quenching provides nonradiative pathways to the ground state but does not induce significant changes to the radiative decay rate. In contrast, changes in the radiative rates may arise from the interactions of fluorophores with nearby particles through the interactions of the incident light and the fluorophore's oscillating dipole with the nearby metal surface, leading to increased fluorescence. The fluorescence enhancement of the fluorophores on the metal surface is called surface enhanced fluorescence (SEF). Researchers have demonstrated that Cu, Ag, and Au NPs are effective substrates for SEF mainly because of their great resonance oscillation with light in the UV-visible region.[7–16]

The local electromagnetic (EM) environment of fluorophores on a metal surface is an important factor for controlling their fluorescence intensity. By taking advantage of the interaction of the fluorophore with its surroundings, dramatic improvements in its fluorescence can be achieved. The effect of the surrounding media on the emission properties of fluorophores was first demonstrated using free atoms in a high-Q cavity.[17] These improvements in fluorescence emission have been further realized in various systems such as micropillars and microdiscs and more recently in photonic crystal defect nanocavities.[18–22]

A crucial challenge in SEF is the surface itself, which is designed to control the fluorophore emission and to induce the maximum amount of fluorescence in the direction of the detector. The surface also modifies the excitation rate of a fluorophore through altering its local EM field. Thus, a specifically designed surface together with a precise excitation of optical geometry is another crucial aspect of SEF. By altering the structure of a metal's surface, one can control the properties of surface plasmons, in particular their interaction with light. Surface plasmons are waves that propagate along the surface of a conductor, usually a metal. When a conductor interacts with light waves, its free electrons respond collectively by oscillating in resonance with the light wave. The resonant interaction between the surface charge oscillation and the EM field of the light constitutes the surface plasmon and gives rise to its unique properties. Due to their high sensitivity to geometry and surroundings, surface plasmons allow researchers to direct and focus light with subwavelength optics.[23] Enhancements of the EM fields through surface plasmons have been demonstrated in a variety of optical applications, including non-linear optics.[24–26]

In this chapter, we describe the impact of the interactions of fluorophores with metal NPs on their fluorescence. The roles that the nature of the metal surface and the distance of the fluorophores from it play in determining the fluorescence are discussed from a theoretical aspect. We also emphasize the detection of a number of analytes, including DNA, proteins, and metal ions, using metal NPs containing fluorophores. The remarkable practical potential of metal NPs-fluorophore sensing systems is described. With their high sensitivity, these sensing systems are extremely demonstrated useful for medical diagnostics.

10.2 Theory

The interactions of fluorophores with metallic surfaces can cause increases or decreases in their fluorescence. Fluorescence decreases are due to energy transfer quenching by metals such as Au and Ag, which can be understood by the damping of the dipole oscillators by the nearby metal.[27] On the other hand, SEF is responsible for increased fluorescence, mainly because fluorophores are coupled to propagating surface plasmons near metal NPs.

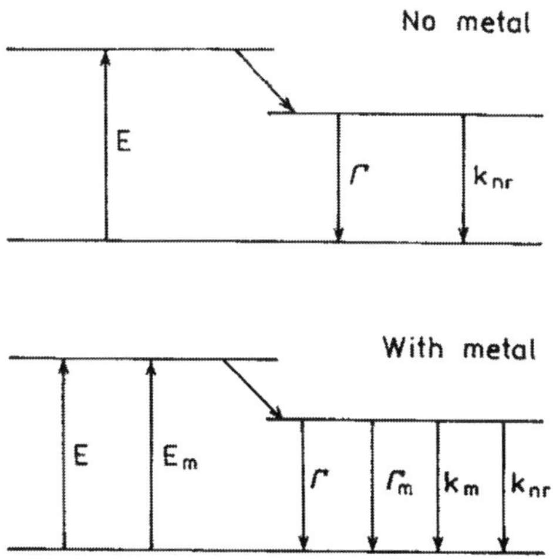

Figure 10.1 Jablonski diagram without (top) and with (bottom) the effects of near metal surfaces. For distances over 50 Å the effect of quenching by the metal (k_m) is expected to be minimal. Reprinted with permission from Ref. 28.

Figure 10.1 depicts the Jablonski diagrams of a fluorophore in the absence and presence of a metal.[28] The magnitudes of the radiative rate (Γ) and the sum of the nonradiative decay rates (k_{nr}) govern the quantum yield (Q_s) and lifetime (τ_0) of a fluorophore. First, we consider how Γ affects Q_s and τ_0 of a fluorophore in the absence of a metal surface. The Q_s of the fluorophore in the absence of other quenching interactions is given by

$$Q_s = \Gamma/(\Gamma + k_{nr}) \tag{10.1}$$

Q_s is the fraction of the excited fluorophores which decay through emission (Γ) relative to the total decay ($\Gamma + k_{nr}$). A fluorophore with a higher radiative rate has a higher quantum yield and a shorter lifetime. Γ is determined by the oscillator strength (extinction coefficient) of the electronic transition. The extinction coefficient of a fluorophore is only slightly dependent on its environment, and thus Γ is essentially constant for any given fluorophore. In other words, Q_s is only controlled by varying k_{nr}; Q_s increases upon decreasing k_{nr}. In the absence of other quenching interactions, τ_0 is given by

$$\tau_0 = (\Gamma + k_{nr})^{-1} \tag{10.2}$$

The sum of the rates that depopulate the excited state determines τ_0. When $k_{nr} = 0$, $\tau_0 = \Gamma^{-1}$. In this case, we often use τ_N (the natural lifetime of a fluorophore) to represent τ_0. Like Q_s, τ_0 is dependent on k_{nr}; τ_0 decreases as k_{nr} increases. Almost invariably, Q_s and τ_0 increase or decrease together.

When a fluorophore is placed on a metal surface, its fluorescence properties are also dependent on the metal species. Nearby metal can increase the intrinsic radiative decay rate of the fluorophore, which is not similar to fluorescence spectroscopy.[28] Assume the presence of a nearby metal surface increases the radiative rate by addition of a new rate Γ_m (see Fig. 10.1, bottom). For the present discussion, we will not consider the quenching effect of the metal (k_m). In this case, the quantum yield (Q_m) and lifetime (τ_m) of the fluorophore near the metal surface are given by

$$Q_m = \frac{\Gamma + \Gamma_m}{\Gamma + \Gamma_m + k_{nr}} \tag{10.3}$$

$$\tau = (\Gamma + \Gamma_m + k_{nr})^{-1} \tag{10.4}$$

As the value of Γ_m increases, Q_m increases while τ_m decreases. It is informative to compare the effects of increasing values of Γ_m with increased quenching of the fluorescence intensity of a fluorophore. Figure 10.2 shows this comparison in terms of the Stern-Volmer plots. The Stern-Volmer equation is $\frac{F_0}{F} = 1 + k_q[Q_u]$, in which F_0 and F are the fluorescence intensities in the absence and presence of the quencher, respectively. The effects of the rate Γ_m are dramatically different from the effects of the collision quenching rate k_q $[Q_u]$, in which k_q is the collision quenching constant and $[Q_u]$ is the quencher concentration. In the case of collision quenching, both the lifetimes and quantum yields decrease (see Fig. 10.2). On the other hand, increases in Γ_m in the presence of metallic colloids cause a decrease in τ_m but an increase in Q_m.

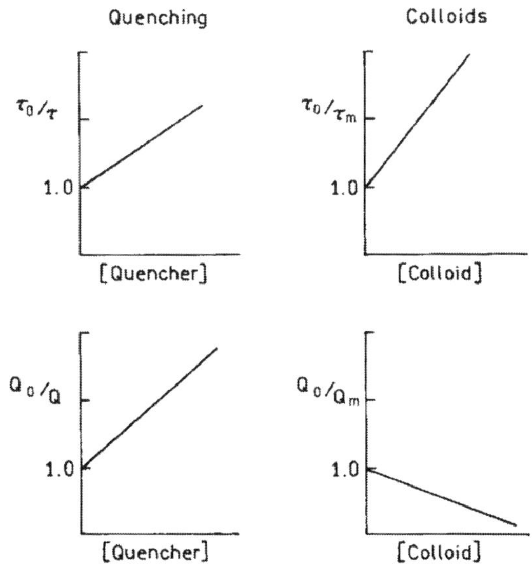

Figure 10.2 Comparison of Stern–Volmer plots for collisional quenching and colloids which enhance Γ_m. Reprinted with permission from Ref. 28.

In addition to quenching, an enhanced local field and an increase of the radiation decay rate of the fluorophore affect the Q_m of a fluorophore near a metal surface. When these two effects are considered, we use the apparent quantum yield (Y) to substitute for Q_m.

$$Y = |L(\omega_{ex})|^2 Z(\omega_{em}) \tag{10.5}$$

The first term $L(\omega_{ex})$ describes the local intensity that is proportional to the product of the quantum yield without a metal present and the amplification of the incident field. Since the light intensity is proportional to the square of the local electric field, a metal can induce a significant enhancement in the local excitation intensities. The second term $Z(\omega_{em})$ describes the partition of energy into the radiative and nonradiative decay pathways near a metal surface. The production and its effect on the decay rate of a fluorophore with enhanced local fields have been demonstrated in the presence of ellipsoidal particles with a maximum enhancement of the magnitude about 140.[29]

Metallic spheroids affect the spectral properties of nearby fluorophores.[30–33] Figure 10.3 illustrates the changes in the radiative rates for a fluorophore at various distances from the surface of a Ag particle and for different orientations of the fluorophore transition moment.

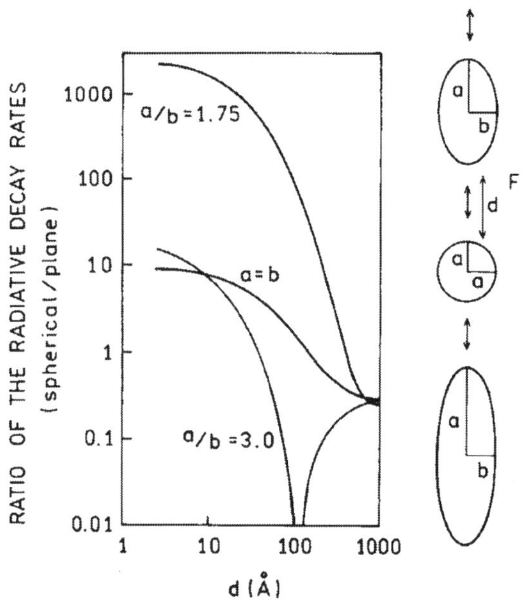

Figure 10.3 Effect of a metallic spheroid on the radiative decay rate of a fluorophore. The resonant frequency of the dye is assumed to be 25,600 cm^{-1}, approximately equal to 391 nm. The volume of the spheroids is equal to that of a sphere with a radius of 200 Å. Reprinted with permission from Ref. 28.

In this study, the Ag particle is an ellipsoid with an aspect ratio of a/b, in which a and b are the long and short axes, respectively. The fluorophore is located outside the particle on the long axis at a distance r from the center of the spheroid and a distance d from the surface. The orientation of the fluorophore can be parallel or perpendicular to the metallic surface. The most remarkable effect is observed when a fluorophore is perpendicular to the surface of a spheroid with $a/b = 1.75$ with an enhancement factor of 1000-fold or greater. The dominant effect of the perpendicular orientation is likely due to an enhancement of the local field along the long axis along the particle; the fluorophore's dipole and the dipole in the metal are synergistic. The effect is smaller for a sphere ($a/b = 1.0$) or a more elongated spheroid ($a/b = 3.0$) when the optical transition is not in resonance with the particle.

10.2.1 Fluorescence Quenching

Fluorescence quenching of a fluorophore by a quencher (Q_u) is related to its biomolecular rate constant k_q that decreases the quantum yield (Q) according to:

$$Q = \Gamma / \left(\Gamma + k_{nr} + k_q [Q_u]\right) \tag{10.6}$$

In the presence of a quencher, τ of the quenched fluorophore decreases due to an additional nonradiative path to the ground state with a rate $k_q\,[Q_u]$:

$$\tau = \left(\Gamma + k_{nr} + k_q [Q_u]\right)^{-1} \tag{10.7}$$

To understand how a metal causes fluorescence quenching of a fluorophore, we first provide the basic concept of Förster resonance energy transfer (FRET) that physically originates from the weak electromagnetic coupling of two dipoles. One can imagine that the FRET limit can be circumvented by introducing additional dipoles, providing more coupling interactions. To understand the consequences of this physical interaction, we must invoke the Fermi Golden Rule in the dipole approximation of energy transfer.[34] The Golden Rule approximation relates the energy transfer rate (k_{FRET}) to a product of the interaction elements of the donor (F_D) and acceptor (F_A): $k_{FRET} \approx F_D F_A$. These interaction elements can be simplified such that their separation distance (r) dependencies are sole functions of their geometric arrangement. Because FRET consists of two single dipoles ($F \approx 1/r^3$), its energy transfer rate (k_{FRET}) is easily derived from this rule: $k_{FRET} \approx F_D F_A \approx (1/r^3)(1/r^3) \approx 1/r^6$. More commonly, the relationship between k_{FRET} and r in FRET is written as:

$$k_{\mathrm{FRET}} = \frac{1}{\tau_0}\left(\frac{R_0}{r}\right)^6 \tag{10.8}$$

In which R_0 is the Förster radius that is a function of the oscillator strengths of the donor and acceptor molecules and their mutual energetic resonance. Typically a detectable distance is limited to <50 Å in FRET.

Using a similar formalism of FRET, we can describe the rate of energy transfer from a dipole to a metallic surface interband transition.[35-37] Instead of k_{FRET}, a surface energy transfer (SET) rate (k_{SET}) is used for a fluorophore near a metal surface: $k_{\mathrm{SET}} \approx F_{\mathrm{D}}F_{\mathrm{A}} \approx (1/d^3)(1/d) \approx 1/d^4$. Herein, d is the distance between a fluorophore and the metal surface. Thus, energy transfer to a surface follows a very different distance trend and magnitude of interaction from that in FRET. The exact form of the dipole-surface energy transfer is:

$$k_{\mathrm{SET}} = \frac{1}{\tau_0}\left(\frac{d_0}{d}\right)^4 \tag{10.9}$$

The characteristic distance length is

$$d_0 = \left(0.525\frac{c^3 Q_{\mathrm{D}}}{\omega^2 \omega_f k_f}\right)^{1/4} \tag{10.10}$$

In which Q_{D} is a function of the donor quantum efficiency, ω is the frequency of the donor electronic transition, ω_{f} is the Fermi frequency, and k_{f} is the Fermi wave vector of the metal. The interaction of fluorophores with metal surfaces is different, depending on the distance regime. At very close distances (<10 Å), radiative rate enhancement is observed; at intermediate distances (20–300 Å), energy transfer is the dominant process; and at very large distances (>500 Å), fluorescence oscillations due to dipole-mirror effects occur. The quantum efficiency (Φ_{SET}) of the energy transfer between a fluorophore and a metal can be expressed as:

$$\Phi_{\mathrm{SET}} = \frac{1}{1+\left(\frac{d}{d_0}\right)^n} \tag{10.11}$$

In which n is 4. Recall that n is 6 in FRET. Thus, interrogation of the slope of a plot of the energy transfer efficiency versus the separation distance of the donor and acceptor allows for the identification of the nature of the energy transfer mechanism.

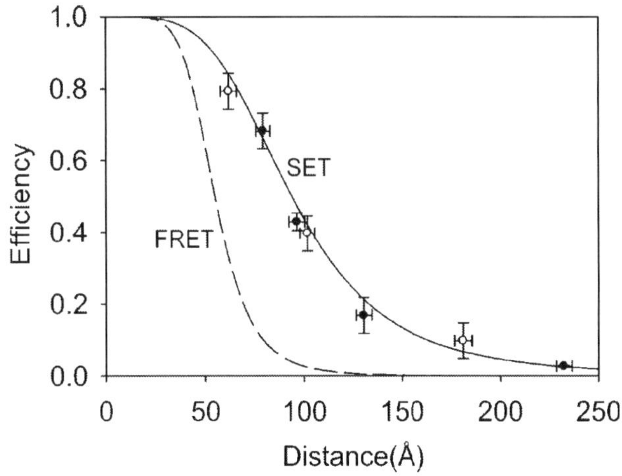

Figure 10.4 Energy transfer efficiency plotted versus separation distance between FAM and Au NPs. Filled circles (•) represent DNA lengths of 15 bp, 20 bp, 30 bp, and 60 bp. The measured efficiencies of these strands with the addition of *M. EcoRI* are represented by the open circles (∘). The dashed line is the theoretical FRET efficiency, while the solid line is the theoretical SET efficiency. Reprinted with permission from Ref. 34.

What will be the dominant quenching mechanism when a metal NP (diameter 1–100 nm) is used as the acceptor? Will the metal NP behave more like a dipole and be therefore FRET-like, or will it behave more like a metal surface and be SET-like? The distance dependence of the quenching efficiency between Au NPs and a donor dye (succinimidyl ester modified fluorescein; FAM) can answer the question.[34] A plot of the energy transfer efficiency versus the separation distance of a FAM-Au NP illustrates the distance-dependent behavior for the energy transfer from a molecular dipole to a NP (see Fig. 10.4). The theoretical energy transfer efficiency curves for a pure dipole–dipole (FRET) and dipole–surface (SET) energy transfer process are also displayed in Fig. 10.4. The curves facilitate calculations of R_0 and d_0, using Förster's equation and Persson and Lang's equation, respectively. The values of R_0 and d_0 are 59 Å and 94.3 Å, respectively. Comparison of the quenching efficiency and slope indicates poor agreement with a Förster mechanism ($1/R^6$) and precise agreement with the ($1/d^4$) plot, indicating the energy transfer process follows a SET route. To assess the trend in distance independently from the theoretical predictions, different values of r_0 and n as fitting parameters were used. For the six replicated experiments, the average value of n was 4.0 with an average r_0 of 92 Å at 50% quenching efficiency. These results are in good agreement (<2% error) with the theoretically calculated values for a SET mechanism (d_0 = 94.3 Å) while the strong discrepancy between the fit and the FRET model in terms of slope and distance eliminates FRET as the quenching mechanism. Therefore, the mechanism of fluorescence quenching for an organic dye near a metal NP is almost entirely due to the energy transfer to the metal surface, and thus the quenching efficiency is an $1/d^4$ distance dependence.

10.2.2 SEF

10.2.2.1 Surface plasmons

Use of the proper surface structures to resonantly couple the surface plasmon polariton (SPP) modes into radiative emission and to recover the energy is an important aspect of SEF. There are two main momentum matching techniques that are used to couple the SPP modes to photons. The first increases the momentum of the photon by using high index materials with specific optical geometries. The second technique involves breaking the translational invariance of a smooth metallic surface through corrugated or roughened surfaces. We discuss these techniques below.

10.2.2.1.1 *Flat metallic surfaces*

Coupling between propagative light and SPP on flat surfaces enhances both the excitation and the emission processes of the fluorophores. Because the evanescent EM field associated with SPP has its maximum at the surface, excitation processes are enhanced. Subsequently, the energy given to the SPP by near-field coupling with the fluorophore is recovered due to the enhancement of the emission processes. Therefore, fluorophore coupling with propagating SP plays a crucial role in SEF.

Using a Kretschmann configuration, surface plasmons on the front side of a metallic film (i.e., the fluorophore side) can be excited by the rear side. The Kretschmann configuration indicates that the index of refraction of the material on the rear side is higher than the one on the front side as shown in Fig. 10.5(A).

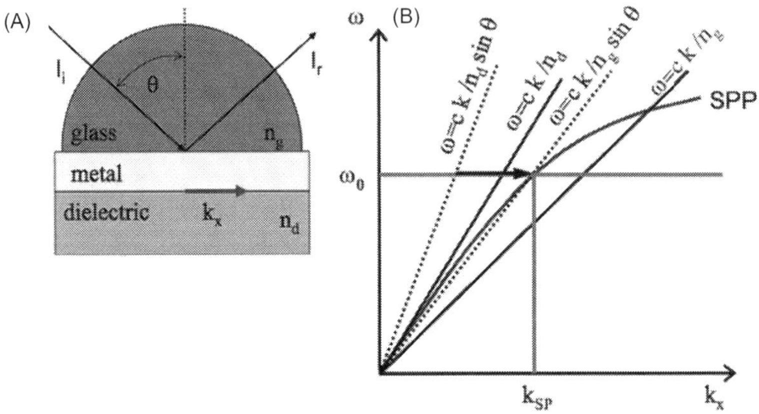

Figure 10.5 (A) A schematic representation of the Kretschmann optical configuration for the three layer stacking glass/metal/dielectric. The index of refraction of the glass prism n_g is higher than the one of the dielectric n_d. (B) Dispersion curves for the Kretschmann configuration showing that the resonant coupling between light and SPP is possible when the light cone crosses the SPP dispersion curve. The in-plane momentum for a given incident angle θ is increased by Δk, in which $\Delta k = \omega(n_g - n_d)/c$, ω is the angular frequency and c is the speed of light. Reprinted with permission from Ref. 13.

When illuminating the metallic thin film at an angle θ_0, the light in-plane wave vector is $k_{||} = n_g\, k_0 \sin\theta_0$, in which n_g and k_0 are the index of refraction of the glass prism and the momentum in free space, respectively. The dispersion relation for the SPPs propagating on the opposite side of the metallic thin film can thus be satisfied for a given incident angle θ_{SP} as shown in Fig. 10.5(B). The excitation of the SPP occurs at the minimum of the reflected intensity. At the resonant angle for SPP excitation, the reflected intensity equals zero for a specific thickness d_c of the metallic thin film.[38] At the same time, the EM field reaches its maximum at the metallic surface on the opposite side. The field can be significantly enhanced when compared to that with a similar configuration without the metal.[39]

In order to represent the enhanced factor of the EM field both with and without using a metal, enhancement (G) is used. G is defined as the ratio of the transmitted intensity of the EM field T_{metal} on the opposite side of the metallic thin film to the transmitted intensity without the metal $T_{\text{w/metal}}$. G is obtained using Fresnel's equation for a three layer stacking of glass/metal/dielectric:[40]

$$G = \frac{T_{\text{metal}}}{T_{\text{w/metal}}} = \frac{t_{\text{p}}^{\text{gm}} t_{\text{p}}^{\text{md}}}{1 + r_{\text{p}}^{\text{gm}} r_{\text{p}}^{\text{md}} \exp\left(2ik_{\text{zm}}d\right)} \tag{10.12}$$

where t_p^{ij} and r_p^{ij} (g – glass; m – metal; d – dielectric) are the Fresnel's transmission and reflection coefficients in p-polarization, respectively, for the boundary between media i and j when light is incident from i to j; d is the thickness of the metal thin film; and k_{zm} is the component of the wave vector in the metal normal to the surface. The resonant excitation of the SPP on one side of the metal thin film induces a charge oscillation that results in an enhanced EM field at the metal–dielectric interface. The EM field increases throughout the film thickness to reach a maximum at the metal–dielectric interface.[38] The calculated G values of the EM field at λ = 634 nm for an optimized film thickness of about d = 50 nm are 14.3 for Ag and 5.9 for Au.

10.2.2.1.2 *Corrugated surfaces*

SPPs are usually nonradiative because their wave vector (momentum) is greater than those of free photons of the same frequency, resulting from the fact that the real part of the SPP effective refractive index (n_{SPP}) is slightly larger than the refractive index of the dielectric medium. We note that $n_{\text{SPP}} = \sqrt{\varepsilon_{\text{d}}\varepsilon_{\text{m}}/\left(\varepsilon_{\text{d}} + \varepsilon_{\text{m}}\right)}$, in which ε_{d} and ε_{m} are the relative permittivities of the medium and that of the metal surface, respectively. Instead of a specific illumination condition, this momentum excess can be overcome using a textured metallic surface.

Patterning the metallic surface with a periodic wavelength scale corrugation provides an elegant solution for the excess of the momentum. Breaking the translational invariance of a thin film allows investigators to relax the momentum conservation restriction. For a periodic modulation of period z, the momentum conservation is now given by $k'_{\text{SP}} = k_{\text{SP}} \pm n\, g_{\text{B}}$ where g_{B} is the grating or Bragg wave vector that is equal to $2\pi/z$ and n is an integer. Figure 10.6 shows a typical example of the effective enhancement factor plotted as a function of the emission angle θ for a corrugated metal-clad waveguide sample versus a non-corrugated one.[41] With this corrugated metal-clad waveguide sample, the directionally scattered bound-mode features are clearly visible. The emission features can be attributed to the out-coupling of the three waveguide modes (two transverse magnetically polarized modes and one transverse electrically polarized mode). The prominent sharp peak at $\theta \approx 15°$ is associated with the SPP mode (i.e., the lowest transverse magnetic-polarized-polarized mode). The direction of the light beam is highly directional, following the moment conservation relation that can be quite interesting to increase signal to noise ratios.

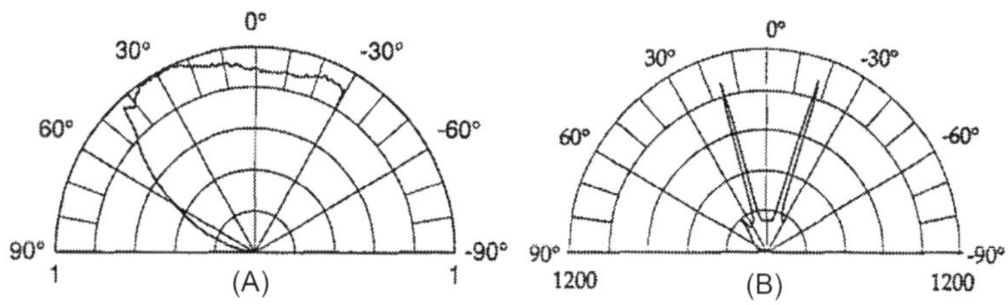

Figure 10.6 Measured effective enhancement factor versus emission angle θ for a corrugated metal-clad sample. The excitation angle is $\theta_{exc} = 45°$. The metal-clad waveguide is composed of glass/Ag/LiF/dye/air. The LiF thickness is $d = 300$ nm. (A) On a uncorrugated sample. (B) On a corrugated sample, the grating period is 640 nm and the grating depth is about 100 nm. Reprinted with permission from Ref. 41.

The efficiency with which a light beam can be recovered by scattering from a corrugated surface can be as high as 80% for the SPP propagating normal to the grooves.[42] This efficiency reaches an average value of 60% independent of the SPP direction using a bi-grating.[43] Recovering the energy transferred to the SPP modes by using grating couplers effectively increases the yield of light emitting diodes (LED), which necessarily incorporate metal contacts for efficient electron injection.[44,45] The presence of the grating directly affects the spontaneous emission of the emitters themselves since the photonic mode density they experience will necessarily be different from the planar case due to the different boundary conditions. Both the distance dependence of the lifetime and the spatial distribution of the emitted light significantly change upon the introduction of a corrugation quite apart from the Bragg-scattered bound-mode features.[46]

The efficiency of the light cross-coupling can also be enhanced by using corrugated thin films. The fluorescence emission from a structure with a corrugated thin metal film is over 50 times greater than that from a similar planar structure.[47] Samples containing a planar metal film with a corrugated dielectric overlayer have similar properties. The strong fluorescence emission is mediated via coupled SPPs, a factor which is promising for devices such as surface-emitting LEDs.

10.2.2.1.3 *Roughened surfaces*

The coupling of a fluorophore with a corrugated surface is a simpler approach than that with a roughened surface. In other words, roughened surfaces can be considered as multi-corrugated surfaces provided that the roughness is sufficiently small.[38] The emission of GaN quantum wells can be enhanced on rough metallic layers (50 nm thick Ag film) mainly because of the efficient scattering of SPPs into radiative modes.[48] A modulation depth of the Ag surface is approximately 30–40 nm with a length scale of a few hundred nanometers. An enhancement of light emission is generated using a corrugated grating while no enhancement is observed for either an uncoated GaN or a thick Ag film evaporated surface. This measurement suggests that the size of the metal structures determines the SP-photon coupling and light extraction.

The presence of metal nanostructures has a dramatic effect on the redirection of the angular emission of an individual molecule as well as on the enhancement of the excitation rate of the fluorophore. Researchers have experimentally observed the influence of nearby metal NPs on the angular photon emission on a single molecule (carbocyanine dye) for various dipole orientations.[49] For z-oriented molecules the emitted photons are attracted toward the center of the metal coating. For x-oriented molecules an influence is observed only for larger probe-sample separations.

In this section, we show how fluorescence enhancement on a flat surface is improved by surface shaping, additional corrugation, and roughness. Fluorescence is amplified by propagating surface plasmon modes. In the case of highly roughened surfaces, multiple electron scattering induces localization of the surface plasmons. The next section deals with SEF using localized and non-propagating surface plasmons. Successive enhancement processes starting from the simplest nanometric objects (single particles) to more complex surfaces will be described.

10.2.2.2 Localized enhancements

The EM field of a fluorophore can be significantly enhanced near metal nanomaterials when their sizes are much smaller than the illumination and/or detected wavelengths. When metal objects are much smaller than the wavelength, the EM fields are localized, giving rise to inhomogeneities in the EM field distribution. In fact, any discontinuity between a metal and a dielectric gives rise to inhomogeneities in the EM field distribution, a factor which is useful for the specific excitation of a given fluorophore.[50] Any localization of EM intensity near metal nanomaterials that couples to propagating modes increases the fluorescence of a fluorophore by several orders of magnitude. These high EM effects have been realized in various non-linear phenomena such as second harmonic generation[51–54] and Raman scattering.[55]

Researchers have studied the spatial localization of light in a number of metal systems, including single metal NPs, metal aggregates, and metal films.[56–58] Each system has its specific enhancement properties linked closely to its geometry. Single metal ellipsoids, for instance, are sources for generating an exceptionally large fluorescence enhancement (up to 50-fold). The fluorescence of a given fluorophore can be increased by more than 2 orders of magnitude by varying the gap (usually less than 50 nm) between two metal NPs, a procedure which is also wavelength dependent. Inhomogeneous metal films, given their random nature, are expected to enhance the fluorescence of various fluorophores simultaneously, allowing multiple fluorescence imaging.

In addition to the composition and shape, the size of the NPs plays an important role in determining SEF. There are many different interactions that have dramatically different effects on SEF, which are dependent on the fluorophore emission frequency (ω), on the distance (d) between the fluorophore and the metal, and on the size of the metal NPs.[59]

(i) When distance d is on the order of 1 nm, for the low frequency regime, $\omega \leqq \omega_{SP}$, where ω_{SP} is the surface plasmon frequency. The dominating phenomenon is Landau damping,[60] an efficient damping of the fluorescence.

(ii) When $d \geqq 1$ nm, for $\omega \approx \omega_{SP}$, coherent excitation of the surface plasmon occurs on metal NPs that act as a nanoantenna, enhancing the strength of the dipole oscillator and inducing enhanced fluorescence. It is worth noting that these enhancements can be applied to a variety of optical effects in which the signal is usually very low, for instance in surface enhanced Raman scattering (SERS)[25,61] and surface plasmon amplification by stimulated emission of radiation.[62]

(iii) When $d \geqq 1$ nm, for $\omega \approx \omega_{SP}$, besides the surface plasmon resonance, the propagating modes of SPPs are excited on a metal with macroscopic extension. In this case, the metal system acts as an optical antenna that propagates the excitation of the fluorophore to the far field, leading to an increase in the fluorescence efficiency and intensity but to a shorter fluorescence lifetime.[63]

The present section deals with the localization of light around metal nanomaterials when illuminated by an EM wave and how these localizations enhance the fluorescence. In the following sections, we will show how single particle and multiple particles interact strongly with light, leading to increased fluorescence. The differences in fluorescence enhancement among single objects, aggregates, and non-continuous films will be discussed.

10.2.2.2.1 *Single metal particles*

When the localized surface plasmon resonance of metal NPs couples with the emission of a fluorophore (the dipole), four interesting phenomena arise:[64]

(i) Close to a plasmon resonance, maximum radiative and nonradiative emission intensities may occur at various wavelengths.

(ii) The apparent quantum yield tends to be zero at the plasmon resonance frequency or when the distance between the fluorophore and the metal particle is close to zero.

(iii) The local field factor and the fluorescence enhancement reach a maximum at a wavelength slightly longer than the plasmon wavelength.

(iv) The fluorescence enhancement factor is much higher when the transition dipole is along the main axis of the metal NP (when the particle is not strictly symmetric).

Some interesting phenomena have been proved experimentally. It has been suggested that the dipole approximation neither strongly overestimates the quantum yield at short distances nor predicts fluorescence quenching while giving a fairly good estimate of the excitation rate.[65] In order to obtain a more accurate description of the nonradiative rate, higher multipole orders are necessary. A multiple multipole method is useful to correctly describe the observed variation of the fluorescence rate with respect to the particle-molecule distance.[66] The fluorescence enhancement of Nile blue dye achieves a maximum at a distance of 5 nm from the surface of 80 nm diameter Au NPs. When a laser with $\lambda = 637$ nm irradiates the Au NPs, the fluorescence enhancement of Nile blue is strongest at its fluorescence wavelength of 680 nm and weakest at another of its fluorescence wavelengths of 485 nm, showing the redshift of the excitation frequency with respect to the localized surface plasmon resonance of the Au NPs.

10.2.2.2.2 *Multiple metal NPs*

When two or more NPs are close to each other, the overall system is similar to an ensemble of elementary NPs. Contrary to a complex object having a spherical symmetry, polarization of the incident light is crucial when more than two NPs are close.[67,68] When two NPs are close enough to each other, the dipole of each NP induces a dipole on the other. This dipole–dipole interaction essentially hybridizes the elementary localized surface plasmon resonance. To achieve a narrow width of the localized surface plasmon resonance and increase the field enhancement, use of several NPs forming a chain-like structure is essential. The enhancement of the electric field can be calculated by using the electrostatic approximation.[69] If each particle enhances its applied field by a factor α, the cumulative effect of the chain of particles results in an enhancement factor of α^{n} where n is the number of NPs in the chain. However, it is difficult to prepare such a chain-like structure.

For specific shapes of NPs, the electromagnetic coupling inside the gap can lead to huge enhancements of 4 orders of magnitude.[70–72] For example, Au NPs have been used for producing nonlinear, optical four-wave mixing. By decreasing the interparticle distance from a large separation to that of touching contact, we can increase the 4 four-wave mixing yield by 4 orders of magnitude mainly because of the shift of the localized surface plasmon resonance to infrared wavelengths as the dimer forms. In a similar way as antennas in the radio wave regime, nanostructures are designed to increase the radiation efficiency of the fluorescent particle. For example, the interaction of a single quantum dot with a bowtie antenna enhances visible light.[73] When scanned over the quantum dot, the photoluminescence enhances while the excited state lifetime decreases, showing that the relaxation channels of a single quantum emitter can be controlled by coupling it to an efficiently radiating metallic nanoantenna. We point out that the optimum coupling requires impedance matching, depending on the wavelength and polarization of the light involved. Because the dielectric function of metal in the visible regime and in the radio wave regime differs significantly with respect to ohmic losses and plasmon resonance, the optimized antennas are significantly different in the two regimes.

In a mixture of metal NPs of various sizes, localized surface plasmon (LSP) resonance occurs at various photon energies, depending on the wavelength and the polarization of the incident light. Because of different LSP resonances, EM fields couple only within distances of less than 10 nm. However, coupling of LSP with long range interactions through the propagative modes of SPP can occur in random (semicontinuous) films.[74,75] The peculiarity of semicontinuous films lies in the range of accessible shapes and sizes of metal NPs on the surface. They are usually prepared by thermal evaporation of a metal on a dielectric surface followed by annealing. Metal evaporation ends around the percolation threshold when the first continuous electric path between opposite sides of the substrate appears. Around the percolation threshold, almost every size of metal NPs is present in the film, giving rise to resonances all over the film from the visible to the far infrared. In such films, the propagation of SPP enhances the resonant effect of LSP, leading to higher intensities of the propagating SPP waves. Not only does the random nature of the LSP modes broaden the accessible launching angles for SPP, but the various shapes of NPs also increase the number of accessible resonance wavelengths and polarizations.

The localization of light can also be carried out on rough Au films, aggregates, and colloidal films.[56–58] The size of the high intensity peaks, called hot spots, at which light is localized is much smaller than the wavelength of light. The predicted wavelength dependence of localized optical excitations has been experimentally shown.[76] A slight change in the wavelength or in the polarization properties of light allows changes in the position of these hot spots. Because of their strong nonlinear properties, random metal films are especially important for nonlinear, optical applications.[54,77] The local distribution of the EM field allows dramatic increases in nonlinear effects[51,53] that are used for multiphoton enhanced fluorescence.[78]

10.3 Analytical Applications

Depending upon the distance and geometry, a metal surface can result in the quenching of fluorescence or its enhancement by factors of up to 1000. As a result, fluorophores on metal surface can be employed in developing sensitive detection systems. In order to make the systems practical, recognition molecules such as antibody, enzymes, DNA, and ligands must be introduced. We now focus on their applications in protein immunoassays, DNA analysis, cell imaging, and metal ion detection.

10.3.1 Protein Immunoassays

Homogeneous and competitive fluorescence quenching immunoassays are sensitive for the analysis of proteins. One example is the use of Au NP/polyelectrolyte-coated polystyrene particles for the determination of the presence of biotin. Figure 10.7 shows a schematic illustration of a competitive fluorescence quenching immunoassay using a suspension of Au NP/PE-coated latexes.[79]

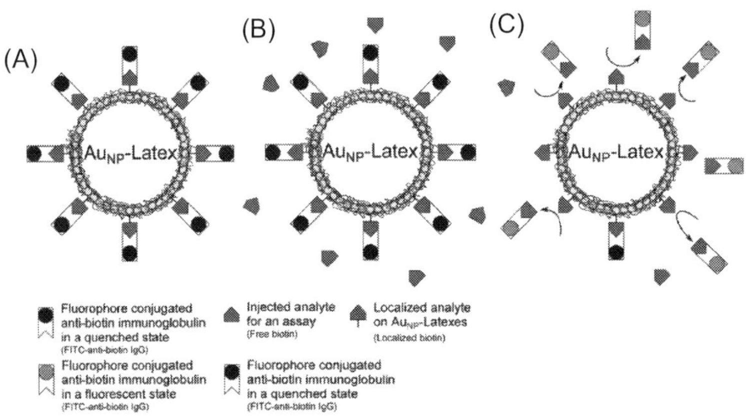

Figure 10.7 Schematic illustration of competitive immunoassays using a suspension of Au NP/PE-coated latexes. (A) Fluorophore-labeled antibodies are quenched before injection of analyte (biotin). (B) Injection of analyte. (C) Fluorophore-labeled antibodies fluoresce after being competitively released by biotin. Reprinted with permission from Ref. 79.

The sensing film is prepared on glass or quartz substrates with a layer-by-layer (LbL) technique. In this sensing system, Au NP/polyelectrolyte-coated polystyrene particles of 488 nm diameters act as quenching agents for a fluorescein isothiocyanate (FITC) that is labeled with anti-biotin immunoglobulin (anti-biotin IgG). Biotin molecules localize on the Au NP/polyelectrolyte-coated polystyrene particles by depositing a layer of biotinylated poly(allylamine hydrochloride), and FITC-anti-biotin IgGs are subsequently bound to the particles through interaction with the biotin. Transmission electron microscopy and quartz crystal microgravimetry confirm the multilayer formation on latex particles and planar Au surfaces, respectively. The biotin-functionalized Au NP/polyelectrolyte-coated polystyrene particles terminated by FITC-anti-biotin IgG exhibit a dynamic sensing range of 1–50 nmol for biotin.

Researchers have also developed a unique, sensitive, and highly specific fluoroimmunoassay system for antigen detection using Au NPs and magnetic NPs.[80] The assay is based on the fluorescence quenching of FITC caused by Au NPs coated with monoclonal antibody. To demonstrate its analytical capabilities, magnetic nanoparticles coated with anti-α-fetoprotein polyclonal antibodies, which specifically bind with α-fetoprotein, are used. Au NPs coated with anti-α-fetoprotein monoclonal antibodies sandwich the α-fetoprotein captured by the magnetic NP probes. A magnetic field can then be applied to separate the sandwich-type immunocomplex formed on the surface of the magnetic NPs. The supernatant liquid, which contains the unbound Au NPs probes, quenches the fluorescence. The fluorescence intensity of FITC at 516 nm is proportional to the α-fetoprotein concentration. This approach provides an LOD of 0.17 nM for α-fetoprotein.

Aptamer-conjugated Au NPs (Apt-Au NPs) are useful sensors for the detection of proteins. In these sensors, the Apt-Au NPs act as fluorescence quenchers. An Apt-Au NP-based molecular light switching sensor has been demonstrated for the analysis of platelet-derived growth factor (PDGF) and their receptors in homogeneous solutions.[81] Increases in the concentrations of PDGFs are associated with a variety of disorders, including atherosclerosis; fibroproliferative diseases of the lungs, kidneys, and joints; and neoplasia.[82,83] PDGFs also play important roles in cell transformation and tumor growth and progression.[84,85] The PDGF binding aptamer has a unique structure with a triple helical conformation that allows *N,N*-dimethyl-2,7-diazapyrenium dication (DMDAP) and PDGF bindings. The fluorescence of DMDAP is almost completely quenched by Apt-Au NPs when it intercalates with the aptamers. Once PDGFs bind to the Apt-Au NPs, the DMDAP molecules are released from the NP surfaces into the bulk solution, leading to increased fluorescence. Owing to the large magnitudes of these increases (up to 40-fold) in the turn-on fluorescence signals of DMDAP/Apt-Au NPs upon PDGFs binding, this approach is highly sensitive for the detection of PDGFs.

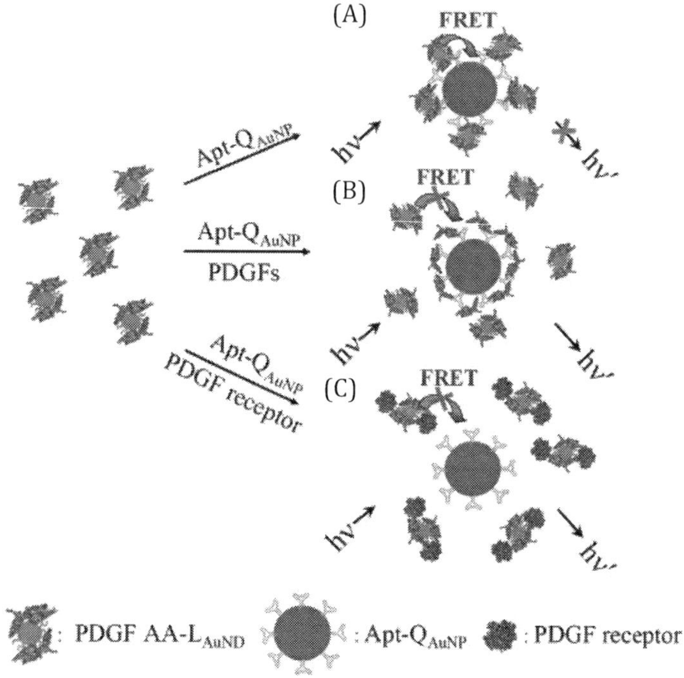

[a] h, Planck's constant; ν, frequency of light.

Figure 10.8 Schematic representations of PDGF and PDGF receptor nanosensors that operate based on the modulation of the photoluminescence quenching between PDGF AA-L$_{AuND}$ and Apt-Q$_{AuNP}$. Reprinted with permission from Ref. 86. See also Color Insert.

Use of two differently sized Au NPs, acting separately as donors and acceptors, in homogeneous photoluminescence quenching assays are sensitive for the analysis of proteins.[86] Introduction of a breast cancer marker protein, PDGF AA, to a solution of 11-mercaptoundecanoic acid-protected 2.0 nm photoluminescent Au nanodots (L_{AuND}) leads to the preparation of PDGF AA-L_{AuND} as the donor (see Fig. 10.8). Thiol derivative PDGF binding aptamers and 13 nm spherical Au NPs are used to synthesize the Apt-Q_{AuNP} acceptor. The photoluminescence of PDGF AA-L_{AuND} at 520 nm decreases when photoluminescence quenching occurs between Apt-Q_{AuNP} and PDGF AA-L_{AuND}. The PDGF AA-L_{AuND}/Apt-Q_{AuNP}-based molecular light switching system is useful for the analyses of PDGFs and PDGFα-receptor in separate homogeneous solutions with LODs of 80 pM and 0.25 nM respectively. In the presence of PDGFs, the interaction between Apt-Q_{AuNP} and PDGF AA-L_{AuND} decreases as a result of competitive reactions between the PDGFs and Apt-Q_{AuNP}. Similarly, the interaction between Apt-Q_{AuNP} and PDGF AA-L_{AuND} decreases as a result of competitive reactions between PDGFα-receptor and PDGF AA-L_{AuND}. When using the Apt-Q_{AuNP} as a selector for the enrichment of PDGF AA and the removal of matrixes possessing intense background fluorescence from cell media and urine samples, this approach provides an LOD for PDGF AA as low as 10 pM.

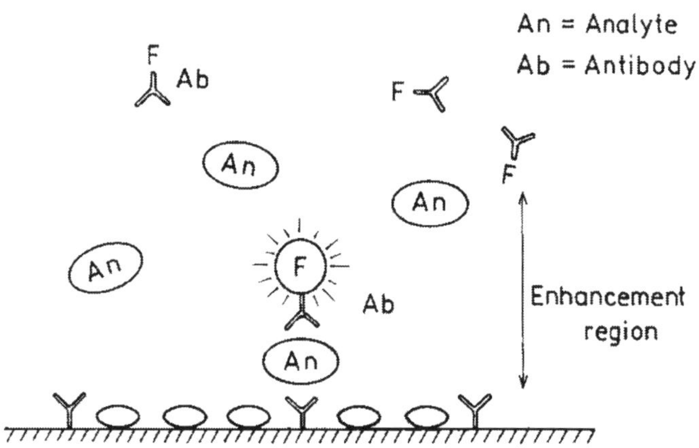

Figure 10.9 Sandwich immunoassay with low quantum yield fluorophores. Reprinted with permission from Ref. 28.

At present investigators usually strive to use fluorophores with the highest quantum yields to achieve greater sensitivity. However, these fluorophores sometimes may not be available or may not be suitable for the detection systems and/or labeling involved in specific experiments. When using metal surfaces, it may be desirable to use fluorophores with low quantum yields. Consider the schematic immunoassay displayed in Fig. 10.9. Assume that a capture antibody is covalently bound to the surface near the metal particles. The presence of the analyte (An) results in surface binding of a second antibody that is labeled with a nonfluorescent chromophore. Upon binding to the antigen the previously nonfluorescent species emits due to increases in the radiative rate. The unbound species that are located at longer distances from the metal site will not interfere because they do not fluoresce. The nonfluorescent species becomes a molecular switch, emitting only when close to the metal particles. Similarly, a sandwich-type immunoassay has been used for the determination of the cardiac marker myoglobin.[10] Myoglobin is first captured on silver-island films and glass surfaces coated with anti-myoglobin antibodies; the surfaces are then incubated with rhodamine Red-X-labeled anti-myoglobin antibodies. The fluorescence emission from the rhodamine Red-X-labeled antibody on the silver-island films is about 10–15-fold that on the glass substrate alone. This approach provides an LOD of 50 ng/mL for myoglobin, a value much lower than the clinical cut-off concentrations for myoglobin in healthy patients (100 ng/mL).

Indocyanine green is widely used in medical imaging and testing because of its safety in use and has been approved by the U.S. Food and Drug Administration. Indocyanine green-labeled human serum albumin that is bound to a noncontinuous coating of silver particles on a glass substrate increases its intensity approximately 20-fold and decreases the concomitant decay time.[87] Since the rate of photobleaching does not increase, indocyanine green-silver particle complexes can yield at least 20-fold more photons per indocyanine green molecule for improved medical imaging. The signal of a fluorophore can be further improved on Ag colloid coated surfaces that have elongated colloid aggregates. When a monolayer of Texas Red-labeled bovine serum albumin is separately deposited on the surfaces of noncontinuous coating of Ag particles and Ag colloid coated surfaces, the last provides a fluorescence signal approximately twice as strong under the same experimental conditions.[88] The last surface is also more efficient for the intensity decays of the fluorophore and does not provide the residual long-component of the intensity. Similar results are also found in fluorescein over-labeled human serum albumin deposited on the two surfaces.[88]

Variable shapes of nanomaterials such as Ag nanorods and triangular Ag NPs are also useful for SEF. The absorption spectra for Ag nanorods are somewhat different than their spherical Ag NPs, similarly showing a ~420 nm transverse absorption band with an additional ~580 nm longitudinal absorption. Ag nanorod-coated surfaces show density dependent fluorescence enhancements when coated with monolayers of human serum albumin labeled with indocyanine green with greater than 11-fold fluorescence enhancements.[89] The absorption spectra of Ag triangles differ from Ag nanorods and spherical Ag NPs, showing two SPR bands at about 450 and 550 nm. Ag triangle-coated surfaces also show density dependence of the fluorescence but provide greater enhancements of the monolayer of human serum albumin labeled with indocyanine green for similar surface optical densities.[90]

In addition to Ag NPs, Au and Cu NPs are also useful materials for SEF.[14–16] Au NPs with 40 and 200 nm diameters that are deposited onto glass substrates have been used to observe angular dependent fluorescence emission of fluorescein-human serum albumin.[14] The emission intensity of fluorescein-human serum albumin is 2.5-fold brighter than the emission on bare glass substrates at an angle of 270° due to factors explained by the Radiating Plasmon Model wherein the mixing system of the fluorophore and Au NPs emits following the photophysical characteristics of the fluorophore after the excitation. In addition, partial radiationless energy transfer occurs between the excited states of the fluorophore and the surface plasmons of the Au NPs. The fluorescence enhancement of 200 nm Au NPs is greater than that of 40 nm Au NPs due to the increased contribution of the scattering portion. When compared to Ag NPs, Au NPs offer more stable surfaces for applications requiring longer term storage and use. Cu NPs also provide similar SEF effects. Although surfaces coated with Cu NPs are not as stable as those coated with Au, they are cheaper.[16]

10.3.2 DNA Analysis

Completion of the human genome sequence is driving development of a wide variety of approaches to DNA analysis, including DNA arrays or gene chips, PCR-based assays, and hybridization assays.[91–94] Many of these assays are based on FRET. In the case of hybridization assays, the length of the sequence needs to be small enough to position the donors and acceptors within the Förster distance in order to achieve efficient FRET efficiencies, leading to great sensitivity.[93,94] This limitation may be overcome by conducting the assays on metal surfaces. Since the transfer distance can be increased 10-fold by a metal particle, the FRET assays can be performed if the donors and acceptors are 150 base pairs apart rather than the more typical 15 base pair difference. Alternatively, metal-enhanced FRET may be used to probe longer range structures in DNA, RNA, and ribosomes.

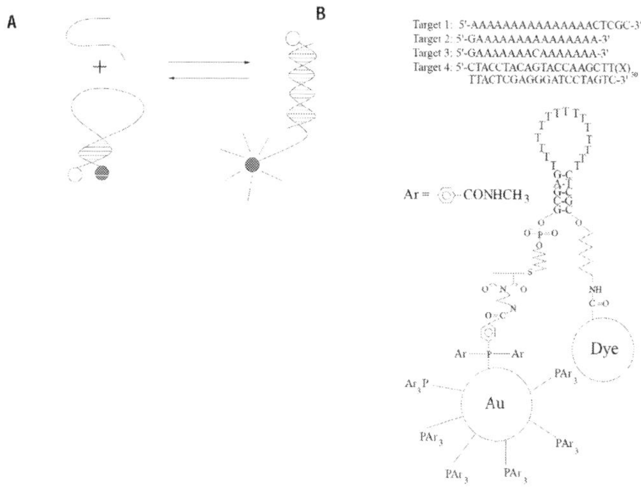

Figure 10.10 (A) Schematic drawings of the two conformations of the dye–oligonucleotide–Au conjugate and of the Au-quenched molecular beacon. (B) The oligonucleotide has a chain of 15 thymidines embedded into two complementary 5-nucleotide-long segments. The two hybridized segments form a hairpin stem with the probe sequence located in the hairpin loop. The maleimide of a monofunctional Au cluster that is 1.4 nm in diameter and passivated with on average 12 phosphine ligands is covalently linked to the 5′-terminal phosphate through a $(CH_2)_6$-SH group. The dye is linked to the 3′-hydroxyl group by a $(CH_2)_7$-NH_2 linker. Reprinted with permission from Ref. 96.

Molecular beacons (MBs) are commonly used for the detection of nucleic acids.[95] Generally, MBs are DNA sequences composed of one target-recognition region of about 15–30 bases flanked by two short complementary stem sequences, which force the entire sequence to form a stem-loop structure in the absence of a target. To allow the monitoring conformation changes in MBs upon reactions with targeted DNA, a fluorophore and a quencher are covalently conjugated at the termini of each MB strand. MBs act as FRET-based switches that are normally in the closed or fluorescence off state but that switch to the open or fluorescence on state in the presence of target (complimentary) DNA strands. However, a drawback of MBs is the limited quenching efficiency of the molecular quencher. When the molecular quencher is replaced with Au NPs, the quenching is much more efficient, resulting in more sensitive probes. As shown in Fig. 10.10, detection of target DNA can be performed by using a hybrid system containing a 1.4 nm Au NP, a single-stranded DNA molecule, and a fluorophore (rhodamine 6G) that is highly quenched by the NP through a distance dependent process.[96] When the single-stranded DNA (ssDNA) binds to complementary DNA, the fluorescence of this system increases by a factor of more than several thousand, resulting in sensitivity improvements up to 100-fold. The ability of this approach to detect a single mismatch within a strand of DNA is 8-fold greater than that of conventional MBs. Detection of DNA using DNA functionalized 2.5 nm Au NPs has been realized; the Au NP functions as both a nanoscaffold and a nanoquencher (an efficient energy acceptor).[97] Attached to this core are oligonucleotide molecules labeled with a thiol group at one end and a fluorophore at the other. This hybrid bioinorganic interaction spontaneously assembles into a constrained arch-like conformation on the particle surface. The binding of the target molecules results in a conformational change, which restores the fluorescence of the quenched fluorophore. Unlike conventional MBs with stem-and-loop structures, the NP probes do not require a stem, and their background fluorescence increases little with temperature. Researchers have demonstrated a novel fluorescent assay for DNA hybridization using Au NPs based on the electrostatic properties of DNA.[98] This assay takes advantage of the fact that ssDNA is adsorbed on negatively charged Au NPs while double-stranded DNA (dsDNA) is not. The fluorescence of dye-tagged (rhodamine red or Cy-5) probe sequences is efficiently quenched when they are mixed with Au NPs unless they hybridize with components of the analyte. This assay can detect sub-femtomole quantities of untagged target molecules in minutes.

DNA hybridization assays based on SEF are useful for the detection of DNA. When fluorescein-labeled complementary oligonucleotide is captured with thiolated-oligonucleotides that are bound to Ag NPs on a glass substrate, the fluorescence intensity increases 12-fold.[99] This effect is thought to result from the decreased fluorescence lifetime and SEF near metallic Ag NPs. The effects of SEF on Ag NP-coated glass surfaces have been measured for two dyes commonly used in DNA microarrays, Cy3 and Cy5.[12] Biotinylated, singly labeled 23 bp DNAs bind to avidin-coated silver surfaces, resulting in a fluorescence enhancement that is dependent on the DNA spotting concentration. Below ~12.5 μM, SEF fluorescence increases linearly, and at larger concentrations, SEF fluorescence remains at a constant maximum of 28-fold for Cy5 and 4-fold for Cy3 when compared to those on avidin-coated glass substrates. A detection system consisting of DNA-modified Ag NPs and a fluorophore-labeled complementary DNA is useful for the detection of DNA (see Fig. 10.11).[100]

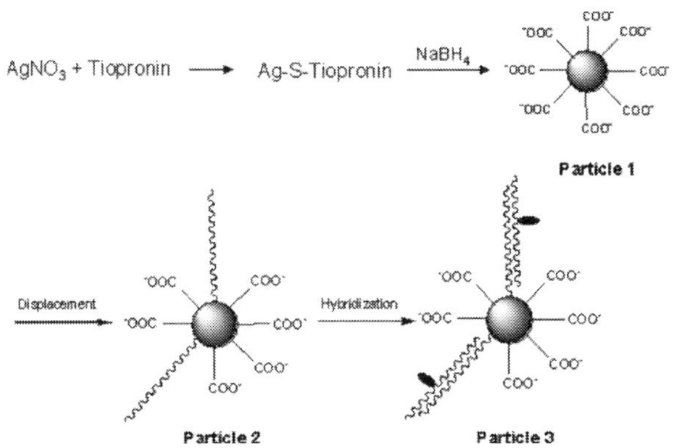

Figure 10.11 Preparation, displacement by thiolate oligonucleotides, and hybridization with fluorescein-labeled complementary oligonucleotides of tiopronin-monolayer protected Ag NPs. Reprinted with permission from Ref. 100.

Single-stranded oligonucleotides displace *N*-(2-mercaptopropionyl)- glycine (tiopronin) monolayer-protected Ag NPs through ligand exchanges. The oligonucleotide-displaced particles can then be hybridized with complementary fluorescein-labeled oligonucleotides. Both the oligonucleotide-displaced and hybridized particles form aggregates via electrostatic interactions with salt (10 mM KCl) in buffer solution. Because the aggregates display enhanced luminescence from fluorescein, DNA can be detected.

All presently used DNA assays rely on extrinsic probes (labeling) that are used to impart strong fluorescence to intrinsically nonfluorescent DNA. Because this labeling usually requires time consuming processes and produces undesirable byproducts, techniques that allow for the detection of DNA though its intrinsic fluorescence are desired. When DNA is adjacent to a metal surface, its radiative decay rate increases after being excited by UV light, leading to the enhanced intrinsic emissions of DNA.[28] There are several commercial UV lasers for this purpose, including Ar ion lasers, ArF excimer lasers, Nd:YAG lasers, and several others. One problem with using UV lasers for excitation is the fluorescence interference from sample matrixes such as proteins. In addition, UV lasers are usually more expensive, and their maintenance is usually more necessary and costly. These problems can be overcome by using visible or NIR lasers when applying two-photon or multiphoton excitation. Metal NPs can accelerate two-photon or multiphoton excitation due to enhanced local EM fields.

10.3.3 Other Applications

Fluorescence microscopy is a prevalent technique for cell imaging. Although systems for obtaining high resolution cell images are available, systems that allow for the simultaneous monitoring of a number of cells are still necessary when statistical investigations are conducted. Such systems require both low magnification to obtain a reliable statistical population and high contrast to obtain an accurate diagnosis of the nature of the cells' perturbation. Because microscopic objectives with low magnification generally yield low collection efficiency, such studies are limited by the fluorescence signal weakness. To overcome this technological bottleneck, metal-coated substrates that enhance the fluorescence process and improve collection efficiency in epifluorescence observations are used in commercial microscopes.[101] The presence of a reflective surface modifies both the excitation and emission processes and additionally reshapes the fluorescence emission images. This system produces increased fluorescence signal from a layer of Cy3 dye on a substrate by a factor ~30. Metal plasmon-coupled probes have been demonstrated for the fluorescence imaging of HEK 293 A and

T-lymphocytic cells with single cell resolution.[102,103] The fluorescent metal plasmon-coupled probes are Alexa Fluor 647-labeled concanavalin A (con A) bound to *N*-(2-mercapto-propionyl)glycine-coated Ag NPs. Imaging results demonstrate that cells labeled by this probe are 20-fold brighter than those labeled with free con A.

The quenching properties of Au NPs have been applied to develop a Hg^{2+} sensor in aqueous solution. When the dye rhodamine B (RB) is adsorbed onto Au NPs surfaces, quenching occurs, leading to weak fluorescence. However, in the presence of Hg^{2+} ions, RB molecules are quickly replaced and released to the bulk solution, leading to increased florescence of the RB in the 10 minute window (see Fig. 10.12).[104]

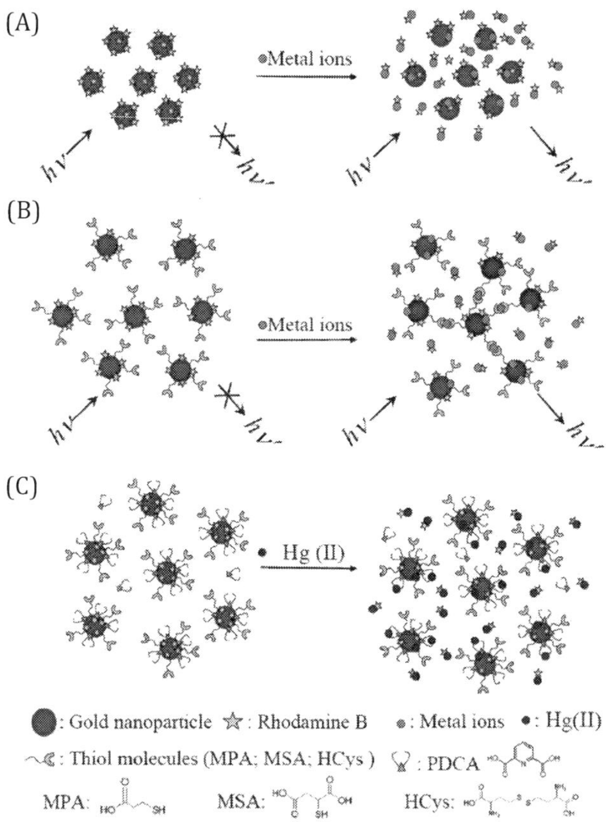

Figure 10.12 Schematic representations of Hg(II) nanosensors that operate on the basis of modulation of the FRET between RB and Au NPs. Reprinted with permission from Ref. 104.

The selectivity of the probe for Hg^{2+} ions can be further improved by adding a chelating ligand (2,6-pyridinedicarboxylic acid) to the sample solutions when using Au NPs capped with mercaptopropionic acid. This approach provides an LOD of 2.0 ppb for Hg^{2+} ions, a selectivity 50 times that of other metal ions.

Use of DNA-functionalized Au NPs and OliGreen, a dye that binds specifically to DNA, is selective and sensitive for the detection of Hg^{2+} ions. When OliGreen binds to DNA on the Au NPs surfaces, its fluorescence is weak as a result of Au NP quenching. Once Hg^{2+} ions interact with the thymidine units of the DNA molecules on the Au NPs, the conformations of these DNA derivatives change from linear to hairpin structures (see Fig. 10.13).[105]

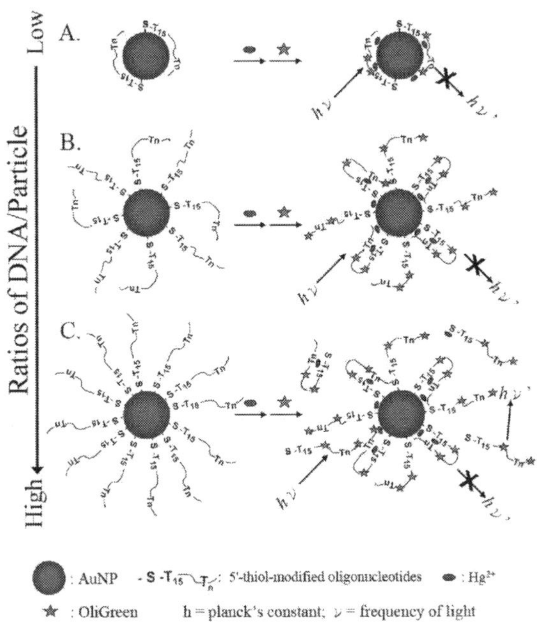

Figure 10.13 Schematic representation of Hg^{2+} nanosensors at various DNA-to-Au NPs molar ratios: <30 (A), 30–50 (B), and >60 (C). Reprinted with permission from Ref. 105.

As a result, some of the DNA-OliGreen complexes release from the surface of the Au NPs into the bulk solution, leading to increased fluorescence. This system is the first that allows for the detection of Hg^{2+} ions based on the release of DNA molecules induced by conformational changes on Au NP surfaces. The sensitivity of this approach is highly dependent upon the surface DNA density. Under optimum conditions, this approach provides an LOD at the nanomolar level for Hg^{2+} ions.

10.4 Conclusions and Outlook

Fluorescence quenching and SEF using novel metals have proved themselves sensitive techniques for the detection of proteins, DNA, and small solutes. Whether metal surfaces and NPs possess quenching effects or SEF is highly dependent on the distance between a fluorophore and the metal object. When the distance is less than 50 Å, fluorescence quenching occurs. On the other hand, when the distance is between 70–100 Å, SEF most likely takes place. Fluorescence quenching by metal NPs shows fourth order distance dependence, which differs from FRET. SEF efficiency can be controlled by tailoring the EM field of the fluorophore by carefully varying the surface morphology of the metal surfaces. Metallic nanostructured surfaces (corrugated or rough surfaces) provide much greater SEF efficiencies when compared to those obtained on flat metal surfaces. When metal NPs are used, SEM effects can be controlled by varying their sizes and shapes as well as the distance between them. SEF does not only amplify the molecular fluorescence emission but also modifies the fluorescence lifetime, photobleaching, intermolecular coupling, and emission patterns.

Although SEF techniques are not as popular as fluorescence quenching and surface enhanced Raman spectroscopy in the present analytical environment, its use has been recognized in the detection of DNA and proteins. In addition, specific illumination configurations (e.g., Kretschmann's configuration) allow for the efficient excitation of fluorophores in certain local areas through the excitation of plasmon modes, which are of particular interest for local probing such as cell imaging. The processes described in SEF are readily applicable to other molecular luminescence techniques such as chemiluminescence, electroluminescence, and phosphorescence.

The advanced nanotechnology research has spurred the preparation of many nanomaterials, including Au-Ag nanrods, Au nanowires, Ag nanoflowers,[106–111] and many others, which possess great potential for developing highly sensitive SEF techniques. Nanoparticles can be advantageously coupled to fluorophores to locally enhance their fluorescences when deposited on surfaces or as free probes. In addition, surfaces that have well defined patterns and structures on the nanometric scale (e.g., two-dimensional photonic crystal slabs) can provide increased fluorescence intensities by a factor of up to 100 as opposed to smooth surfaces.[112] Along with advanced nanotechnology, we can foresee that SEF techniques soon will become popular and powerful techniques for the analysis of trace amounts of analytes and for cell imaging.

Acknowledgments

This work was supported by the National Science Council of Taiwan under contracts NSC 98-2113-M-002-011-MY3 and NSC 99-2113-M-018-005-MY2. We would like to thank those who provided preprints that were used in this article.

References

1. A. Hagfeldt, and M. Grätzel, *Acc. Chem. Res.*, **33**, 269 (2000).
2. M. Quintana, T. Edvinsson, A. Hagfeldt, and G. Boschloo, *J. Phys. Chem. C*, **111**, 1035 (2007).
3. P. K. Sudeep, B. I. Ipe, K. G. Thomas, and M. V. George, *Nano Lett.*, **2**, 29 (2002).
4. D. M. Adams, L. Brus, C. E. D. Chidsey, S. Creager, C. Creutz, C. R. Kagan, P. V. Kamat, M. Lieberman, S. Lindsay, R. A. Marcus, R. M. Metzger, M. E. Michel-Beyerle, J. R. Miller, M. D. Newton, D. R. Rolison, O. Sankey, K. S. Schanze, J. Yardley, and X. Zhu, *J. Phys. Chem. B*, **107**, 6668 (2003).
5. F. Cannone, M. Collini, L. D'Alfonso, G. Baldini, G. Chirico, G. Tallarida, and P. Pallavicini, *Nano Lett.*, **7**, 1070 (2007).
6. C. Li, X. Liu, M. Yuan, J. Li, Y. Guo, J. Xu, M. Zhu, J. Lv, H. Liu, and Y. Li, *Langmuir*, **23**, 6753 (2007).
7. C. D. Geddes, and J. R. Lakowicz, *J. Fluoresc.*, **12**, 121 (2002).
8. C. D. Geddes, A. Parfenov, and J. R. Lakowicz, *Appl. Spectrosc.*, **57**, 526 (2003).
9. J. R. Lakowicz, C. D. Geddes, I. Gryczynski, J. Malicka, Z. Gryczynski, K. Aslan, J. Lukomska, E. Matveeva, J. Zhang, R. Badugu, and J. Huang, *J. Fluoresc.*, **14**, 425 (2004).
10. K. Aslan, I. Cryczynski, J. Malicka, E. Matveeva, J. R. Lakowicz, and C. D. Geddes, *Curr. Opin. Biotechnol.*, **15**, 55 (2005).

11. M. Kawasaki, and S. Mine, *Chem. Lett.*, **34**, 1038 (2005).
12. C. R. Sabanayagam, and J. R. Lakowicz, *Nucleic Acids Res.*, **35**, e13 (2007).
13. E. Fort, and S. Grésillon, *J. Phys. D: Appl. Phys.*, **41**, 013001 (2008).
14. K. Aslan, S. N. Malyn, and C. D. Geddes, *J. Fluoresc.*, **17**, 7 (2007).
15. J. Zhang, and J. R. Lakowicz, *Opt. Express*, **15**, 2598 (2007).
16. Y. Zhang, K. Aslan, M. J. R. Previte, and C. D. Geddes, *Appl. Phys. Lett.*, **90**, 173116 (2007).
17. E. M. Purcell, *Phys. Rev.*, **69**, 681 (1946).
18. J. M. Gérard, B. Sermage, B. Gayral, B. Legrand, E. Costard, and V. Thierry-Mieg, *Phys. Rev. Lett.*, **81**, 1110 (1998).
19. P. Michler, A. Kiraz, C. Becher, W. V. Schoenfeld, P. M. Petroff, L. Zhang, E. Hu, and A. Imamoglu, *Science*, **290**, 2282 (2000).
20. P. Lodahl, van D. A. Floris, I. S. Nikolaev, A. Irman, K. Overgaag, D. Vanmaekelbergh, and W. L. Vos, *Nature*, **430**, 654 (2004).
21. A. Kress, F. Hofbauer, N. Reinelt, M. Kaniber, H. J. Krenner, R. Meyer, G. Bohm, and J. J. Finley, *Phys. Rev. B*, **71**, 241304 (2005).
22. M. Nomura, S. Iwamoto, T. Yang, S. Ishida, and Y. Arakawa, *Appl. Phys. Lett.*, **89**, 241124 (2006).
23. W. L. Barnes, A. Dereux, and T. W. Ebbesen, *Nature*, **424**, 824 (2003).
24. A. M. Glass, A. Wokaun, J. P. Heritage, J. G. Bergman, P. F. Liao, and D. H. Olson, *Phys. Rev. B*, **24**, 4906 (1981).
25. M. Moskovists, *Rev. Mod. Phys.*, **57**, 783 (1985).
26. C. C. Schatz, in *Handbook of Vibrational Spectroscopy*, Ed. R. P. Van Duyne (Wiley, New York, 2002).
27. A, Champion, A. R. Gallo, C. B. Harris, H. J. Robota, and P. M. Whitmore, *Chem. Phys. Letts.*, **73**, 447 (1980).
28. J. R. Lakowicz, *Anal. Biochem.*, **298**, 1 (2001).
29. J. Gersten, and A. Nitzan, *J. Chem. Phys.*, **75**, 1139 (1981).
30. M. R. Philpott, *J. Chem. Phys.*, **62**, 1812 (1975).
31. R. R. Chance, A. Prock, and R. Silbey, *Adv. Chem. Phys.*, **37**, 1 (1978).
32. D. A. Weitz, S. Garoff, J. I. Gersten, and A. Nitzan, *J. Chem. Phys.*, **78**, 5324 (1983).
33. H. Chew, *J. Chem. Phys.*, **87**, 1355 (1987).
34. C. S. Yun, A. Javier, T. Jennings, M. Fisher, S. Hira, S. Peterson, B. Hopkins, N. O. Reich, and G. F. Strouse, *J. Am. Chem. Soc.*, **127**, 3115 (2005).

35. B. Persson, and N. Lang, *Phys. Rev. B*, **26**, 5409 (1982).

36. A. P. Alivisatos, D. H. Waldeck, and C. B. Harris, *J. Chem. Phys.*, **82**, 541 (1985).

37. K. Kuhnke, R. Becker, M. Epple, and K. Kern, *Phys. Rev. Lett.*, **79**, 3246 (1997).

38. H. Raether, in *Surfaces Plasmons on Smooth and Rough Surfaces and on Gratings* (*Springer Tracts in Modern Physics vol 111*) (Springer, Berlin, 1988).

39. J. Enderlein, and T. Ruckstuhl, *Opt. Express*, **13**, 8856 (2005).

40. M. Born, in *Principles of Optics* 7th *edn*, Ed. E. Wolf (Cambridge University Press, Cambridge, 1999).

41. K. G. Sullivan, O. King, C. Sigg, and D. G. Hall, *Appl. Opt.*, **33**, 2447 (1994).

42. J. Moreland, A. Adams, and P. K. Hansma, *Phys. Rev. B*, **25**, 3340 (1982).

43. W. L. Barnes, *J. Mod. Opt.*, **45**, 661 (1998).

44. J. M. Lupton, B. J. Matterson, I. D. W. Samuel, M. J. Jory, and W. L. Barnes, *Appl. Phys. Lett.*, **77**, 3340 (2000).

45. A. Kock, W. Beinstingl, K. Berthold, and E. Gornik, *Appl. Phys. Lett.*, **52**, 1164 (1988).

46. P. Andrew, and W. L. Barnes, *Phys. Rev. B*, **64**, 125405 (2001).

47. S. Wedge, and W. L. Barnes, *Opt. Express*, **12**, 3673 (2004).

48. K. Okaoto, I. Niki, A. Shvartser, Y. Narukawa, T. Mukai, and A. Scherer, *Nature Mater.*, **3**, 601 (2004).

49. H. Gersen, M. F. García-Parajó, L. Novotny, J. A. Veerman, L. Kuipers, and N. F. Van Hulst, *Phys. Rev. Lett.*, **85**, 5312 (2000).

50. J. J. Bowman, in *Electromagnetic and Acoustic Scattering by Simple Shapes*, Ed. T. B. A. Senior and P. L. E. Uslenghi (Hemisphere, Bristol, 1987).

51. G. T. Boyd, Th Rasing, L. R. R. Leite, and Y. R. Shen, *Phys. Rev. B*, **30**, 519 (1984).

52. I. I. Smolyaninov, A. V. Zayats, and C. C. Davis, *Phys. Rev. B*, **56**, 9290 (1997).

53. C. Anceau, S. Brasselet, J. Zyss, and P. Gadenne, *Opt. Lett.*, **28**, 713 (2003).

54. M. I. Stockman, D. J. Bergman, C. Anceau, S. Brasselet, and J. Zyss, *Phys. Rev. Lett.*, **92**, 057401 (2004).

55. F. Brousers, S. Lacher, A. N. Lagarkov, A. K. Sarichev, P. Gadenne, and V. M. Shalaev, *Phys. Rev. B*, **55**, 13234 (1997).

56. S. I. Bozhelvolni, B. Vohnsen, I. I. Smolyaninov, and A. V. Zayats, *Opt. Commun.*, **117**, 417 (1995).

57. S. N. Bozhelvolnyi, V. A. Markel, V. Coello, W. Kim, and V. M. Shalaev, *Phys. Rev. B*, **58**, 11441 (1998).

58. P. Shang, T. L. Haslett, C. Douketis, and M. Moskovits, *Phys. Rev. B*, **57**, 15513 (1998).

59. R. Carminati, J. J. Greffet, C. Henkel, and J. M. Vigoureux, *Opt. Commun.*, **261**, 368 (2006).

60. I. A. Larkin, M. I. Stockman, M. Achermann, and V. I. Kilmov, *Phys. Rev. B*, **69**, 121403 (2004).

61. D. A. Weitz, T. J. Gramila, A. Z. Genack, and J. I. Gersten, *Phys. Rev. Lett.*, **45**, 355 (1980).

62. D. J. Bergman, and M. I. Stockman, *Laser Phys.*, **14**, 409 (2004).

63. R. M. Roth, N. C. Panoiu, M. M. Adams, R. M. Osgood, C. C. Neacsu, and M. B. Raschke, *Opt. Express*, **14**, 2921 (2006).

64. M. Thomas, J. J. Greffet, R. Carminati, and J. R. Arias-Gonzalez, *Appl. Phys. Lett.*, **85**, 3863 (2004).

65. P. Anger, P. Bharadwaj, and L. Novotny, *Phys. Rev. Lett.*, **96**, 113002 (2006).

66. L. Novotny in *Principles of Nano-Optics*, Ed. B. Hecht (Cambridge University Press, Cambridge, 2006).

67. E. Hao, and C. C. Schatz, *J. Chem. Phys.*, **120**, 357 (2004).

68. J. P. Kottmann, and O. J. F. Martin, *Opt. Express*, **8**, 655 (2001).

69. K. Li, M. I. Stockman, and D. J. Bergman, *Phys. Rev. Lett.*, **91**, 227402 (2002).

70. E. Cubukcu, E. A. Fort, K. B. Crozier, and F. Capasso, *Appl. Phys. Lett.*, **89**, 093120 (2006).

71. M. Danckwerts, and L. Novotny, *Phys. Rev. Lett.*, **98**, 026104 (2007).

72. T. Sondergraad, and S. Bozhevolnyi, *Phys. Rev. B*, **75**, 073402 (2007).

73. J. N. Farahani, D. W. Pohl, H. J. Eisler, and B. Hecht, *Phys. Rev. Lett.*, **95**, 017402 (2005).

74. A. V. Zayats, and I. I. Smolyaninov, *J. Opt. A: Pure Appl. Opt.*, **5**, S16 (2003).

75. P. Gadenne, in *Nonlinear Optics of Nanostructured Random Media*, Ed. J. C. Rivoal (Springer, Berlin, 2002) P183.

76. S. Ducourtieux, *Phys. Rev. B*, **64**, 165403 (2001).

77. V. M. Shalae, in *Nonlinear Optics of Random Media-Fractal Composites and Metal-Dielectric Films* (Springer, Berlin, 2000).

78. W. Wenseleers, F. Stellacci, T. Meyer-Friedrichsen, T. Mangel, C. A. Bauer, S. J. K. Pond, S. R. Marder, and J. W. Perry, *J. Phys. Chem. B*, **106**, 6853 (2002).

79. N. Kato, and F. Caruso, *J. Phys. Chem. B*, **109**, 19604 (2005).

80. L. Ao, F. Gao, B. Pan, R. He, and D. Cui, *Anal. Chem.*, **78**, 1104 (2006).

81. C.-C. Huang, S.-H. Chiu, Y.-F. Huang, and H.-T. Chang, *Anal. Chem.*, **79**, 4798 (2007).

82. J. S. Huang, and S. S. Huang, *Cell*, **39**, 79 (1984).

83. R. Ross, E. W. Raines, and D. F. Bowen-Pope, *Cell*, **46**, 155 (1986).

84. A. Greco, E. Roccato, C. Miranda, L. Cleris, F. Formelli, and M. A. Pierotti, *Int. J. Cancer*, **92**, 354 (2001).

85. R. H. Alvarez, H. M. Kantarjian, and J. E. Cortes, *Mayo Clin. Proc.*, **81**, 1241 (2006).

86. C.-C. Huang, C.-K. Chiang, Z.-H. Lin, K.-H. Lee, and H.-T. Chang, *Anal. Chem.*, **80**, 1497 (2008).

87. J. Malicka, I. Gryczynski, C. D. Geddes, and J. R. Lakowicz, *J. Biomed. Opt.*, **8**, 472 (2003).

88. J. Lukomska, J. Malicka, I. Gryczynski, and J. R. Lakowicz, *J. Fluoresc.*, **14**, 417 (2004).

89. K. Aslan, Z. Leonenko, J. R. Lakowicz, and C. D. Geddes, *J. Phys. Chem. B*, **109**, 3157 (2005).

90. K. Aslan, J. R. Lakowicz, and C. D. Geddes, *J. Phys. Chem. B*, **109**, 6247 (2005).

91. T. L. Ferea, and P. O. Brown, *Curr. Opin, Genet. Dev.*, **9**, 715 (1999).

92. C. A. Harrington, C. Rosenow, and J. Retief, *Curr. Opin. Microbiol.*, **3**, 285 (2000).

93. L. E. Morrison, Detection of energy transfer and fluorescence quenching. In *Nonisotopic Probing, Blotting and Sequencing*, Ed. L. J. Kricka (Academic Press, New York, 1996), p. 429.

94. K. M. Parkhurst, and L. J. Parkhurst, *J. Biomed. Opt.*, **1**, 435 (1996).

95. K. Wang, Z. Tang, C. J. Yang, Y. Kim, X. Fang, W. Li, Y. Wu, C. D. Medley, Z. Cao, J. Li, P. Colon, H. Lin, and W. Tan, *Angew. Chem. Int. Ed.*, **37**, 2 (2008).

96. B. Dubertret, M. Calame, and A. J. Libchaber, *Nat. Biotechnol.*, **19**, 365 (2001).

97. D. J. Maxwell, J. R. Taylor, and S. Nie, *J. Am. Chem. Soc.*, **124**, 9606 (2002).
98. H. Li, and L. J. Rothberg, *Anal. Chem.*, **76**, 5414 (2004).
99. J. Malicka, I. Gryczynski, and J. R. Lakowicz, *Biochem. Biophys. Res. Commun.*, **306**, 213 (2003).
100. J. Zhang, J. Malicka, I. Gryczynski, and J. R. Lakowicz, *Anal. Biochem.*, **330**, 81 (2004).
101. E. L. Moal, E. Fort, S. Lévêque-Fort, F. P. Cordelières, M. P. Fontaine-Aqpart, and C. Ricolleau, *Biophys. J.*, **92**, 2150 (2007).
102. J. Zhang, Y. Fu, and J. R. Lakowicz, *Bioconjugate Chem.*, **18**, 800 (2007).
103. J. Zhang, Y. Fu, D. Liang, K. Nowaczyk, R. Y. Zhao, and J. R. Lakowicz, *Nano Lett.*, **4**, 1179 (2008).
104. C.-C. Huang, and H.-T. Chang, *Anal. Chem.*, **78**, 8332 (2006).
105. C.-W. Liu, C.-C. Huang, and H.-T. Chang, *Langmuir*, **24**, 8346 (2008).
106. C.-C. Huang, Z. Yang, and H.-T. Chang, *Langmuir*, **20**, 6086 (2004).
107. Z. Yang, and H. T. Chang, *Nanotechnology*, **17**, 2304 (2006).
108. Y.-F. Huang, Y.-W. Lin, and H.-T. Chang, *Nanotechnology*, **17**, 4885 (2006).
109. K.-H. Lee, K.-M. Huang, W.-L. Tseng, T.-C. Chiu, Y.-W. Lin, and H.-T. Chang, *Langmuir*, **23**, 1435 (2007).
110. Z. Yang, Z.-H. Lin, C.-Y. Tang, and H.-T. Chang, *Nanotechnology*, **18**, 255606 (2007).
111. Z.-H. Lin, Z. Yang, and H.-T. Chang, *Langmuir*, **24**, 365 (2008).
112. N. Ganesh, W. Zhang, P. C. Mathias, E. Chow, J. A. N. T. Soares, V. Maylyarchuk, A. D. Smith, and B. T. Cunningham, *Nat. Nanotechnol.*, **2**, 515 (2007).

Chapter 11

Surface-Enhanced Raman Scattering Based on Noble Metal Nanoparticles

Li-Lin Tay* **and John E. Hulse**
National Research Council Canada, 1200 Montreal Road, Ottawa Ontario K1A0R6, Canada
*lilin.tay@nrc-cnrc.gc.ca

Surface-enhanced Raman scattering (SERS) is a powerful spectroscopic technique that leverages the enormous electromagnetic field enhancement caused by the excitation of an intense, sharp and localized surface plasmon resonance of metal nanostructures. The effect can provide rich structural and chemical information for molecules adsorbed on or bonded to SERS active nanometer-sized metal structures. Recent advances in nanotechnology and nanofabrication techniques have enabled researchers to design SERS active colloidal nanoparticle (NP) systems with optimized electromagnetic enhancements engendering a large variety of SERS-based bioanalytical and bioimaging applications. The advantages of SERS over standard fluorescent labeling techniques lie not only in its multiplexing capability and superior photostability, but also in the potential multimodal functionality provided by the other intrinsic properties of the metal NPs, such as the photothermal response which enable its therapeutic role in the treatment of cancer.[1] This

From Bioimaging to Biosensors: Noble Metal Nanoparticles in Biodetection
Edited by Lai-Kwan Chau and Huan-Tsung Chang

ISBN 978-981-4267-24-3 (Hardcover), 978-981-4303-10-1 (eBook)
www.panstanford.com

chapter reviews the enhancement mechanisms that lead to SERS and discuss the important methods used to strengthen the effect. The chapter then focuses on recent reports of the achievements of metal NP-based SERS in bioanalytical applications with specific attention given to its use in pathogen detection and bioimaging.

11.1 Introduction

Raman spectroscopy is a vibrational technique which provides a wealth of information on the molecular species under interrogation. Its many fields of application include identification and structural characterization of semiconductor materials, authentication of artifacts and legal documentations, quality control in pharmaceutical manufacturing, and the development of new biophysical tools for disease diagnosis and health monitoring. A major disadvantage of Raman spectroscopy is the inherently small scattering cross section of the Raman process, which is typically 12–14 orders of magnitudes smaller than fluorescence cross-sections. This was why the observation of an unexpectedly large Raman signals from pyridine adsorbed on roughened Ag electrode surprised researchers in the field. In 1974, Fleischmann *et al.* reported intense Raman scattering from pyridine adsorbed onto a Ag electrode roughened through repeated oxidation–reduction cycles in an attempt to develop an *in situ* monitoring tool that is chemically specific.[2] The authors attributed the large pyridine Raman signal to the increase in number of molecules adsorbed on the increased surface area of the roughened Ag electrode. In 1977, Van Duyne *et al.* recognized that the large intensity observed could not be accounted for by the increase in the number of scatterers and proposed an electric field enhancement model to account for their observation.[3] Ultimately, it was the 1978 report by Moskovits, in which he put forward an interpretation in terms of electromagnetic resonances in the form of a localized surface plasmon resonance (LSPR) in noble metal nanostructures that paved the way for the electromagnetic enhancement theory as it is currently understood.[4] In that same report, Moskovits also predicted that a similar intense SERS signal would be observable in colloid metal NPs. Concurrently, Albrecht and Creighton in their 1977 report speculated that resonance Raman scattering from molecular electronic states, broadened by their interaction with metal surface, could be responsible for the increased intensity.[5]

11.1.1 Electromagnetic Enhancement Mechanism

The collective excitation of the conduction electron is known as surface plasmon. A small spherical NP whose dimension is much smaller than the wavelength of incident radiation will sustain oscillating surface plasmon multipole. For a sufficiently small particle (i.e., on the scale of the wavelength of the incident radiation), the electric field is approximately uniform across the entire particle and the LSPR can be approximated as a dipole, p_0. When the excitation radiation matches the energy of the plasmon dipole, the nanoparticle (NP) will radiate characteristic plasmonic radiation which can be easily monitored by absorption and scattering spectroscopic techniques. The following description of the EM mechanism is adapted from the theoretical model presented in Kerker *et al.*[6]

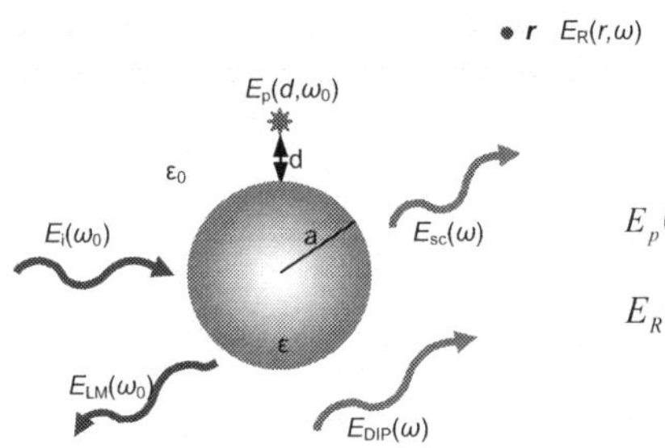

$$E_p(d,\omega_0) = E_i(d,\omega_0) + E_{LM}(d,\omega_0)$$

$$E_R(r,\omega) = E_{DIP}(r,\omega) + E_{sc}(r,\omega)$$

Figure 11.1 A schematic view of the SERS relevant electric fields near a spherical NP of radius a, and dielectric function ε immersed in a medium with a dielectric constant ε_0. An adsorbate molecule is placed at a distance d away from the sphere. An observation point r located in the far-field is associated with field E_R. At the incident frequency ω_0, there are the incident, Lorenz-Mie and primary field denoted as $E_i(\omega_0)$, $E_{LM}(\omega_0)$, $E_p(\omega_0)$ respectively. At the Raman shifted frequency, ω, there are the dipole, scattered, and Raman fields denoted as $E_{DIP}(\omega)$, $E_{SC}(\omega)$, $E_R(\omega)$, respectively.[6] Reprinted with permission from Ref. 6. See also Color Insert.

It is instructive to consider this enhancement mechanism in the framework of a molecule situated at a distance d away from a spherical metal NP as depicted in Fig. 11.1. The particle has a radius a and dielectric function of $\varepsilon(\omega)$ and is surrounded by a medium with dielectric constant ε_0. Upon irradiation with a plane wave of frequency ω_0, the molecule (treated as a classic electric dipole) will irradiate at the Raman shifted frequency ω with a dipole moment

$$p(d,\omega) = \alpha_M E_p(d,\omega_0); \tag{11.1}$$

where α_M is the molecular Raman polarizability. The primary field at $E_p(d,\omega_0)$ is composed of two parts.

$$E_p(d,\omega_0) = E_i(d,\omega_0) + E_{LM}(d,\omega_0); \tag{11.2}$$

with $E_i(d,\omega_0)$ being the incident field and $E_{LM}(d,\omega_0)$ the elastically scattered field derived from Lorenz-Mie theory. The electric field associated with the Raman-shifted radiation at an observation point r is given by $E_R(r,\omega)$ which also composed of two components.

$$E_R(r,\omega) = E_{DIP}(r,\omega) + E_{sc}(r,\omega); \tag{11.3}$$

where E_{DIP} is the field of the oscillating dipole p in the absence of the metal NP and E_{sc} is the field scattered by the sphere at the Raman-shifted frequency ω. The Raman scattering intensity, I_R, is the square of the far-field amplitude of E_R and the SERS enhancement factor G is defined as

$$G = \frac{I_R}{I_R^0} \tag{11.4}$$

where I_R^0 is the Raman intensity in the absence of the metal NP.

In the regime where the size of the NP is sufficiently small compared to the excitation wavelength λ_0, the NP will exhibit a dipole moment, p_0

$$p_0 = g_0 a^3 E_i(d,\omega_0) \tag{11.5}$$

where $g_0 = (\varepsilon_0 - 1)/(\varepsilon_0 + 2)$ and is essentially the field enhancement averaged over the surface of the particle brought on by the incident light excitation of the metal NP. This dipole moment, p_0, is also responsible for the surface enhanced Rayleigh radiation. A molecule located at a distance d away from the metal NP exhibits a dipole moment, p_1 which is induced by E_p

$$p_1 = \alpha_M E_p(d,\omega_0) \tag{11.6}$$

The secondary scattered field E_{sc} also induces a dipole moment

$$p_2 = g a^3 E_{DIP}(d,\omega) \tag{11.7}$$

where $g = (\varepsilon - 1)/(\varepsilon + 2)$ and thus represent the field enhancement of the Raman scattered radiation in the presence of the metal NP. In the configuration with a molecule on the surface of the NP and the polarization of the incident and scattered radiation perpendicular to the scattering plane, the SERS enhancement factor is given by Kerker *et al.*[6] as

$$G = 5\left|1 + 2g_0 + 2g + 4gg_0\right|^2 \tag{11.8}$$

The quantity g or g_0 becomes large when Re(ε) approaches −2 which occurs at the surface plasmon resonance. Under this condition, $G \approx 80\left|gg_0\right|^2$. Thus, for a low-wavenumber Raman vibrational band where $g \sim g_0$, the enhancement factor G is proportional to the fourth power of the enhancement of the local incident near field, i.e., $|g|^4$ or $|E_L|^4$. Experimentally, Van Duyne *et al.*[7] has define the SERS enhancement factor G as

$$G = \frac{I_R(\omega)/N_{surf}}{I_R^0(\omega)/N_{vol}} \tag{11.9}$$

where N_{surf} is the number of molecules bound to the enhancing metallic substrates and N_{vol} is the number of molecules in the excitation volume. The enhancement factor is often used as a gauge to assess the enhancing ability of various SERS active substrates.

In summary, there are three oscillating induced dipoles, p_0, p_1, and p_2; where p_0 arises from the collective oscillation of the NP with frequency ω_0 while p_1 and p_2 are both induced dipoles oscillating with a Raman shifted frequency ω. The observed Raman scattering from a molecule positioned near a spherical NP is associated with the two oscillating dipoles p_1 and p_2 both related to the induced molecular dipole. The p_1 dipole induces its own new local dipolar field E_{DIP} which in turn induces a dipole p_2 in the sphere. The readers who are interested in a more comprehensive overview of the EM mechanism are encouraged to a number of excellent reviews by Moskovits[8–10] and the original report by Kerker.[6,11]

11.1.2 Consequences of Electromagnetic Enhancement

The EM enhancement mechanism has led to the understanding of many characteristic SERS effects. We outline a few of the direct consequences of the EM enhancement mechanisms in this section. According to the EM model, the largest SERS signals are expected when both the frequency of the incident and Raman scattering frequency approach the surface plasmon resonance conditions, e.g., Re(ε) approaches −2 if the ambient medium is vacuum. The metals that provided the largest enhancement should exhibit large Re(ε) and small Im(ε) which immediately singled out the noble metals as best enhancers for excitation with visible light sources. The LSPR of small Ag and Au particles are extremely sensitive to composition, morphology, geometry, degree of aggregation, and dielectric properties of the ambient as demonstrated in the calculations depicted in Fig. 11.2.

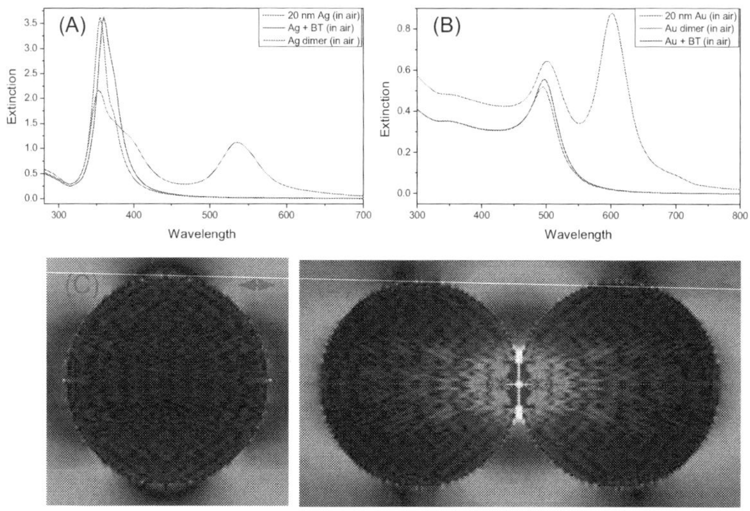

Figure 11.2 Extinction spectra of Ag and Au NPs and their corresponding dimers. (A) Ag NP in air (green), Ag NP coated with a monolayer of benzenethiol (blue) and a pair of Ag NP separated by 1 nm gap (red). (B) Au NP in air (green), Au coated with a monolayer of benzenethiol (blue), and a coupled Au NP dimer separated by 1 nm gap (red). See also Color Insert.

In Fig. 11.2, the LSPR of 20 nm Ag and Au particles are estimated to lie at 355 nm and 500 nm, respectively, from a Mie scattering calculation.[12] In the presence of a monolayer of benzenethiol, the extinction spectra showed a slight red-shifted of the resonances, whereas a substantial red-shift is observed when particles aggregated into a dimer (red spectra, Fig. 11.2A,B). Note that the dimer calculation was carried out using the Discrete Dipole Approximation (DDA) computer codes of Draine *et al.*[13,14] This sensitivity allows one to design nanostructures and tailor their LSPR for particular SERS applications. For example, nanorods, nanoshells, and nanoprisms can all be tuned by controlling aspect ratio,[15–18] shell-radius ratio,[19,20] and edge-sharpness,[21] respectively.

Another outcome of the electromagnetic enhancement theory is the predicted distance dependence built into the SERS enhancement factor, G, which is proportional to $(a + d)^{-12}$. This inherently restricts the SERS effect to adsorbate molecules that are situated either directly on the surface or in the immediate vicinity of the NP. This has also had an impact on the design of SERS-based sensors.[22] The EM theory also predicted that additional significant enhancements can be produced through tight coupling of NPs as a result of coupling of surface plasmon dipoles from the individual NP. Consider the simplest coupled-NP systems as a set of two NPs (dimer) separated by a small inter-particle distance. Theoretical calculation[23,24] has demonstrated that a simple dimer excited with light polarized parallel to the inter-particle axis showed enormous optical field strength in the inter-particle gap and the expected SERS enhancement exceeded 10^{11}. Figure 11.2 shows field amplitude images calculated by DDA for a single NP (Fig. 11.2C), and a coupled NP dimer separated by a distance of 1 nm (Fig. 11.2D). The differential field enhancement (normalized to the incident field) for a coupled dimer to a single spherical NP was ~6 orders of magnitude in this case, with the highest field amplitude located at the center of the gap between particles. Hence, a molecule situated in the inter-particle gap of dimer particles excited with a light polarized parallel to the inter-particle axis will benefit from the intense field enhancement, thus enabling detection of very few to even a single molecule by SERS.[25–28] The overall enhancement of dimer particles, however, depends strongly on the separation distances as illustrated in References 23 and 27. The enhancement by dimer particles also exhibited strong dependence on the polarization of the incident radiation with the strongest enhancement being observed for light polarized parallel to the inter-particle axis. Conversely, dimers excited with light polarized perpendicular to the inter-particle axis, had a region of highest localized optical fields at the two separate polar regions of the NP while the field in the inter-particle gap was depleted, forming a "cold spot."

A final result of the EM theory is an imposed size-limitation of the nanostructure for the overall enhancement of the SERS active system. SERS-active systems must ideally possess structures in the 5–100 nm range. The upper limit is dictated by the dipole plasmon approximation for the particular wavelength used to excite the NP. At the other end of the dimensional scale, diminishing conductivity of the metal NPs as a result of electronic scattering processes at the particle's surface will reduce the quality of the LSPR and also the SERS enhancement.[10]

11.1.3 Chemical Enhancement

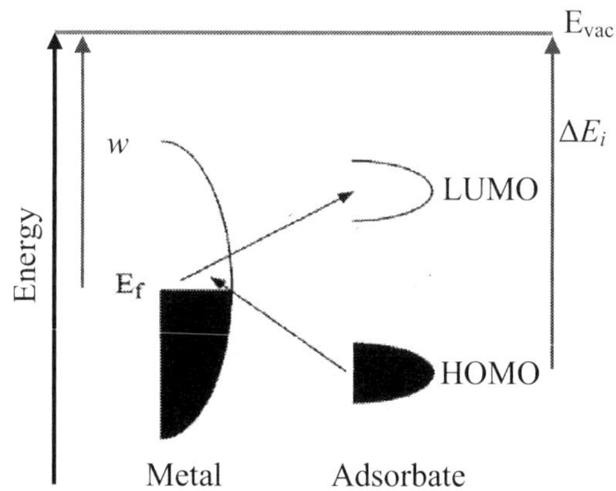

Figure 11.3 Energy level diagram for a molecule adsorbed on a metal surface. The occupied (HOMO) and unoccupied (LUMO) molecular orbitals are broadened into resonances by their interaction with the metal states; orbital occupancy is determined by the Fermi energy. The molecule-to-metal charge transition is indicated by the black arrows. Work function (*w*) of the metal and ionization potential (ΔE_i) of adsorbate molecules are depicted with blue arrows. Reproduced with permission from Ref. 30 with permission. See also Color Insert.

Another contribution to the observed SERS intensity is generally referred to as "chemical enhancement."[5] This usually applies to the adsorbates strongly bond (chemisorbed) to the metal surface so that the Raman scatterer is essentially an adsorbate-surface complex, analogous to a metal–ligand or coordination complex. The creation of the surface complex not only increases the Raman scattering cross-section, it also leads to resonances in the visible region of the spectrum due to a metal-to-molecule or molecule-to-metal transitions. Figure 11.3 describe this process in a pictorial form. In many molecules, the Fermi energy of the noble metal surfaces is conveniently situated in between the HOMO and LUMO of the intramolecular transition. Thus, the new energy states can contribute resonantly to the Raman scattering cross-section of the surface complex, increasing its magnitude. A theoretical account of the chemical enhancement process is summarized in Lombardi *et al.*[29]

11.1.4 SERS Bioanalytical Applications

There are two different approaches to applying the NP-based SERS detection techniques in bioanalysis: label-free or labeled. The label-free methods rely on the species of interest adsorbing directly to the SERS active surfaces. In the label-free detection scheme, NPs are introduced into the biological system of interest. Because of the strong distance-dependent characteristics of the SERS effect, this approach provides vibrational information of the nano-environment surrounding the NPs. It has been applied to the study of cellular imaging[31–34] and microorganism identifications. The label-free detection has been applied with success in pathogen detection which requires high sensitivity, rapid response, and benefits from the elimination of extrinsic labeling steps as well as SERS' ability to differentiate species and strains of different pathogens.[35–42] This can be simply achieved by introducing the pathogen cells to a colloidal metal sol that subsequently adsorbs on the cell surface rendering each pathogen cell SERS-active as shown in Fig. 11.4. Of note, the cell Raman spectrum implicitly samples all of the biomolecules of the entire cell make-up whereas the SERS spectrum only probes the cell surface composition due to the distance-dependent nature of SERS. Since the cell surface of different pathogen contains different marker proteins, the chemically specific SERS spectra allow one to discern the different types of bacteria through chemometric analysis.

Although label-free detection is a convenient approach, it also has a number of issues that one must be aware of. One of the biggest problems in the label-free approach lies in the non-selective nature of SERS. Using pathogen detection as an example, Zeiri *et al.* has pointed out that SERS spectra obtained from identical strains of bacteria can produce very different SERS response from different laboratories.[40–42] Because of the non-selective and distance-dependence nature of SERS, often, only the molecule that is situated in the SERS active hot-site will receive optimal enhancement. This applies to the biomolecules present on the cell wall or cell membrane of the microorganism but the technique is not immune to interference from a large number of biomolecules used in the bacteria culture. This points out the short fall of the label-free detection.

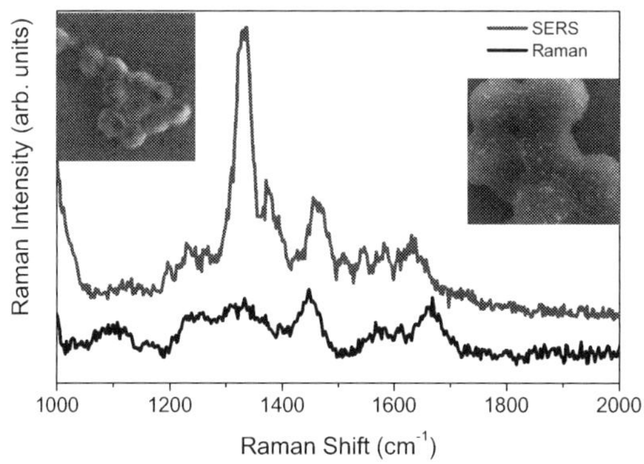

Figure 11.4 Raman (black) and SERS (blue) spectra of *Staphylococcus aureus* cells. Left inset, a small cluster of *S. aureus* cells. Right inset, *S. aureus* cells incubated with colloidal Ag sol. The cells are well decorated with Ag NPs. SERS spectra of *S. aureus* cells shows a distinct sugar vibration at 1330 cm^{-1}. Cell Raman and SERS spectra were acquired with 60 and 1 s acquisition time, respectively. See also Color Insert.

In the labeled detection scheme, a Raman active reporter molecule is adsorbed on the surface of NPs that are co-functionalized with recognition (e.g., antibody) and passivation molecules to enable detection of a specific target and reduce nonspecific bonding events with unwanted biomolecules as shown in the schematics of Fig. 11.5B. There are large number of examples of SERS-labeled detection with target species including neurotransmitters,[43] nucleic acids,[44,45] proteins,[46–49] enzymes,[50–53] cellular organelles,[54] microbes,[55,56] spores,[57–59] and diseased cells.[60–62] As very high SERS enhancements are attainable through small NP aggregates, it is desirable to design functional SERS NP assemblies with such SERS "hot spots" built into each unit.[55] This approach relies on a controlled aggregation of NPs that are subsequently protected with either passivation molecules or inorganic shells. This approach is particularly suitable when designing multiplexed experiments in which multiple targets are to be identified with different SERS probes carrying different Raman labels.

An example of such a NP assembly, called nanoaggregate embedded beads (NAEB), is outlined in the next section. Since the sensitivity of SERS rivals or surpasses that of fluorescence, labeled SERS detection can be used in almost all circumstances that a fluorophor is used. The Raman reporter molecule used in the SERS-labeled detection should, ideally, have a strong Raman cross section, and a well-characterized and simple SERS spectrum. Although common dye molecules have been used extensively in designing NP assemblies for labeled SERS detection owing to their large cross sections, their spectral complexity and photosensitivity renders spectral deconvolution problematic. Many thiol-phenyl derivatives are much more suitable candidates as SERS reporter molecules.

11.2 NAEB: A Novel SERS-Active Nanoparticle Assemblies

In this section, we describe one particular NP assembly called nanoaggregate embedded beads (NAEB) and its application in pathogen detection. NAEB is fabricated by controlled formation of small Au NP aggregates adsorbed with reporter molecules and subsequent encapsulation of these SERS active moieties in a protective silica shell as outlined in Fig. 11.5A and detailed in References 55 and 56. NAEB fully utilize the advantage of LSPR coupling of aggregated NPs thus rendering each nano-sized bead as an ultrahigh sensitivity SERS nanoprobe. In principle, any organic molecule with well-characterized Raman spectrum can be incorporated into NAEB. Specifically, in the example presented below the Raman reporter molecules (R6G) were incorporated into the nanoaggregate during the formation process to give each NAEB a unique Raman signature. Bioconjugation and surface passivation is performed on the glassy silica shell to enable target-specific detection.

Noble metal NPs co-functionalized with Raman reporter and bio-recognition molecules have been used extensively as biosensors. However, NAEB has the added advantage of stability. Without the protective silica shell, even passivated Au or Ag NPs immersed in biological buffers are prone to parasitic signals from adsorption of the molecules in the biological fluids or loss of signals due to the desorption of the Raman reporter molecule. In the fabrication of NAEB, controlled aggregation is achieved by carefully balancing the pH of the colloidal sol and the molecular adsorbate concentration during the encapsulation process. Formation of nanoaggregates in the colloidal Au sol was demonstrated by a change in color and in extinction response as shown in Fig. 11.6A. Monodispersed 12 nm Au NPs exhibit an absorption maximum at 520 nm prior to the addition of Raman reporter molecule, R6G. The extinction response of NAEB in Fig. 11.6A showed an additional peak at 640 nm indicative of the nanoaggregates structure. A transmission electron microscopy (TEM) image of the NAEB (Fig. 11.6C) shows that a majority of the NAEB are made of 2–5 NPs encapsulated in a dense silica shell and have a typical dimension of ~150 nm. A typical SERS spectrum of R6G-NAEB is shown in Fig. 11.6B.

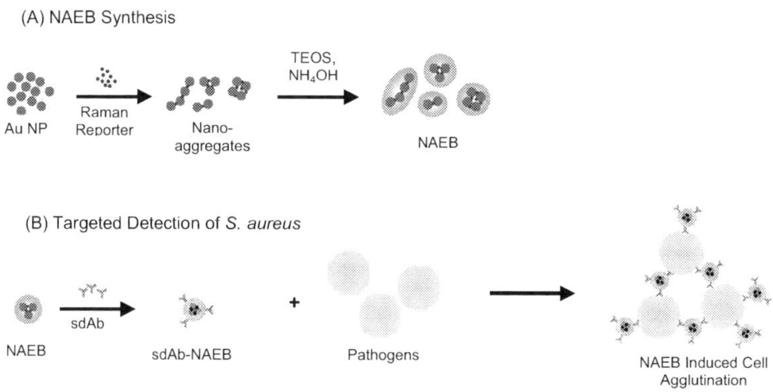

Figure 11.5 (A) Schematic depiction of NAEB fabrication; (B) Targeted detection of *S. aureus* by NAEB conjugated to *S. aureus* specific sdAb. Reproduced from Ref. 56 with permission.

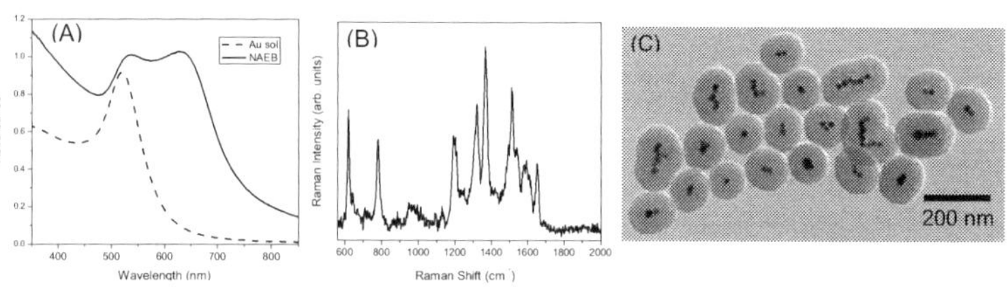

Figure 11.6 (A) Bulk extinction spectra of 12 nm colloidal Au sol (dash) and R6G-NAEB; (B) SERS spectrum of R6G-NAEB; (C) TEM image of NAEB. Reproduced from Ref. 56 with permission.

To achieve target-specific detection of *S. aureus*, a selected antibody must exhibit both good binding affinity and specificity to the desired antigen. Protein A is a virulence factor which is naturally expressed on the cell wall of *S. aureus* in great abundance (tens of thousands/cell).[63] It is highly specific to the *S. aureus* species and thus serves as a key marker for this pathogen. A small protein unit, single domain antibody (sdAb), derived by panning a V_H phage display library against protein A[64,65] is conjugated onto the silica shell of NAEB which enables target-specific recognition (Fig. 11.5B). Raman imaging of the *S. aureus* cells treated with sdAb-NAEB is shown in Fig. 11.7. Here, two sets of sdAb-NAEB-labeled *S. aureus* cells are visible in the SEM image of Fig. 11.7A. The upper set consists of a group of 3 cells while the lower set is a single cell. Both sets of cells were well decorated with sdAb-NAEB which is indicative of the positive binding response between the sdAb-NAEB and the targeted pathogen. An optical image of the same area is shown in Fig. 11.7B. The false-colored Raman intensity map (Fig. 11.7C) is constructed from the integrated intensity of the 1196 cm^{-1} and 1238 cm^{-1} vibrational bands of R6G. Two bright regions were observed in the Raman intensity maps, demonstrating good spatial correlation to the cells observed in the optical (Fig. 11.7B) and SEM (Fig. 11.7A) images. Figure 11.7D is a full SERS spectrum of the R6G-NAEB taken from the single cell (lower bright spot) region. The single cell from the Raman intensity map is clearly resolved and detected through sdAb-NAEB labeling. The specificity of the sdAb and the ultrahigh sensitivity of NAEB render targeted detection of *S. aureus* at single cell level easily attainable.

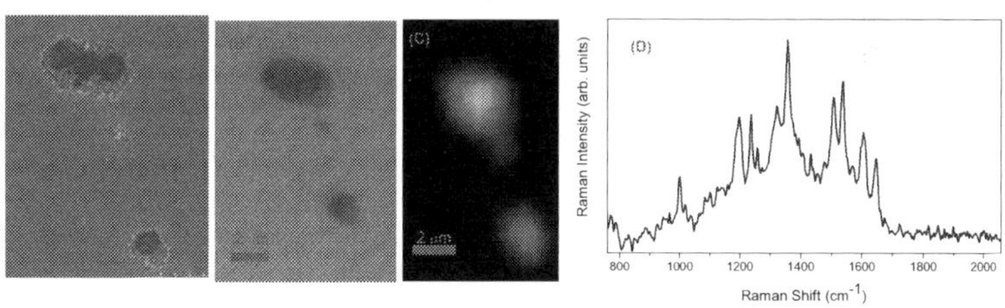

Figure 11.7 SEM (A), Optical (B), and SERS intensity map (C) of NAEB-labeled *S. aureus* cells. (D) SERS spectrum of a single *S. aureus* cell labeled with NAEB. Reproduced from Ref. 56 with permission. See also Color Insert.

It is possible to introduce different reporter molecules into NAEB and couple it with different antibodies to enable multiplexed detection of different types of pathogen. However, in such operations, care must be exercised in selecting reporter molecules with a minimal amount of spectral overlap and similar scattering cross sections. The latter criterion is particularly important when fluorescent molecules are used as Raman reporter. The Raman cross section of fluorophors can be very different when excited on and off electronic resonance thus resulting in orders of magnitude difference in the observed SERS intensity.

11.3 SERS-Based Bioimaging with Multifunctional Nanoparticles

An important frontier in molecular imaging is the utilization of the inordinate sensitivity of SERS to achieve target-specific detection of cellular proteins *in vivo*. SERS microscopy applied in cellular imaging has been used to study the localization of HER2 and CD10 on cell membranes,[62] to examine the over-expression of phospholipid Cγ1 in human embryonic kidney (HEK293) cells,[61] to image the EGFR expression in human hepatoma (Huh7.5) cells,[66] and to locate the β-adrenergic receptors in cardiac myocyte (H9C2) cells.[67] It has also been applied to study the cell surface receptors in mammalian cells[68] as well as for tissue immunohistological assay in cancer pathology.[69] In every regards, SERS labels rival that of fluorescent contrasting agents and can be adapted to most of the fluorescent detection schemes. In this section, we outline SERS imaging of cell surface receptors in mammalian cells as well as in a localization study of receptor-driven aggregation.

Figure 11.8 shows a cartoon representation of the generic cell-labeling method. NPs designed for cellular imaging must meet the following criteria. They must be water-soluble, highly specific, biocompatible, and stable toward substitution. Also, they must not alter the biochemistry of host cells as nontoxic metals are known to do. Ideally, the size of the particles should be comparable to the proteins and receptors they target on cell surfaces — typically less than 20 nm in diameter. Many of the core-shell type of SERS probes reported in the literature are larger than this ideal dimension which limits their applications for the cellular imaging. It is possible to use NP assemblies composed of smaller NPs so that the overall dimension of the assembly stays in the ideal window as outlined in reference.[67] Another possibility is to work with small NPs functionalized with

Raman reporter molecules and target-specific antibody as described in Fig. 11.8. Although SERS enhancement diminishes as the size of particles decreases, it is still possible to generate detectable SERS upon aggregation of relatively small NPs. As demonstrated in Reference 67 which NPs labeled with a secondary antibody targeting the β-adrenergic receptors are used to label mouse cardiac myocytes. The authors carefully passivated the NPs and relied upon the receptors-mediated aggregation to produce a detectable SERS signal. Because these receptors are known to form signaling domains of ~140 nm in size which typically containing ~15 dimerized receptor units, NP labeling allowed the authors to obtain a complete receptor map on the cell surface.

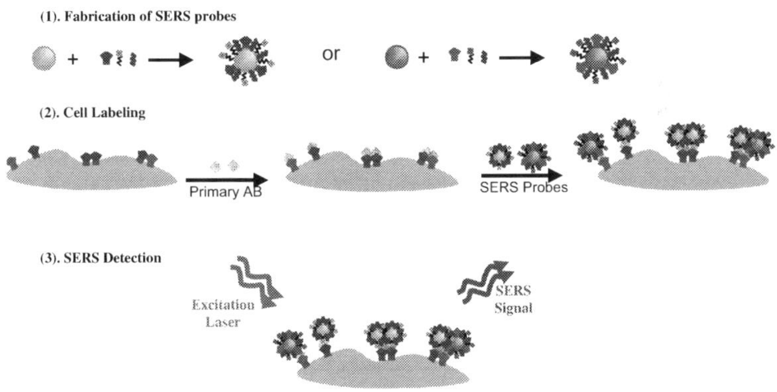

Figure 11.8 Schematics representation of the SERS-based cell microscopy. (1) SERS active probes are fabricated through co-labeling of Raman reporter molecule, secondary antibody, and passivation molecules. (2) Receptors on the cells are first labeled with primary antibody before being exposed to SERS nanoprobes. (3) SERS detection of receptors. See also Color Insert.

Figure 11.9A shows an optical image of HeLa cells expressing the transmembrane domain of the platelet-derived growth factor receptor (TM) which has been labeled with NPs co-functionalized with a nitrile-reporter molecule and a target-specific recognition unit. The nitrile vibrational group uniquely falls in a spectroscopically quiet region which enables its ease of detection. The SERS intensity map shown in Fig. 11.9B revealed three SERS active sites marked as I, II, and III. These SERS-active regions are further characterized in SEM in Fig. 11.9C,D. The three observed SERS hot-sites are made of tetramer (spot I), trimer (spot II), and dimer (spot III). Although SEM revealed other regions that are labeled by NPs, these monomeric particles do not support strong SERS signals and thus were not detected. SERS spectra taken from spot III also revealed a much weaker nitrile vibration compared to the other two. As spot III is made up of a coupled rod-sphere structure, it is quite possible that the surface plasmon resonance of the coupled structure shifted to the red and could no longer be excited effectively at the excitation wavelength (632.8 nm) used in this study. Of note, it is important to point out that because the NPs were not deliberately induced into aggregation in this type of labeling study, the observation of SERS signals will entirely rely on the receptor-mediated aggregation. Membrane proteins often cluster onto micro-domains called rafts, which help facilitate aggregation of NPs upon labeling thus producing strong SERS signals.

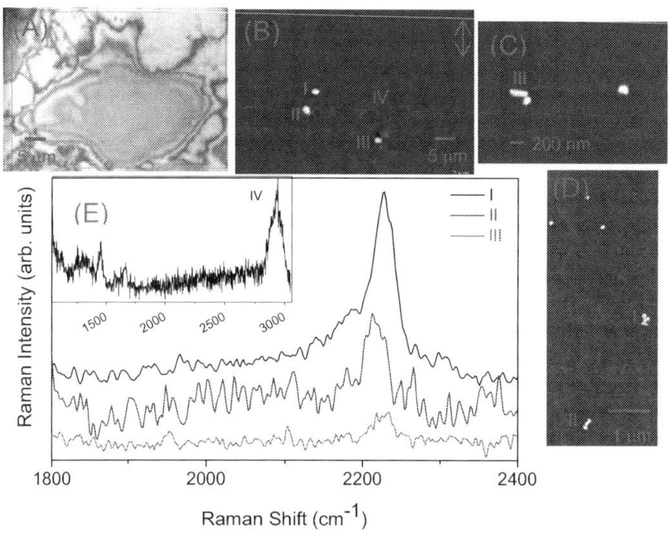

Figure 11.9 (A) Optical image of a HeLa cell co-labeled with Raman-reporter and target-specific molecules. (B) SERS intensity map of the nitrile vibrational band with three SERS hot spots I, II, and III identified. (C) and (D) SEM image of the corresponding area showed SERS activity. (E) SERS spectra of the three spots identified in the intensity map. Inset of (E) shows the cell Raman spectrum taken from the nucleus region labeled as spot IV.[68] See also Color Insert.

In the same study, the authors also pointed out that NP-labeled cells can result in light-induced damage when exposed to a tightly focused laser beam. NP-induced photothermal heating of cells is well characterized and has been proposed as an effective route to deliver therapeutic treatments in cancer research.[1,70] In addition, NPs can be used as a vehicle to deliver therapeutic molecules as payloads in cellular endocytotic events as demonstrated in reference.[66] It is also possible to design a SERS transducer that contains a built-in redox reaction by carefully selecting the reporter molecules that support such reactions. This allows one to monitor the pH value of the nanoscale environment as demonstrated in reference.[71] All of these added functionalities enable the NP-based SERS imaging as a potentially useful monitoring, diagnostic, and therapeutic tool for biomedical research community.

11.4 Summary and Outlook

Since been discovered in the late 1970s, studied intensely in the 80s, and rejuvenated by the advances of the nanotechnology, theoretical modeling tools and single molecule detection capabilities have demonstrated in the last 15 years that SERS has reached the maturity to embark on a program of development that goes beyond simple academic curiosity and ventures into the real-world applications.

SERS has demonstrated enormous sensitivity as an active optical transducer in local environment sensing. This local environment can either be the intrinsic and complex environment of a living organism or specific reporter molecules with well-characterized Raman signature as in the labeled detection scheme. Properly designed SERS active nanostructures such as the NAEB outlined in this chapter have sensitivities rivaling that of fluorescent tag with superior stability and are better suited for conjugating to the desired target molecules. More importantly, the narrow Raman vibrational signature coupled with the availability of a large number of reporter molecules renders this type of probe highly desirable for the multiplexed detection.

In SERS-based cell surface receptor imaging, noble metal NPs co-labeled with target-specific antibody, Raman reporter molecule and passivating ligands are used to label the desired cell surface receptors and rely on the receptor-driven aggregation event to generate a detectable SERS signal. In these studies, the metal NP serves as a contrasting agent in identifying the location of cell surface receptors under the electron microscope. Care in selecting an NP dimension for a close match to the receptor dimension allows one to estimate the number of receptors present on the cell surface. In addition to the role as a transduction unit, the metal NP can be rendered multifunctional through its photothermal properties or act as a payload carrier in delivering therapeutic reagents into the organisms.

While there are numerous demonstrations of SERS-based bioanalytical applications and many research groups actively involved in improving the designs of high sensitivity and reproducibility SERS nanoprobes, the emphasis on its performance and design in the interface layer with biomolecules will play a key role into its successful deployment into clinical and commercial settings. For example, adapting a functional layer of ZnS on the surface of the NAEB SERS nanoprobe enables strong conjugation with antibodies that contain the His-tag and retain the strong SERS signal opens the door for NAEB to many affinity assay applications.[72] Incorporating other functionality such as the SERS-active magnetic nanoprobes also open the door for additional functionality.

SERS research continues at a rapid pace. The fundamental aspects of this phenomenon are now understood. Three decades of intense fundamental researches have laid a solid foundation for this technique. Together with the advances in instrumental developments achieved in the past few decades, one can envision a compact, high throughput portable spectrometer enabled with high quantum efficiency CCD detector and coupled microscope capable of operating in confocal or even near-field modes poised to launch this technique into practical real-world environments.

Acknowledgments

We would like to thank those who provided the permission for the artwork and figures used in this article. We are greatly indebted to our colleagues and collaborators for the published and unpublished materials and their valuable discussions in putting together this chapter: Dr. Ping-Ji Huang, Prof. Lai-Kwan Chau, Dr. Jamshid Tanha, Ms. Shannon Ryan, Dr. Qingyan Hu, Dr. David Kennedy, and Dr. John Paul Pezacki.

References

1. L. R. Hirsch, R. J. Stafford, J. A. Bankson, S. R. Sershen, B. Rivera, R. E. Price, J. D. Hazle, N. J. Halas, and J. L. West, *Proc. Natl. Acad. Sci. U.S.A.*, **100**, 13549 (2003).
2. M. Fleischman, P. J. Hendra, and A. J. McQuillan, *Chem. Phys. Lett.*, **26**, 4 (1974).
3. D. L. Jeanmaire, and R. P. V. Duyne, *J. Electroanal. Chem.*, **84**, 1 (1977).
4. M. Moskovits, *J. Chem. Phys.*, **69**, 4159 (1978).
5. M. G. Albrecht, and J. A. Creighton, *J. Am. Chem. Soc.*, **99**, 5215 (1977).
6. M. Kerker, D.-S. Wang, and H. *Chew, Appl. Opt.*, **19**, 4159 (1980).
7. A. D. McFarland, M. A. Young, J. A. Dieringer, and R. P. Van Duyne, *J. Phys. Chem. B*, **109**, 11279 (2005).
8. M. Moskovits, *Rev. Mod. Phys.*, **57**, 783 (1985).
9. M. Moskovits, L. L. Tay, J. Yang, and T. Haslett, in *Optical Properties of Nanostructured Random Media*, Vol. 82, p. 215 (2002).
10. M. Moskovits, *J. Raman Spectrosc.*, **36**, 485 (2005).
11. M. Kerker, O. Siiman, and D. S. Wang, *J. Phys. Chem.*, **88**, 3168 (1984).
12. C. F. Bohren, and D. R. Huffman in *Absorption and Scattering of Light by small Particles,* New York: Wiley-Interscience (1983).
13. B. T. Draine, and P. J. Flatau, *J. Opt. Soc. Am. A,* **11**, 1491 (1994).
14. B. T. Draine, and P. J. Flatau, http://arxiv.org/abs/0809.0337 (2009).
15. S. Link, and M. A. El-Sayed, *J. Phys. Chem. B,* **103**, 8410 (1999).
16. Y. Y. Yu, S. S. Chang, C. L. Lee, and C. R. C. Wang, *J. Phys. Chem. B,* **101**, 6661 (1997).
17. C. J. Murphy, and N. R. Jana, *Adv. Mater.*, **14**, 80 (2002).
18. C. J. Murphy, T. K. San, A. M. Gole, C. J. Orendorff, J. X. Gao, L. Gou, S. E. Hunyadi, and T. Li, *J. Phys. Chem. B,* **109**, 13857 (2005).
19. S. J. Oldenburg, R. D. Averitt, S. L. Westcott, and N. J. Halas, *Chem. Phys. Lett.*, **288**, 243 (1998).
20. J. B. Jackson, and N. J. Halas, *J. Phys. Chem. B,* **105**, 2743 (2001).
21. R. C. Jin, Y. W. Cao, C. A. Mirkin, K. L. Kelly, G. C. Schatz, and J. G. Zheng, *Science,* **294**, 1901 (2001).
22. K. E. Shafer-Peltier, C. L. Haynes, M. R. Glucksberg, and R. P. Van Duyne, *J. Am. Chem. Soc.*, **125**, 588 (2003).
23. H. X. Xu, J. Aizpurua, M. Kall, and P. Apell, *Phys. Rev. E,* **62**, 4318 (2000).

24. H. X. Xu, and M. Kall, *Chem. Phys. Chem.*, **4**, 1001 (2003).
25. S. M. Nie, and S. R. Emery, *Science*, **275**, 1102 (1997).
26. K. Kneipp, Y. Wang, H. Kneipp, L. T. Perelman, I. Itzkan, R. Dasari, and M. S. Feld, *Phys. Rev. Lett.*, **78**, 1667 (1997).
27. H. X. Xu, E. J. Bjerneld, M. Kall, and L. Borjesson, *Phys. Rev. Lett.*, **83**, 4357 (1999).
28. A. M. Michaels, M. Nirmal, and L. E. Brus, *J. Am. Chem. Soc.*, **121**, 9932 (1999).
29. J. R. Lombardi, R. L. Birke, T. Lu, and J. Xu, *J. Chem. Phys.*, **84**, 4174 (1986).
30. A. Campion, and P. Kambhampati, *Chem. Soc. Rev.* **27**, 241 (1998).
31. K. Kneipp, H. Kneipp, I. Itzkan, R. R. Dasari, and M. S. Feld, *J. Phys. Condensed Mat.*, **14**, R597 (2002).
32. K. Kneipp, *et al.*, *Appl. Spectrosc.*, **56**, 150 (2002).
33. J. Kneipp, H. Kneipp, M. McLaughlin, D. Brown, and K. Kneipp, *Nano Lett.*, **6**, 2225 (2006).
34. J. Kneipp, H. Kneipp, A. Rajadurai, R. W. Redmond, and K. Kneipp, *J. Raman Spectrosc.*, **40**, 1 (2009).
35. R. M. Jarvis, and R. Goodacre, *Anal. Chem.*, **76**, 40 (2004).
36. W. R. Premasiri, D. T. Moir, M. S. Klempner, N. Krieger, G. Jones, and L. D. Ziegler, *J. Phys. Chem. B*, **109**, 312 (2005).
37. L. Zeiri, B. V. Bronk, Y. Shabtai, J. Eichler, and S. Efrima, *Appl. Spectrosc.*, **58**, 33 (2004).
38. L. Zeiri, B. V. Bronk, Y. Shabtai, J. Czege, and S. Efrima, *Colloids Surfaces A*, **208**, 357 (2002).
39. R. M. Jarvis, A. Brooker, and R. Goodacre, *Faraday Discuss.*, **132**, 281 (2006).
40. S. Efrima, and L. Zeiri, *J. Raman Spectrosc.*, **40**, 277 (2009).
41. L. Zeiri, and S. Efrima, Isr. *J. Chem.*, **46**, 337 (2006).
42. L. Zeiri, and S. Efrima, *J. Raman Spectrosc.*, **36**, 667 (2005).
43. R. J. Dijkstra, W. Scheenen, N. Dam, E. W. Roubos, and J. J. ter Meulen, *J.Neurosci. Methods*, **159**, 43 (2007).
44. Y. W. C. Cao, R. C. Jin, and C. A. Mirkin, *Science*, **297**, 1536 (2002).
45. R. C. Jin, Y. C. Cao, C. S. Thaxton, and C. A. Mirkin, *Small*, **2**, 375 (2006).
46. C. D. Keating, K. M. Kovaleski, and M. J. Natan, *J. Phys. Chem. B*, **102**, 9404 (1998).

47. D. S. Grubisha, R. J. Lipert, H. Y. Park, J. Driskell, and M. D. Porter, *Anal. Chem.*, **75**, 5936 (2003).

48. J. Ni, R. J. Lipert, G. B. Dawson, and M. D. Porter, *Anal. Chem.*, **71**, 4903 (1999).

49. M. D. Porter, R. J. Lipert, L. M. Siperko, G. Wang, and R. Narayanana, *Chem. Soc. Rev.*, **37**, 1001 (2008).

50. E. J. Bjerneld, Z. Foldes-Papp, M. Kall, and R. Rigler, *J. Phys. Chem. B*, **106**, 1213 (2002).

51. P. Scodeller, V. Flexer, R. Szamocki, E. J. Calvo, N. Tognalli, H. Troiani, and A. Fainstein, *J. Am. Chem. Soc.*, **130**, 12690 (2008).

52. Z. S. Wu, G. Z. Zhou, J. H. Jiang, G. L. Shen, and R. Q. Yu, *Talanta,* **70**, 533 (2006).

53. S. P. Xu, X. H. Ji, W. Q. Xu, B. Zhao, X. M. Dou, Y. B. Bai, and Y. Ozaki, *J. Biomed. Opt.*, **10** (2005).

54. O. F. Karatas, E. Sezgin, O. Aydin, and M. Culha, *Colloids Surfaces B* **71**, 315 (2009).

55. P. J. Huang, L. K. Chau, T. S. Yang, L. L. Tay, and T. T. Lin, *Adv. Funct. Mater.*, **19**, 242 (2009).

56. P. J. Huang, L. L. Tay, J. Tanha, S. Ryan, and L. K. Chau, *Chem. Eur. J.*, **15**, 9330 (2009).

57. X. Y. Zhang, J. Zhao, A. V. Whitney, J. W. Elam, and R. P. Van Duyne, *J. Am. Chem. Soc.*, **128**, 10304 (2006).

58. J. K. Daniels, T. P. Caldwell, K. A. Christensen, and G. Chumanov, *Anal. Chem.*, **78**, 1724 (2006).

59. X. Y. Zhang, M. A. Young, O. Lyandres, and R. P. Van Duyne, *J. Am. Chem. Soc.*, **127**, 4484 (2005).

60. X. M. Qian, *et al.*, *Nat. Biotechnol.*, **26**, 83 (2008).

61. S. Lee, S. Kim, J. Choo, S. Y. Shin, Y. H. Lee, H. Y. Choi, S. H. Ha, K. H. Kang, and C. H. Oh, *Anal. Chem.*, **79**, 916 (2007).

62. J. H. Kim, *et al.*, *Anal. Chem.*, **78**, 6967 (2006).

63. G. Kronvall, P. G. Quie, and R. C. Williams, *J. Immunol.*, **104**, 273 (1970).

64. J. Tanha, G. Dubuc, T. Hirama, S. A. Narang, and C. R. MacKenzie, *J. Immunol. Methods,* **263**, 97 (2002).

65. J. Tanha, P. Xu, Z. G. Chen, F. Ni, H. Kaplan, S. A. Narang, and C. R. MacKenzie, *J. Biol. Chem.*, **276**, 24774 (2001).

66. D. C. Kennedy, D. R. Duguay, L. L. Tay, D. S. Richeson, and J. P. Pezacki, *Chem.Commun.*, 6750 (2009).

67. D. C. Kennedy, L. L. Tay, R. K. Lyn, Y. Rouleau, J. Hulse, and J. P. Pezacki, *ACS Nano,* **3**, 2329 (2009).
68. Q. Y. Hu, L. L. Tay, M. Noestheden, and J. P. Pezacki, *J. Am. Chem. Soc.*, **129**, 14 (2007).
69. S. Schlucker, B. Kustner, A. Punge, R. Bonfig, A. Marx, and P. Strobel, *J. Raman Spectrosc.*, **37**, 719 (2006).
70. D. P. O'Neal, L. R. Hirsch, N. J. Halas, J. D. Payne, and J. L. West, *Cancer Lett.*, **209**, 171 (2004).
71. S. W. Bishnoi, C. J. Rozell, C. S. Levin, M. K. Gheith, B. R. Johnson, D. H. Johnson, and N. J. Halas, *Nano Lett.*, **6**, 1687 (2006).
72. L.-L. Tay, P.-J. Huang, J. Tanha, S. Ryan, X. Wu, J. Hulse, and L.-K. Chau, *Chem. Comm.*, **48**, 1024 (2012).

Chapter 12

Mass Spectrometric Bioanalysis Assisted by Noble Metal Nanoparticles

Yen-Hsiu Lin and Wei-Lung Tseng*
Department of Chemistry, National Sun Yat-sen University, Lien-hai Road, Kaohsiung, Taiwan
*tsengwl@mail.nsysu.edu.tw

The chapter reviews recent developments in the application of noble metal nanoparticles (NPs) to laser desorption/ionization mass spectrometry (LDI-MS), secondary ion MS (SIMS), and inductively coupled plasma MS (ICP-MS). Metal NPs as matrices in LDI-MS enable the selective and sensitive detection of biomolecules such as proteins, peptides, aminothiols, drugs, and carbohydrates. Metal NPs act as both signal enhancers and target concentrators in SIMS when they are attached to a well-controlled surface such as self-assembled monolayers. ICP-MS is well suited to determine the concentration of metal NPs that have been conjugated to antibody. Besides, metal NPs are capable of serving as affinity and concentrating probes for target analytes prior to LDI-MS. A table summarizes the applications of metal NPs to the analysis of a variety of analytes in LDI-MS.

From Bioimaging to Biosensors: Noble Metal Nanoparticles in Biodetection
Edited by Lai-Kwan Chau and Huan-Tsung Chang

ISBN 978-981-4267-24-3 (Hardcover), 978-981-4303-10-1 (eBook)
www.panstanford.com

12.1 Introduction

Over the past few years, nanoparticles (NPs) and NP-based materials have a great impact on the field of analytical chemistry, such as biosensing, molecular spectrometry, separation, sample preparation, and microdevices. They offer several advantages, including size-dependent optical, electric, and magnetic properties, long-term stability, high surface area-to-volume ratio, as well as ease of chemical modification.[1,2] Mass spectrometry (MS) is a powerful technology for the determination of molecular weight and structure of biomolecules, with the advantages of sensitivity, precision, accuracy, precision, small sample volumes.[3] When coupled to nanomaterials, a variety of MS techniques — including, laser desorption/ionization MS (LDI-MS), secondary ion MS (SIMS), and inductively coupled plasma MS (ICP-MS) — have been demonstrated to be useful for diverse applications: (1) the analysis of low molecular weight analytes in LDI-MS, such as neutral carbohydrate, aminothiols, and olefins-containing compounds; (2) the improvement of spot-to-spot reproducibility in LDI-MS; (3) the extension of mass range in SIMS; (4) the determination of enzyme activity and its inhibition in SIMS; (5) simultaneous detection of multiple antigens in ICP-MS. The scope of this review is narrowed to the use of noble metal NPs in MS-related techniques, including LDI-MS, SIMS, and ICP-MS. We also include the use of noble metal NPs to enrich and extract the target analytes in LDI-MS. Although other nanomaterials, for example, carbon nanotube and Fe_3O_4 NPs, are commonly coupled to LDI-MS, they are not discussed herein.

12.2 Nanomaterials in LDI-MS

Since its invention in 1987, matrix-assisted LDI MS (MALDI-MS) developed by Karas and Hillemkamp[4] has proven to be useful for the analysis of medium-size molecules (500–10,000 Da) such as proteins, peptides, and nucleic acids.[5] Organic matrices having a strong absorption at the chosen laser wavelength act as efficient energy mediators to facilitate analyte ionization transfer, leading to the production of minimum fragmentation. Unfortunately, the ionization of organic matrix also occurs under the laser irradiation and results in a high background signal in the low-mass region

(<500 Da).[6] Therefore, MALDI-MS has not been extensively used for the characterization of low molecular weight compounds. Moreover, although the co-crystallization of the analytes and organic matrix is prerequisite for a successful MALDI-MS analysis, the inhomogeneous distribution of sample spot requires sweet-spot searching.[7] This phenomenon leads to poor shot-to-shot and sample-to-sample reproducibility.[8]

To circumvent these problems, matrix-free LDI-MS has been developed using porous silicon as a sample target for the sensitive detection of small molecules such as peptides, drugs, surfactants, and carbohydrates.[9] This well-known technique is called desorption/ionization on porous silicon.[10] Other approaches associated with matrix-free LDI-MS include sol-gels,[11] carbon-based microstructures,[12] silicon nanowires-based silicon wafers,[13] Au-plated silicon wafers,[14] and germanium nanodots-based chips.[15] For more information associated with matrix-free LDI MS, the reader is referred to excellent reviews by Peterson,[9] Huck,[12] and Mrksich.[14]

Alternatively, several groups have introduced different types of matrices for the determination of analytes ranging from small organic molecules to biopolymers. Early in 1988, Tanaka *et al.* first reported that 30 nm cobalt NPs (suspended in glycerol) served as matrices for the detection of proteins with molecular weights greater than 20000 Da.[16] Sunner *et al.* also utilized micrometer-sized graphite particles mixed with glycerol for the analysis of peptides and proteins, and named this method surface-assisted laser desorption/ionization (SALDI).[17] This method can reduce background in the low mass region while maintaining the advantages of MALDI. Encouraged by these results, a series of inorganic micro- and nanomaterials — such as graphite particles,[18] titanium dioxide NPs,[19] silicon NPs,[20] carbon nanotubes,[12] gold NPs (AuNPs), silver NPs (AgNPs), and platinum NPs (PtNPs) — have been extensively studied as potential inorganic matrices. Compared to organic matrices, the use of inorganic materials as matrices can provide several advantages, including high surface areas, better detection reproducibility, easy sample preparation, flexibility in the sample deposition conditions, and no dependence on the irradiation wavelength. Moreover, the high molar matrix-to-analyte ratio (10^7 to 10^9 analytes/particle) is obtained using nanomaterials as LDI matrices and thus contributing to high efficient ionization.[21] Table 12.1 lists different kinds of noble metal nanomaterials that have been used as LDI matrices.

Table 12.1 NPs used in LDI-MS without enrichment of analyte

Nps	Capping agent[a]	Size (nm)	Analyte[b]	LOD	Ref.
Au	Citrate	2, 5, 10	Substance P	100 fmol	21
Au	Citrate	13	Neutral steroid	188–641 nM	22
Au	Citrate	13	Carbohydrate	1.3–0.7 μM	22
Au	Citrate	13	Angiotensin I	5.1 μM	22
Au	Citrate	13	Indoleamine	46 nM	22
Au	Citrate	20–30	Angiotensin I	<0.7 fmol	23
Au	Citrate	20–30	Cytochrome c	<5 pmol	23
Au	Citrate	20–30	Insulin	<5 pmol	23
Au	Citrate	20–30	DDAC	$<10^{-7}$ mg/mL	23
Au	Citrate	20–30	Pyrene	$<10^{-5}$ mg/mL	23
Au	4-ATP	5	Cytochrome c	NG	24
Au	4-MBA	10	Angiotensin I	NG	25
Au	CHCA	20	Protein digest	NG	26
Au	No	12	Carbohydrate	82–151 nM	27
Au	No	12	α-, β-, and γ-CD	0.25–0.5 μM	28
Au	No	12	Insulin	<100 μM	28
Au	Substrate	10	Glycosyl transferase	NG	29
Au	No	Nanorod	Bradykinin	<650 fmol	30
Au	No	Nanorod	Insulin	<2 pmol	30
Au	Citrate	14	Aminothiol	1.0–1.3 μM	32
Au	Aptamer	13	ATP	2.1 μM	33
Ag	Citrate	160	Bradykinin	<0.1 mg/mL	41
Ag	Citrate	160	Angiotensin I	<0.5 mg/mL	41
Ag	NG	20, 60	Olefin	<274 pmol	42
Ag	No	10, 20	Aminothiol	7–22 nM	43
Ag	Octadecanethiol	<50	Gramicidin in urine	0.13 μM	46
Ag	Octadecanethiol	<50	Ubiquitin	<25 nM	46
Ag	Octadecanethiol	<50	BSA	<1 μM	46
Ag	Citrate	34	Estrogens	NG	48

Nps	Capping agent[a]	Size (nm)	Analyte[b]	LOD	Ref.
Pt	No	Nanoflower	Angiotensin I	<0.7 fmol	49
Pt	No	Nanoflower	Insulin	<5 fmol	49
Pt	No	Nanoflower	Cytochrome c	<20 fmol	49
Pt	No	<2–5	Substance P	<2.5 pmol	50
Pt	No	<2–5	Angiotensin I	<2.5 pmol	50

[a]4-ATP, 4-aminothiophenol; 4-MBA, 4-mercaptobenzoic acid; CHCA, α-cyano-4-hydroxycinnanic acid; NG, not given.

[b]DDAC, dimethyldioctadecylammonium chloride; CD, cyclodextrin; ATP, adenosine triphosphate; BSA, bovine serum albumin.

In addition to the use of inorganic materials as matrices, surface-functionalized micro- and nanomaterials have also been widely used as affinity probes to simultaneously enrich and isolate the target species through Columbic interaction, hydrophobic adsorption, and/or molecular biorecognition. Flocculated and trapped mixtures can be either directly detected using nanomaterials or mixed separately with organic molecules, such as sinapinic acid and 2,5-dihydroxybenzoic acid. Thus, the type of NPs and suspended liquids play important roles in determining the MS sensitivity and selectivity. In the following sections, we introduce different kinds of noble metal nanomaterials and their successful examples in LDI-MS.

12.2.1 Gold

Because the preparation of citrate-capped AuNPs (citrate-AuNPs) is easy, low-cost, and reproducible, they are one of the most popular materials for LDI-MS. Russell *et al.* examined the effect of the size of citrate-AuNPs on the ionization efficiency of peptides.[21] It is found that small AuNPs (~2 nm) could afford high sensitivity and low background interferences (i.e., Au-clusters species) for peptides compared to large AuNPs (5 and 10 nm). Tseng *et al.* have demonstrated that citrate-AuNPs possess high-salt tolerance for the analysis of biomolecules by LDI-MS.[22] This observation can be extended to the analysis of small molecules in urine samples. In contrast to dried-droplet method, layer-by-layer self-assembled multilayers films of citrate-AuNPs on a silicon wafer could increase detection sensitivity and mass range, thus making it possible to detect subfemtomoles angiotensin I and cytochrome c (12 kDa).[23]

This high detection sensitivity is mainly due to strong absorption of the UV laser light, lower thermal conductivity, and increased surface roughness. Because the mass spectra obtained by citrate-AuNPs contain abundant alkali adducted analyte ions, Russell *et al.* modified citrate-AuNPs with the ionization enhancing ligand, 4-aminothiolphenol.[24] The use of this kind of NPs resulted in a drastic enhancement in the $[M + H]^+$ ion signal, a decrease in the number of interfering peaks from Au clusters, and an increase in the useful analyte mass range. The similar phenomena have been reported in the case of the use of 4-mercaptobenzoic acid- and α-cyano-4-hydroxy-cinnamic acid (CHCA)-capped AuNPs as matrices.[25,26] Cheng *et al.* further discovered that the presence of glycerol in sample solution can improve the dispersion of CHCA-capped AuNPs, thereby increasing the sample ionization and shot-to-shot reproducibility.[26] Moreover, the presence of citric acid in sample solution can serves as an external proton donor, thereby increasing the $[M + H]^+$ ion signal. In addition to citrate-AuNPs, bare AuNPs have been used for highly sensitive detection of neutral carbohydrates without the need of derivatization steps.[27] Under the optimal concentration of bare AuNPs, the limits of detection (LODs) at a S/N ratio of 3 are 82, 41, 144, and 151 nM for ribose, glucose, cellobiose, and maltose. Figure 12.1 compares the use of different matrices for the analysis of glucose through LDI-MS. The same group also disclosed that a unique sample preparation, in which samples are deposited onto the sample plate prior to bare AuNPs, could offer better detection sensitivity and sample homogeneity when compared to (a) a deposition of a mixture of matrix and sample onto the sample plate and (b) a deposition of bare AuNPs onto the sample plate prior to sample.[28] Except for the cyclic oligosaccharide, this sample preparation method was also applied to the analyses of other biological samples, including neutral carbohydrate and steroid, aminothiols, and peptides as well as proteins. Besides, Nishimura *et al.* reported that AuNP-assisted LDI-MS can be conducted for monitoring glycosyltransferase activity when AuNPs has been modified with substrate.[29] Note that glycosyltransferase can catalyze the transfer of sugars to diverse substrates, such as glycoproteins, glycolipids, and proteoglycans. Once the substrate-decorated AuNPs reacted with glycosyltransferase, the product adsorbed onto the surface of AuNPs can be directly detected by LDI-MS. Interestingly, when visible laser was used in place of UV laser in LDI-MS, Hori *et al.* demonstrated that the detection of low-molecular-weight analytes and peptides has been still successfully achieved using gold nanorod.[30,31]

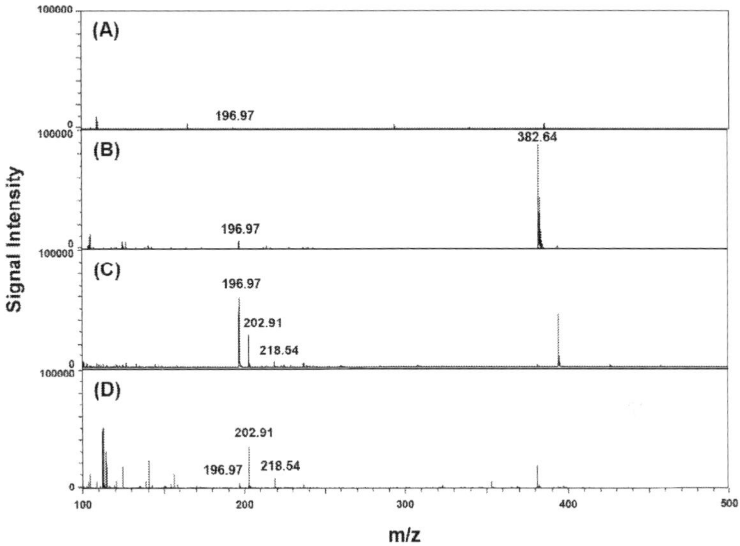

Figure 12.1 Mass spectra obtained for AuNPs with different capping systems: (A) citrate, (B) DDAB, and (C) glucose. (D) Mass spectra of 500 μM glucose was obtained using bare AuNPs as the SALDI matrix. The peaks at m/z = 196.97, 382.64, 202.91, and 218.54 are assigned respectively to the $[Au]^+$, $[DDAB - Br]^+$, $[glucose + Na]^+$, and $[glucose + K]^+$, respectively. A total of 500 pulsed laser shots were applied under a laser influence of 60 μJ. Reprinted with permission from Ref. 27.

On the other hand, AuNPs can serve as affinity probes for the enrichment of target analytes from an aqueous solution prior to LDI-MS. The procedure mainly included three consecutive steps: (a) the capture of analytes using AuNPs, (b) centrifugation and washing of extracts, and (c) AuNP- or matrix-assisted LDI detection of extracts. Citrate-AuNPs decorated with Nile Red were demonstrated to be capable of extracting and enriching aminothiols through the formation of Au-S bonds.[32] When AuNP-assisted LDI-MS was combined with AuNP-based extraction, the LODs for glutathione, cysteine, and homocysteine were down to 25, 54, and 34 nM, respectively. By taking advantage of the Nile-red capped AuNPs as selective and concentrating probes, the analysis of glutathione in red blood cells and of cysteine in plasma has been accomplished. Chang *et al.* described the use of aptamer-modified AuNPs as selective probe and bare AuNPs as LDI matrices for the extraction of anti-aptamer corresponding to adenosine triphosphate.[33] Figure 12.2 summarizes this two-step sample preparation for the analysis of adenosine triphosphate by LDI-MS. The LOD of adenosine triphosphate obtained by this approach is 0.48 μM. They suggested that this method can be applied for monitoring the bioactivity of cells through determinations of the concentrations of adenosine triphosphate and glutathione.

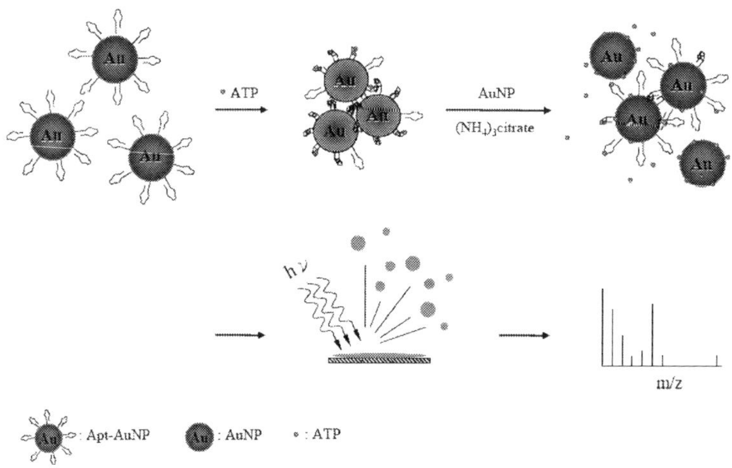

Figure 12.2 Illustration of the use of aptamer-AuNPs for selective extraction of adenosine triphosphate that was then detected using bare AuNPs as LDI matrices. Reprinted with permission from Ref. 33.

Self-assembled multilayer films of citrate-AuNPs could be utilized to extract environmental pollutants dimethyldistearylammonium chloride and pyrene from diluted solutions (concentrations less than 10^{-10} g/L).[23] The integration of magnetic NPs and citrate-AuNPs could selectively trap positively charged proteins and peptides through electrostatic interaction.[34] The analytes adsorbed on the NP surface could be further collected using magnetic field and then detected using organic matrices. The selectivity of this kind of NPs is highly dependent of solution pH. The enrichment of Met- and Leu-enkephalin peptides have been accomplished through the combination of AuNP-assisted single drop extraction and atmospheric pressure MALDI-MS; the lowest concentrations for these peptides were 0.2 and 0.17 μM, respectively.[35] 11-trimethylammonium-undecanethiol and ω-thiol carboxylic acids functionalized AuNPs with 2 nm core diameter were shown to have the ability for selective and efficient extraction of the opposite charged peptides from diluted solutions.[36] When these AuNPs were utilized for the extraction of 250 μL of sample solutions, it is demonstrated that MALDI-MS can detect peptide concentrations as low as 500 pM.

In addition to the use of AuNPs as matrices and/or concentrating probe, AuNPs conjugated to specific alkanethiolate are a versatile and efficient tool for the investigation of cellular uptake of functionalized AuNPs.[37] Alkanethiolate molecules adsorbed on the surface of AuNPs are ionized by LDI, producing the characteristic mass peak. The relative quantities of four kinds of alkanethiolate-capped AuNPs taken up by cells can be simultaneously determined using LDI-MS. When alkanethiolate-capped AuNPs are immersed in the aqueous salt solution such as NaI(aq), ionization of alkanethiolate monolayers by LDI can be further enhanced.[38,39] It is suggested that the mechanism of cation-assisted LDI seems to resemble that observed in the earlier two-laser MS.[40]

12.2.2 Silver and Platinum

Compared to the same size of AuNPs used in LDI-MS, AgNPs possess higher extinction coefficients in the visible region. Nevertheless, little attention has been paid to AgNP-assisted LDI-MS though sensitive detection of peptides,[41] olefins-containing compounds,[42] and thiol-containing compounds.[43] Citrate-capped AgNPs have been demonstrated to be used as matrices for LDI-MS analysis of angiotensin I in the presence of 0.25% SDS.[41] Russell *et al.* found that AgNPs can serve as selective ionization probe for analysis of olefins in the presence of peptides (Fig. 12.3).[42] Also, two carotenoids, β-carotene and phytoene, from a sample of carrot juice were selectively ionized in AgNP-assisted LDI-MS. Wu *et al.* demonstrated bare AgNPs are good LDI matrices for the analysis of aminothiols and sulfur drugs; the LOD for each analyte was down to 7.0 nM.[43] It is found that the detection sensitivity of these analytes obtained by AgNPs is higher than that obtained by AuNPs. LDI-MS analysis of wax compounds on Arabidopsis stem and leaves was successfully accomplished using commercial AgNPs as matrices.[44] Because AgNPs do not form crystals as it dries, good reproducibility of the mass spectral signals is achieved in AgNP-assisted LDI-MS.

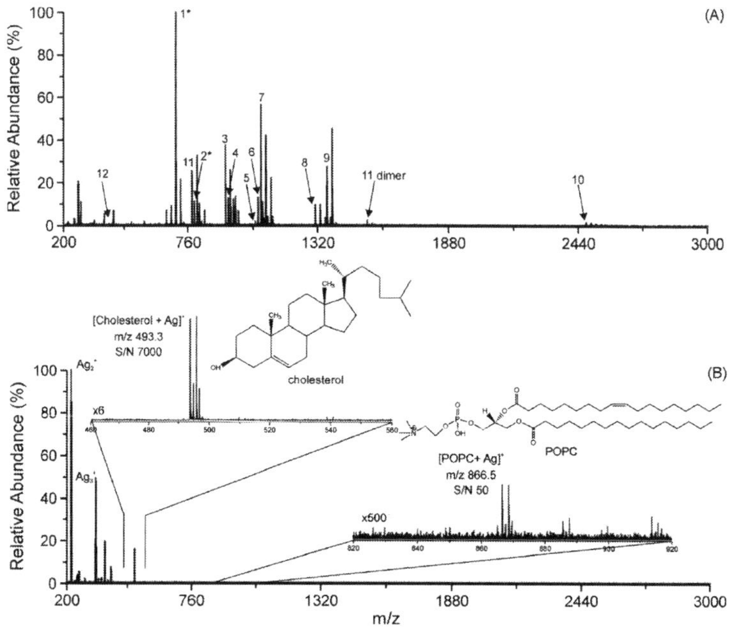

Figure 12.3 MALDI time-of-flight mass spectra of the 12 component mixture obtained using (A) DHB with 120 μM $AgNO_3$ and (B) 20 nm AgNPs. The $[M + H]^+$ or $[M + Na]^+$ (denoted by a "*") ions of each peptide is numbered in the spectrum and identified in Table 12.1. A high abundance of $[M + Na]^+$ ions (unlabeled peaks) are observed owing to the PBS buffer used to prepare the small unilamellar vesicles. Structures for both cholesterol and POPC are provided. Reprinted with permission from Ref. 42.

Very recently, Yeung *et al.* used the same LDI matrices for the direct profiling and imaging of epicuticular waxes on Arabidopsis thaliana leaves and flowers.[45] Because of reproducible spraying of AgNP solution onto the plant's surface, high spatial resolution imaging (~100 μm) of plant surface metabolites has been obtained by LDI-MS. Compared to gas chromatography/MS for the determination of cuticular wax metabolite on flower organs of Arabidopsis, AgNP-assisted LDI-MS has several advantages: (a) sample preparation did not involve in any extraction and derivatization steps; (b) the smaller amounts of sample is required; (c) localization information of metabolites can be preserved.

Moreover, AgNPs are capable of enriching target analytes from the complex matrix. In terms of hydrophobic interaction, AgNPs modified with octadecanethiol can be utilized for liquid–liquid microextraction of peptides and proteins.[46] By the combination of liquid–liquid microextraction and atmospheric pressure — MALDI-MS, the LOD values obtained for gramicidin in water, urine, and plasma were 0.16, 0.13, and 0.16 μM, respectively. However, long extraction time (1.5 h) is required when using this kind of AgNPs. To shorten the extraction time, tetraalkylammonium bromide-capped AgNPs were developed to enrich peptides through electrostatic interaction, followed by atmospheric pressure — MALDI-MS.[47] Interestingly, Chang *et al.* showed that citrate-capped AgNPs can be simultaneously used as extracting agents and LDI matrices in the case of analysis of neutral estrogens.[48] Using this approach, the concentration of estradiol and estriol in a sample of pregnant woman's urine was determined to be 0.16 and 0.83 μM.

In comparison of AuNPs and AgNPs, PtNPs are black and are able to effectively adsorbed laser beam all over the UV-vis region. Thus, PtNPs are a promising matrix in LDI-MS. Yonezawa *et al.* demonstrated that the determination of proteins, peptides, and phospholipids was successfully achieved using Pt nanoflowers as LDI matrices.[49] Because Pt nanoflowers have very high melting temperature, a few Pt clusters was found in the LDI mass spectrum. They also compared four kinds of metal NPs (i.e., Ag, Au, Cu, and Pt) for the determination of peptides by LDI-MS.[50] In terms of detection sensitivity, PtNPs are superior to other metal NPs.

12.3 Nanomaterials in TOF-SIMS

Another MS technique, SIMS, is a powerful method for surface characterization.[51] SIMS used monoatomic primary ions (Ga^+, Cs^+, Au^+) to shot at a sample's surface and then eject the analyte ions from the surface. Once the resulting secondary ions, with either positive or negative charges, are in flight, an electric field directs them into an MS analyzer. TOF instrument starts to dominate this field relative to quadrupole and magnetic-sector instruments. Compared to the other surface techniques such as X-ray photoelectron spectroscopy and angular electron spectroscopy, TOF-SIMS has several advantages, including ultra-high surface sensitivity (information depth is typically 10–15 Å), characteristic molecular fragmentation pattern, high scan rate, and superior spatial resolution. Without sample preparation, TOF-SIMS has been successfully used to record chemical image with submicrometer lateral resolution at the polymer surface.[52,53] However, low secondary ion yields still remain challenge in this research area. To overcome this problem, polyatomic primary ions, such as Au_n^+, Bi_n^+, SF_5^+, C_{60}^+, have been used to replace monoatomic ion beams because they are capable of enhancing detection sensitivity, reducing surface damage, and extending the detectable mass range.[54,55] For example, Schweikert *et al.* first reported that nanomaterials, aluminum monohydrate nanowhiskers, were bombarded with a suite of projectiles (Au^+, Au_3^+, Au_9^+, Au_{400}^{4+}) with kiloelectronvolt energies.[56] The yield of secondary ions is efficient when using a massive projectile like Au_{400}^{4+}. Additionally, the evaporation of a monolayer of noble metal such as Au and Ag onto sample surface, called metal-assisted SIMS, has been found to increase the secondary ion intensities.[57,58] This metallization procedure not only improves the quasi-molecular ion intensities, but also enhances metal-cationized molecules. Also, the lateral resolution of a SIMS was significantly improved by this metallization procedure.[59-61] For example, Piersma *et al.* used metal-assisted SIMS to directly analyze single neuroblastoma cells and rat brain tissue sections, thereby producing high-resolution images of different molecular distributions at cellular resolution.[60] Interestingly, the deposition of gold onto the surface of matrix-coated rat brain also can improve imaging quality and signal intensity in MALDI-MS. Based on the same concept, it is found that the deposition of metal NPs onto sample surface can enhance the yield of secondary ions in TOF-SIMS.[62–64] Without the requirement of metal evaporation, Winograd *et al.* demonstrated that the deposition of citrate-capped AuNPs or AgNPs onto the surface of the polymers can enhance the secondary ion emission and extend the mass range in TOF-SIMS.[62] The obtained signal intensities are comparable to those found using metal evaporation method. Kim *et al.* investigated the effect of the AuNPs and AgNPs on the secondary ion yields of triacontane upon atomic and polyatomic projectiles in SIMS.[63] The yield of secondary ions is strongly dependent on the specific projectile coupled with metal NPs. For instance, under atomic bombardment (Ga^+ and In^+), the characteristic ions increased with increasing the size of the AuNPs; however, with cluster projectiles such as C_{60}^+ and Bi_3^+, the deposition of AuNPs and AgNPs onto the sample surface led to a dramatic decrease in the characteristic ions.

On the other hand, TOF-SIMS can be applied to the determination of the analytes that have been immobilized on a self-assembled monolayer (SAM). The secondary ion yield of the analytes can be efficiently enhanced when the AuNPs were assembled on a SAM. Kim *et al.* reported that the secondary ion emission of peptides adsorbed onto the AuNPs/SAM was significantly increased when compared to that adsorbed onto the SAM.[65] In comparison of the analyte-to-matrix ratio (1: 10^3–10^6) in a matrix-enhanced SIMS, the ratio of analyte to AuNPs/SAM was revealed to be 18–19: 1. Because of this, it is suggested that the AuNPs would allow a more efficient secondary ions generation. Moreover, distinct imaging of peptides and their phosphopeptides adsorbed onto the AuNPs/SAM can be obtained using TOF-SIMS coupled with microfluidic systems. The same group extended this SIMS-based approach to determine the kinase activity and to screen inhibitors.[66]

Through the formation of Au-S bond, cysteine-terminated peptides were conjugated to citrate-capped AuNPs that have been adsorbed onto the 3-aminopropyl triethoxysilane-modified glass. After these peptides reacted with kinase, the resulting phosphopeptides can be easily detected by AuNP-enhanced SIMS approach, including spectrum and imaging. Quantitative assay of kinase activity and its inhibition can be determined by comparing the original unphosphorylated signal with the phosphorylated one within a single spectrum. A label-free, activity-based assay of matrix metalloproteinase and its inhibition can be determined using a similar strategy.[67] Peptide-conjugated AuNPs were electrostatically attached onto the nonbiofoluling poly(oligo(ethylene glycol) methacrylate) films. After these peptides were digested with matrix metalloproteinase, the cleaved peptides fragments were analyzed by AuNP-enhanced TOF-SIMS. The cleavage efficiency of the protease reaction can be estimated by the ratio of the peak intensity of uncleaved peptide to that of cleaved peptide. Figure 12.4 illustrates the entire procedure for the investigation of enzyme activity through AuNP-enhanced TOF-SIMS.

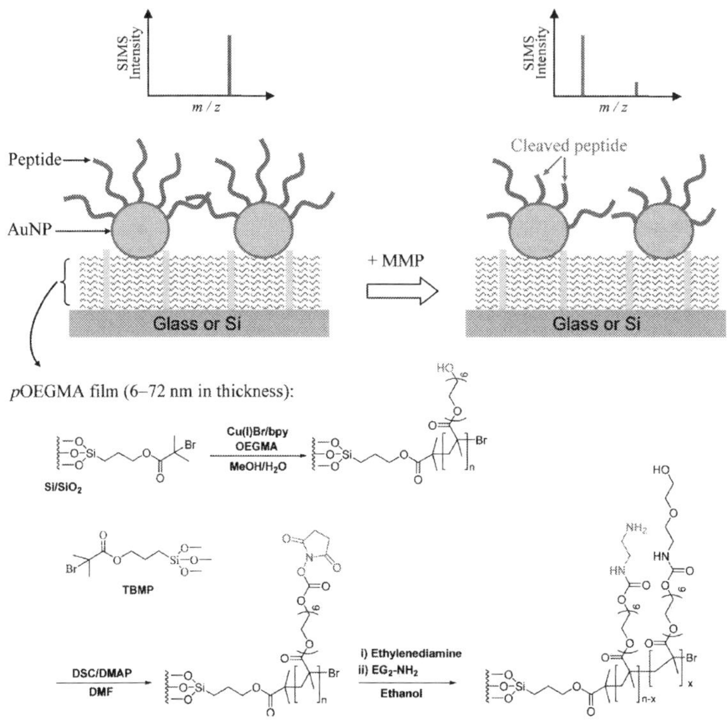

Figure 12.4 Procedure for synthesizing the *p*OEGMA films, and the general principle behind the analysis of matrix metalloproteinase activity using secondary ion mass spectrometry on surfaces containing peptide-conjugated gold nanoparticles. Reprinted with permission from Ref. 67. See also Color Insert.

12.4 Nanomaterials in ICP-MS

It is well known that ICP-MS is an outstanding method for the determination of inorganic element because of its extremely high sensitivity, large dynamic range, low matrix effect, and element specificity. In addition, ICP-MS is capable of simultaneously detecting multiple elements in a few minutes. Thus, by labeling NPs to the biological molecules, simultaneous detection of multiple analytes has been conducted using ICP-MS coupled with immunoassay. Zhang *et al.* reported a novel nonisotopic immunoassay by coupling sandwich-type immunoreaction to ICP-MS.[68] In their study, human immunoglobulin (IgG) immobilized on the solid phase captured rabbit anti-human IgG, which was detected using AuNP-labeled goat-anti-rabbit IgG. After extensive washes, AuNPs were dissociated from the immunocomplex with HNO_3 solution. The collected eluent was subsequently delivered to the ICP-MS for the measurement of elemental Au. An ICP-MS linked immunoassay protocol is illustrated in Fig. 12.5. Using a similar strategy, Baranov *et al.* described an immunoprecipitation method coupled with ICP-MS for the determination of human IgG.[69] The complexes between human IgG and its specific AuNP-modified antibody were precipitated upon the addition of protein A-immobilized sepharose beads. Merkocüi *et al.* utilized ICP-MS for the immunoassay of peptide-conjugated DNA that was immobilized onto nitrocellulose membrane.[70] This analyte was incubated with anti-peptide antibody and then detected by AuNP-modified secondary antibody. Compared to a conventional dot-blot reference method, this ICP-MS-based DNA assay provided a 40-fold improvement in the LOD for the oligonucleotide. Very recently, Zhang *et al.* developed a sandwich-type immunoassay coupled with ICP-MS for the detection of anti-erythropoietin antibody in serum sample.[71]

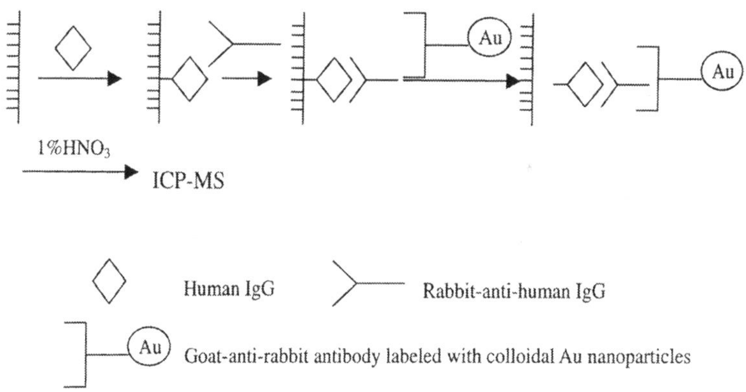

Figure 12.5 An ICP-MS-linked immunoassay protocol. Reprinted with permission from Ref. 68.

Through the combination of AuNP- and Eu^{3+}-labeled antibody with ICP-MS, simultaneous detection of multiple proteins has been introduced by Quinn *et al.*[72] It is demonstrated that this method can provide a linear response to both proteins in the concentration range of 2–100 ng/mL. Because ICP-MS-linked immunoassay cannot be used for microarray detection, Zhang *et al.* reported the detection of multiple proteins — α-fetoprotein IgG, carcinoembryonic antigen, and human IgG — on each spot of the immuno-microarray by laser ablation ICP-MS.[73] Based on sandwich-type immunoreaction, three proteins were detected using Sm^{3+}-labeled α-fetoprotein antibody, Eu^{3+}-labeled carcinoembryonic antibody, and AuNP-labeled goat-anti-human IgG as labeled antibodies; the LODs for α-fetoprotein IgG, carcinoembryonic antigen, and human IgG were 0.20, 0.14, and 0.012 ng/mL, respectively.

12.5 Conclusions

The use of noble metal NPs has been shown to be capable of (a) enhancing ionization efficiency in LDI-MS and SIMS, (b) suppressing background signal of low-mass region in LDI-MS, (c) improving detection reproducibility in LDI-MS, (d) selectively ionizing specific analytes in LDI-MS, and (e) extending the detectable mass range in SIMS. The detection sensitivity of target antigen can be greatly improved when using NP-tagged antibody as a secondary antibody and ICP-MS as a detection and quantification tool. In addition, before the analysis of LDI-MS, metal NPs can act as affinity probes for the extraction of target analytes. However, there are still several areas in which they can be improved. Metal NP-assisted LDI-MS and metal NP-enhanced SIMS are both typically limited to the detection of high molecular weight analytes. If the detectable mass range could be extended to 50,000 or 100,000 Da, these methods would be more suitable for proteomic analysis. In our opinion, the development of new nanomaterials with high energy transfer would be possible to achieve this goal. Moreover, when applying metal NP-assisted LDI-MS and metal NP-enhanced SIMS to the analysis of biological samples such as urine, tear, serum, and cerebrospinal fluids, the detection of target analytes commonly suffer from non-specific adsorption and complex matrix such as high salt and abundant proteins. To circumvent these problems, it is suggested that solid-phase extraction and liquid separation (i.e., liquid chromatography, capillary electrophoresis, etc.) may be required prior to MS analysis. Alternatively, conjugated NPs with high selectivity may be straightforward to simplify analysis procedure. For example, NPs decorated with poly(ethylene glycol) and antibody should provide high selectivity toward target antigen.

Acknowledgment

We thank National Science Council and National Sun Yat-Sen University–Kaohsiung Medical University Joint Research Center for the financial support of this work.

References

1. Z. Wang, and L. Ma, *Coordin. Chem. Rev.*, **253**, 1607 (2009).
2. E. Katz, and I. Willner, *Angew. Chem. Int. Ed.*, **48**, 6042 (2009).
3. D. H. Chace, *Chem. Rev.*, **101**, 445 (2001).
4. M. Karas, D. Bachmann, U. Bahr, and F. Hillenkamp, *Int. J. Mass Spectrom. Ion Proc.*, **78**, 53 (1987).
5. C. Pan, S. Xu, H. Zhou, Y. Fu, M. Ye, and H. Zou, *Anal. Bioanal. Chem.*, **387**, 193 (2007).
6. Z. Guo, Q. Zhang, H. Zou, B. Guo, and J. Ni, *Anal. Chem.*, **74**, 1637 (2002).
7. A. Tholey, and E. Heinzle, *Anal. Bioanal. Chem.*, **386**, 24 (2006).
8. E. Szájli, T. Fehér, and K. F. Medzihradszky, *Mol. Cell Proteomics*, **7**, 2410 (2008).
9. D. S. Peterson, *Mass Spectrom. Rev.*, **26**, 19 (2007).
10. J. Wei, J. M. Buriak, and G. Siuzdak, *Nature*, **399**, 243 (1999).
11. Y. S. Lin, and Y. C. Chen, *Anal. Chem.*, **74**, 5793 (2002).
12. M. Najam-ul-Haq, M. Rainer, Z. Szabó, R. Vallant, C. W. Huck, and G. K. Bonn, *J. Biochem. Biophy. Meth.*, **70**, 319 (2007).
13. E. P. Go, J. V. Apon, G. Luo, A. Saghatelian, R. H. Daniels, V. Sahi, R. Dubrow, B. F. Cravatt, A. Vertes, and G. Siuzdak, *Anal. Chem.*, **77**, 1641 (2005).
14. M. Mrksich, *ACS Nano*, **2**, 7 (2008).
15. T. Seino, H. Sato, A. Yamamoto, A. Nemoto, M. Torimura, and H. Tao, *Anal. Chem.*, **79**, 4827 (2007).
16. K. Tanaka, H. Waki, Y. Ido, S. Akita, Y. Yoshida, T. Yoshida, and T. Matsuo, *Rapid Commun. Mass Spectrom.*, **2**, 151 (1988).
17. J. Sunner, E. Dratz, and Y. C. Chen, *Anal. Chem.*, **67**, 4335 (1995).
18. H. Zhang, S. Cha, and E. S. Yeung, *Anal. Chem.*, **79**, 6575 (2007).
19. C. T. Chen, and Y. C. Chen, *Anal. Chem.*, **77**, 5912 (2005).
20. X. Wen, S. Dagan, and V. H. Wysocki, *Anal. Chem.*, **79**, 434 (2007).

21. J. A. McLean, K. A. Stumpo, and D. H. Russell, *J. Am. Chem. Soc.*, **127**, 5304 (2005).
22. H. P. Wu, C. J. Yu, C. Y. Lin, Y. H. Lin, and W. L. Tseng, *J. Am. Soc. Mass Spectrom.*, **127**, 875 (2009).
23. H. Kawasaki, T. Sugitani, T. Watanabe, T. Yonezawa, H. Moriwaki and R. Arakawa, *Anal. Chem.*, **80**, 7524 (2008).
24. E. T. Castellana, and D. H. Russell, *Nano Lett.*, **7**, 3023 (2007).
25. E. T. Castellana, S. D. Sherrod, and D. H. Russll, *J. Assoc. Lab. Autom.*, **7**, 3023 (2008).
26. J. Duan, M. J. Linman, C. Y. Chen, and Q. J. Cheng, *J. Am. Soc. Mass Spectrom.*, **20**, 1530 (2009).
27. C. L. Su, and W. L. Tseng, *Anal. Chem.*, **79**, 1626 (2007).
28. H. P. Wu, C. L. Su, H. C. Chang, and W. L. Tseng, *Anal. Chem.*, **79**, 6215 (2007).
29. N. Nagahori, and S. I. Nishimura, *Chem. Eur. J.*, **12**, 6478 (2006).
30. L. C. Chen, T. Ueda, M. Sagisaka, H. Hori, and K. Hiraoka, *J. Phys. Chem. C*, **111**, 2409 (2007).
31. L. C. Chen, J. Yonehama, T. Ueda, H. Hori, and K. Hiraoka, *J. Mass Spectrom.*, **42**, 346 (2007).
32. Y. F. Huang, and H. T. Chang, *Anal. Chem.*, **78**, 1485 (2006).
33. Y. F. Huang, and H. T. Chang, *Anal. Chem.*, **79**, 4852 (2007).
34. C. H. Teng, K. C. Ho, Y. S. Lin, and Y. C. Chen, *Anal. Chem.*, **76**, 4337 (2004).
35. P. R. Sudhir, H. F. Wu, and Z. C. Zhou, *Anal. Chem.*, **77**, 7380 (2005).
36. B. N. Y. Vanderpuije, G. Han, V. M. Rotello, and R. W. Vachet, *Anal. Chem.*, **78**, 5491 (2006).
37. Z. J. Zhu, P. S. Ghosh, O. R. Miranda, R. W. Vachet, and V. M. Rotello, *J. Am. Chem. Soc.*, **130**, 14139 (2008).
38. T. K. Ha, T. G. Lee, N. W. Song, D. W. Moon and S. Y. Han, *Anal. Chem.*, **80**, 8526 (2008).
39. K. A. Stumpo, and D. H. Russell, *J. Phys. Chem. C*, **113**, 1641 (2009).
40. J. L. Trevor, D. E. Mencer, K. R. Lykke, M. J. Pellin, and L. Hanley, *Anal. Chem.*, **69**, 4331 (1997).
41. H. J. Lin, and L. G. Chen, *J. Nanopart Res.*, **9**, 1133 (2007).
42. S. D. Sherrod, A. J. Diaz, W. K. Russell, P. S. Cremer and D. H. Russell, *Anal. Chem.* **80**, 6796 (2008).

43. K. Shrivas, and H. F. Wu, *Rapid Commun. Mass Spectrom.*, **22**, 2863 (2008).
44. C. Sluszny, E. S. Yeung, and B. J. Nikolau, *J. Am. Soc. Mass Spectrom.*, **16**, 107 (2005).
45. S. Cha, Z. Song, B. J. Nikolau, and E. S. Yeung, *Anal. Chem.*, **81**, 2991 (2009).
46. K. Shrivas, and H. F. Wu, *Anal. Chem.*, **80**, 2583 (2008).
47. P. R. Sudhir, K. Shrivas, Z. C. Zhou, and H. F. Wu, *Rapid Commun. Mass Spectrom.*, **22**, 3076 (2008).
48. T. C. Chiu, L. C. Chang, C. K. Chiang, and H. T. Chang, *J. Am. Soc. Mass Spectrom.*, **19**, 1343 (2008).
49. H. Kawasaki, T. Yonezawa, T. Watanabe, and R. Arakawa, *J. Phys. Chem. C*, **111**, 16278 (2007).
50. T. Yonezawa, H. Kawasaki, A. Tarui, T. Watanabe, R. Arakawa, T. Shimada, and F. Mafune, *Anal. Sci.*, **25**, 339 (2009).
51. N. Winograd, *Anal. Chem.*, **77**, 142A (2005).
52. A. M. Belu, Z. Yang, R. Aslami, and A. Chilkoti, *Anal. Chem.*, **73**, 143 (2001).
53. P. Sjövall, J. Lausmaa, and B. Johansson, *Anal. Chem.*, **76**, 4271 (2004).
54. D. G.. Castner, *Nature*, **422**, 129 (2003).
55. D. Weibel, S. Wong, N. Lockyer, P. Blenkinsopp, R. Hill, and J. C. Vickerman, *Anal. Chem.*, **75**, 1754 (2003).
56. V. Pinnick, S. Rajagopalachary, S. V. Verkhoturov, L. Kaledin, and E. A. Schweikert, *Anal. Chem.*, **80**, 9052 (2008).
57. A. Delcorte, N. Médard, and P. Bertrand, *Anal. Chem.*, **74**, 4955 (2002).
58. A. Delcorte, J. Bour, F. Aubriet, J. F. Muller, and P. Bertrand, *Anal. Chem.*, **75**, 6875 (2003).
59. H. Nygren, and P. Malmberg, *J. Microsc.*, **215**, 156 (2004).
60. A. F. M. Altelaar, I. Klinkert, K. Jalink, R. P. J. de Lange, R. A. H. Adan, R. M. A. Heeren, and S. R. Piersma, *Anal. Chem.*, **78**, 734 (2006).
61. A. Delcorte, and P. Bertrand, *Appl. Surf. Sci.*, **231–232**, 250 (2004).
62. A. Marcus, and N. Winograd, *Anal. Chem.*, **78**, 141 (2006).
63. Y. P. Kim, E. Oh, M. Y. Hong, D. Lee, M. K. Han, H. K. Shon, D. Won Moon, H. S. Kim, and T. G. Lee, *Anal. Chem.*, **78**, 1913 (2006).
64. N. Wehbe, A. Heile, H. F. Arlinghaus, P. Bertrand, and A. Delcorte, *Anal. Chem.*, **80**, 6235 (2008).

65. K. J. Wu, and R. W. Odom, *Anal. Chem.*, **68**, 873 (1996).
66. Y. P. Kim, E. Oh, Y. H. Oh, D. W. Moon, T. G. Lee, and H. S. Kim, *Angew. Chem. Int. Ed.*, **119**, 6940 (2007).
67. Y. P. Kim, B. S. Lee, E. Kim, I. S. Choi, D. W. Moon, T. G. Lee, and H. S. Kim, *Anal. Chem.*, **80**, 5094 (2008).
68. C. Zhang, Z. Zhang, B. Yu, J. Shi, and X. Zhang, *Anal. Chem.*, **74**, 96 (2002).
69. V. I. Baranov, Z. Quinn, D. R. Bandura, and S. D. Tanner, *Anal. Chem.*, **74**, 1629 (2002).
70. A. Merkoçi, M. Aldavert, G. Tarrasón, R. Eritja, and S. Alegret, *Anal. Chem.*, **77**, 6500 (2005).
71. Y. Lu, W. Wang, Z. Xing, S. Wang, P. Cao, S. Zhang, and X. Zhang, *Talanta*, **78**, 869 (2009).
72. Z. A. Quinn, V. I. Baranov, S. D. Tanner, and J. L. Wrana, *J. Anal. At. Spectrom.*, **17**, 892 (2002).
73. S. Hu, S. Zhang, Z. Hu, Z. Xing, and X. Zhang, *Anal. Chem.*, **79**, 923 (2007).

Index

AB (anti-biotin) 64–65, 92, 172
absorbance 79, 81, 83, 85, 89, 159, 260
acetone 105–6
adenosine 45–46, 51
adenosine triphosphate 48, 171, 275, 278
adhesion 107–8, 113
Ag (silver) 5–8, 42, 51, 65, 135, 140, 151, 160, 182, 191, 213–14, 223, 235, 254, 281–82
Ag nanomaterials 205–6
  anisotropic 33
Ag nanorods 33, 235
Ag NPs (silver nanoparticles) 4, 29, 31–37, 51–52, 64, 149–50, 157, 160, 174–76, 198, 235, 238, 254, 258–59, 273, 279–83
  anisotropic 52
alkanethiol–Au NPs 197
amino acids 33, 36, 166, 168
aminothiols 271–72, 274, 276, 279
analyte concentration 91, 162, 175
analyte mass transport 80, 91
analyte molecules 90, 145
analytes 30, 57–58, 78–79, 81, 85–87, 91–92, 145, 161–62, 169–70, 174–76, 230, 273–74, 277–79, 283, 285–86
  small 45, 48, 162–63, 171, 174
  various 51, 201
angiotensin I 274–75
anisotropic etching 120, 122, 124, 128
anti-biotin (AB) 64–65, 92, 172
antibodies 13, 16–18, 25, 30, 40, 59, 63–64, 70, 92, 141, 152, 161, 181, 265–66, 286
  secondary 69, 263, 286
apolipoprotein AI 169
apolipoprotein B 169
aptamer-conjugated Au NPs 171, 231
aptamers 40, 42–43, 48, 171, 203, 232
assays, small analyte 45, 48
Au (gold) 5–8, 20–23, 28–29, 31–33, 38, 88–89, 160, 181–84, 188, 190–92, 194–98, 201–2, 254, 274, 281–82
Au nanomaterials 205–6
  anisotropic 33
Au nanoparticles (Au NPs) 12–17, 20, 24, 144–46
Au nanorods 17, 20, 23–24, 33, 60, 63, 72, 173, 182
Au nanoclusters 181, 183–89, 191–92, 195, 200, 205
  fluorescent 186–87
  luminescent 184, 188, 191, 205
Au NP aggregates 38, 42, 49
Au NP probes 30, 49
Au NP solutions 162, 199
Au NP surfaces 34, 36, 47, 49–50, 162–63, 169, 172–73, 241
Au NPs (gold nanoparticles) 2–3, 5, 19, 30–34, 36, 38–40, 42–46, 48–51, 62, 68–69, 92, 95, 140–41, 148, 150–52, 157, 162–69, 172–76, 181–84, 186–88, 195–99, 228, 231, 235, 237, 240–41
  aggregation of 40, 43, 46, 49–50, 166, 168–69, 171
  anisotropic 33
  as-prepared 195–96
  bare 276, 278
  capped 166, 183
  conjugated 43, 47
  functionalization of 31, 36
  functionalized 45, 51, 171

large 184, 194–95
small 32, 38, 194
spherical 32, 174, 203, 233
stabilizing 34–35
Au shells 20–21

bovine serum albumin *see* BSA
BSA (bovine serum albumin) 17, 34, 168, 204, 234, 274–75
buffered oxide etch *see* BOE
bulk absorption coefficient 82–84

binding, biomolecular 60–62, 79, 81
bioassays 30–31, 34, 39, 159, 181, 188, 199–200, 206
bioconjugation 11, 14, 36, 51, 200, 259
bioconjugation of noble metal nanoparticles 11–18, 20, 24–26, 28
biodetection 1–2, 4, 6, 8, 10, 14
biofunctional Man-Au NPs 204–5
bioimaging 11, 14, 19, 21, 23–24, 250
biolabeling 11, 19, 21, 23–24
biomolecules 13–14, 16–18, 25, 35–36, 51, 59, 64, 67, 77, 145, 257–58, 266, 271–72, 275
conformation of 17–18
detection of 30–31
biosensing 12, 58, 65–66, 68, 146, 272
biosensor chips 103–4, 106, 108, 110, 112, 114, 116–20, 122, 124, 126, 128, 130–32, 134
fabrication of 103–4, 106, 108, 110, 112, 114, 116, 118, 120, 122, 124, 126, 128, 132, 134
biosensor research 78
biosensors 14, 56, 58, 69, 71, 80–81, 83, 85, 90, 109, 259
nanoparticle-based DNA 68
biotin 36, 40, 61–62, 65, 67–68, 91, 97, 171–72, 230–31
blazed gratings 120–21
BOE (buffered oxide etch) 127
BOE etching 127–28
bonding 118–19, 128, 162, 200
bonding techniques 118–19

calf intestine alkaline phosphatase *see* CIAP
captopril 162–63
cell imaging 24, 31, 157, 176, 181, 183, 206, 211, 230, 239, 242–43
cell surface receptors 262, 265–66
cells
cancer 2, 12, 20
live 12, 14
mammalian 262
normal 171
pathogen 257
single 261
chemical mechanical polishing *see* CMP
chemicals, bifunctional 35–36
chemometric analysis 257
CIAP (calf intestine alkaline phosphatase) 51
citrate 32, 34–35, 183, 277
classical electrostatic model 1, 5–6, 8
CMP (chemical mechanical polishing) 128
co-surfactant system 3
colorimetric assays 30–31, 45, 51, 140, 152, 176
colorimetric bioassay using noble metal nanoparticles 29–30, 32, 34, 36, 38, 40, 42, 44, 46, 48, 50, 52, 54, 56
computed tomography *see* CT
concanavalin A 40, 64, 164
coordination, metal–ligand 39–40
core metal galvanic exchange reactions 191–92
corrugated surfaces 223–25

CT (computed tomography) 14, 19
cysteine 162, 164, 277–78
cytochrome c 274–75

DDA (discrete dipole approximation) 254–55
dendrimers 183–84
detection
  label-free 70, 79, 257–58
  pathogen 205, 250, 257, 259
  real-time 77–78, 89, 96
  sensitive 271, 273, 276, 279
  visual 68, 175
detection limit *see* DL
detection sensitivity 175, 275–76, 279, 281, 286
dextran 36, 164–65
diffraction gratings 119–21, 123
  fabrication of 103, 119, 121, 123, 131
discrete dipole approximation *see* DDA
DL (detection limit) 49, 61–62, 64, 67, 71, 87, 90–93, 97, 140, 150–51, 163
DNA, detection of 30, 47, 171–72, 238–39, 242
DNA Analysis 230, 235
DNA-Au NP aggregation 44, 171
DNA-Au NPs 171, 176
DNA-conjugated Au NPs 42, 47
DNA molecules 47, 50, 241
DNAzymes 49, 150

elastomers 138–39
electrical double layer 142–43
electro-osmotic flow *see* EOF
electrodeposition 112, 114–15
electroforming 112, 114
electronic transitions 183, 194–95, 215, 219
electroplating 112, 114–15
electrostatic interactions 13, 17–18, 24, 47, 200, 238, 278, 281
electrostatic repulsion 32, 35, 50
ELISA (enzyme-linked immunosorbent assay) 58, 69, 78, 92–93
energy transfer efficiency 219–20
enzyme-linked immunosorbent assay *see* ELISA
EOF (electro-osmotic flow) 142
etching depth 127–28
evanescent absorption coefficient 82–83, 85
evanescent wave *see* EW
EW (evanescent wave) 81–82, 127
exposure, holographic 122–23

fiber optic particle plasmon resonance see FO-PPR
fiber optic sensors 84, 124–25
fibrinogen 70, 72, 94, 168–69
FITC (fluorescein isothiocyanate) 231
fluorescein isothiocyanate *see* FITC
fluorescence 4, 14, 23, 39, 100, 148–49, 161, 163–64, 184, 189, 202, 213–14, 225–27, 230–32, 237
fluorescence detection 136, 146, 171
fluorescence enhancement 211–12, 225, 227, 235, 238
fluorescence quenching 202, 204, 211–12, 214, 216, 218, 220–22, 224, 226–28, 230–32, 234, 236, 238, 240, 242
fluorescence spectroscopic detection in microfluidic devices 147, 149
fluorophores 24, 146, 148, 153, 211–19, 221, 225–27, 230, 233–35, 237, 242
  acceptor 146
  excited 148–49, 215
  interactions of 212–14

FO-PPR (fiber optic particle plasmon resonance) 79, 81, 91, 141, 143, 152
FO-PPR biosensor 80–81, 86–87, 92
FO-PPR sensor 85–86, 88–89, 91–94
Förster resonance energy transfer *see* FRET
FRET (Förster resonance energy transfer) 136, 146–48, 153, 218–21, 236, 240, 242
fused silica 127, 129–30

genetically modified organisms *see* GMO
glass 62, 70, 89, 104–5, 127, 137–38, 223, 231, 244
glass transition temperature 117, 119
glucose 164–66, 276–77
glutathione 162, 183, 188, 190, 277–78
glycerol 273, 276
GMO (genetically modified organisms) 68–69
gold 1–2, 4, 21, 37, 59, 64, 67, 69, 85, 93, 95–96, 135, 140, 168, 210
gold-capped nanoparticle layer substrates 65–66, 70
gold nanoparticles *see* Au NPs
gold nanorods 2–3, 14, 63, 71–72, 173
gold nanoshells 4, 64
gray-scale lithography 120–21

hexanethiolates 191–92
holographic gratings 122–23

imaging, cellular 257, 262
immunoassay, competitive fluorescence quenching 230
indium tin oxide *see* ITO
indocyanine green 234–35
injection molding 116, 118, 138–39
interactions
  biomolecular 58, 61, 89, 96–97, 140
  chemical 40, 81
  closed-shell 194
interface, metal–dielectric 223
interparticle 39–40, 52
ITO (indium tin oxide) 94

Kretschmann configuration 221–22

ligand exchange 187, 193, 238
ligand exchange reactions 187–88, 200
lithography 112, 115
  soft 103, 111, 113, 115, 117, 131
localized surface plasmon *see* LSP
localized surface plasmon resonance *see* LSPR
longitudinal plasmon wavelength *see* LPW
LPW (longitudinal plasmon wavelength) 71–72
LSP (localized surface plasmon) 12, 30, 37, 57, 60, 64, 79, 135, 162, 227–29, 249–50
LSPR (localized surface plasmon resonance) 12, 23, 30, 57, 60–61, 66, 72, 79, 135, 149, 151, 162, 227–28, 249–51, 254
LSPR absorptions 37
LSPR bands 38–39, 45, 162, 165
luminescence 23, 182–83, 189–92, 194, 197, 199, 204
luminescence intensity 183, 192, 198, 200, 205

luminescence of luminescent Au NPs 194
luminescence wavelengths 181, 189, 195–96
luminescent Au nanomaterials 206
luminescent Au NPs 181, 183–84, 194–95, 200, 203, 205–6
lysine 166–68

mass analyzers 136, 144
mass spectrometer 143–46
mass spectrometric bioanalysis 271–72, 274, 276, 278, 280, 282, 284, 286, 288, 290
mass spectrometry 98, 137, 144, 152, 187, 190, 202, 271–72, 284
materials
  photo-resistant 113
  plastic 117
matrix metalloproteinase 283–84
MBs (molecular beacons) 146, 236–37
metal coatings 115–16, 225
metal films 66, 226
metal ions 30, 32, 45, 115, 166, 181, 213, 241
metal nanomaterials 226–27
metal nanoparticles 4, 14
  rod-like 1, 4
metal nanorods 3, 5–7
metallic spheroids 217
metallization 282
micro-vortices 142–43
microarray-based LSPR biosensors 70–71
microfluidic channel 90, 94–96
microfluidic chips 69, 89, 96, 136–38, 140, 146
microfluidic devices 135, 137–39, 142–43, 147, 149, 151, 153
microfluidics for biosensor chips 135–36, 138, 140, 142, 144, 146, 148, 150, 152, 154
molecular beacons *see* MBs
multifunctional nanoparticles 262–63
myoglobin 204, 234

nanomaterials 12, 31, 37, 181–82, 235, 242, 272–73, 275, 277, 279, 281–86
nanoparticles 2, 5, 8–9, 11–17, 20, 23–24, 63–65, 67–68, 78–79, 89, 98, 135, 140–42, 146–49, 158
  functionalized 79, 140–41, 153
  metallic 14, 148
nanorod surfaces 17
nanorods 3–4, 14, 63, 71, 166, 254
nanoshells 3–4, 14, 21, 254
nanostructures 21, 60–61, 63–66, 72, 228, 255
nickel 19, 115–16
nitrogen 106, 113, 128
NLS (nuclear-localization signal) 200–1
noble metal nanomaterials 13–14, 16, 182, 273, 275
noble metal nanoparticles 1–8, 10–26, 28, 57, 77–78, 135–37, 146–48, 152, 157–58, 160, 162, 164, 166, 212, 249–50, 259, 265, 270–72, 286
  optical properties of 5, 7
noble metal nanoparticles for PPR detection 152
noble metals 2, 4, 59–60, 135, 139, 151, 182, 254, 256, 282
nuclear-localization signal *see* NLS

optical fiber 77, 79–81, 83–84, 86, 89, 93–94, 124–28, 130–31, 141, 143
optical fiber-based PPR biosensor 86–87, 89, 91
optical fiber windows 124–25, 127–29, 131

manufacture of 124–25, 127, 129
optical imaging 14, 23
optical mask 120–23
optical waveguide 77–80, 82, 84, 86, 88–90, 92, 94, 96, 98, 100, 102, 124–25, 141
organic contaminants 105–6

particle plasmon resonance *see* PPR
particle plasmon resonance detection 139, 141
particles, dimer 255
passivation molecules 258, 263
pathogens 69, 257, 261
PDGFs (platelet-derived growth factor) 39–40, 42–43, 168, 171, 203–4, 231–33, 263
PEG-hybrid gold nanoparticles 19
peptides 16–19, 36, 40, 51, 146, 271–73, 275–81, 283
photolithography 103–5, 107, 131
photoluminescence of gold nanoparticles 181–82, 184, 188, 190, 192, 194, 200, 204, 206, 208, 210
photomasks 108–9
photoresist 104–5, 107–11, 120, 122
  patterned 111
photoresist sensitivity 110
PKA (protein kinase A) 51
planar waveguide 77, 93–95
planar waveguide-based PPR biosensor 93, 95
plasmon absorption 185, 195
plastic chips 119, 138
platelet-derived growth factor *see* PDGFs
platelet-derived growth factors 39, 168, 171, 231
polarizability 7, 159–60
polarization 142, 223, 228–29, 253, 255
poly(vinylpyrollidone) 32–34
polyelectrolytes 21, 34, 36, 52
polymers 32, 34, 107, 112, 130, 177, 184, 187, 206, 282
  light-sensitive 107
PPR (particle plasmon resonance) 77, 79, 135, 137, 140, 143
PPR biosensors 87, 96, 98
PPR spectroscopy 87, 89, 137
propagating surface plasmon resonance *see* PSPR
protein assays 40, 42, 48
protein immunoassays 230
protein kinase A *see* PKA
proteins 16–18, 29–30, 34–36, 40, 42–43, 48, 51, 136, 168–69, 171, 211–13, 261–62, 271–73, 281, 285–86
  analysis of 203, 230, 232
PSPR (propagating surface plasmon resonance) 60

QDs (quantum dots) 14, 24, 185, 206
quantum dots *see* QDs
quencher 215, 218, 237
quenching efficiency 220–21
quenching interactions 214–15

Raman intensity 252, 258, 260–61, 264
Raman reporter molecules 259–60, 263, 265
Rayleigh scattering 151, 158
RB (rhodamine B) 240
RCA clean 106
receptor-analyte pairs 91–92
receptors, immobilized 87, 91–93
recognition molecules 40, 169, 171, 200, 230
refractive index resolution *see* RIR
refractive index sensitivity *see* RIS
reporter molecules 259, 261, 265
resonance light scattering *see* RLS
rhodamine B *see* RB

RIR (refractive index resolution) 86, 88–89, 93, 95, 97
RIS (refractive index sensitivity) 62–64, 94
RLS (resonance light scattering) 157–60, 162, 164, 166–74, 176, 178, 180
RLS approach 162, 164, 166, 168–70, 172, 175
RLS intensity 158, 162–63, 165, 169, 174
RLS peaks 166, 169
RLS techniques 157–59, 161, 163–64, 166, 169, 171, 176
roughness 115–16, 130, 212, 225

salt 48–50, 238
SAM (self-assembled monolayer) 42, 62–63, 146, 148, 150, 271, 283
scattering 4, 7–8, 14, 23, 46, 61, 126, 149, 151–52, 158–60, 162, 164, 224
scattering spectra 1–2, 4–8
SEB (staphylococcal enterotoxin B) 92–93
secondary ions 281–83
SEF (surface enhanced fluorescence) 212–14, 221, 225–26, 235, 238, 242
self-assembled monolayer *see* SAM
sensing systems 48, 213–14, 231
sensitivity 13–14, 30, 43–46, 57, 61, 63, 65–67, 69, 72, 77, 79–81, 87–89, 93–95, 97–98, 173–74
sensors 42, 57, 62, 68, 80–81, 84, 87, 91–94, 101, 125, 131, 134, 153–54, 231, 240
SERS (surface-enhanced Raman scattering) 12, 14, 23, 98, 137, 150–51, 153, 227, 249–60, 262–66, 268, 270
SERS-active nanoparticle assemblies 259, 261
SERS detections, labeled 259
SERS enhancement factor 252–53, 255
SERS-labeled detection 258–59
SERS probes 258, 262–63
SET (surface energy transfer) 17, 219–20
silver nanoparticles *see* Ag NPs
slide-based LSPR biosensors 61, 63, 65, 67, 69
small molecules, analysis of 48, 275
SPCE (surface plasmon-coupled emission) 136, 148–49, 153
spherical Ag NPs 39, 174, 235
SPP (surface plasmon polariton) 60, 66, 221–23, 225, 227, 229
SPR (surface plasmon resonance) 3, 12, 59, 78–79, 139, 212, 227, 253, 264
SPR absorption band 30, 38
SPR sensors 78–80, 87–88, 92
stainless steel 112–13
staphylococcal enterotoxin B *see* SEB
Staphylococcus aureus 258, 260–61
steric stabilization 34–35
streptavidin 36, 40, 61, 64, 68, 87, 91, 93, 97
substrate, polymeric 138
surface energy transfer *see* SET
surface enhanced fluorescence *see* SEF
surface-enhanced Raman scattering *see* SERS
surface plasmon-coupled emission *see* SPCE
surface plasmon polariton *see* SPP
surface plasmon resonance *see* SPR
synthesis of gold nanoparticles 3

TEM (transmission electron microscopy) 45–46, 192, 231, 260

thermal lens detections 136–37
thermoplastics 117–18, 138
thiamazole 162–63
thin film 4, 59, 94, 140, 222–23
thiolates 183, 188, 191, 193, 195, 197
thrombin 43, 48–49
TIR (total internal reflections) 79–80
total internal reflections *see* TIR
TPF (two-photon fluorescence) 24
TPW (transverse plasmon wavelength) 71
transition dipoles 146–47, 227
transitions, interband 188–89, 195
transmission electron microscopy *see* TEM
transverse plasmon wavelength *see* TPW
tubular waveguide 77, 96–97
tubular waveguide-based PPR biosensor 96–97
two-photon fluorescence *see* TPF

wavelength shift response 87
wet chemical approaches 3, 32
wetting agents 115–16

Color Insert

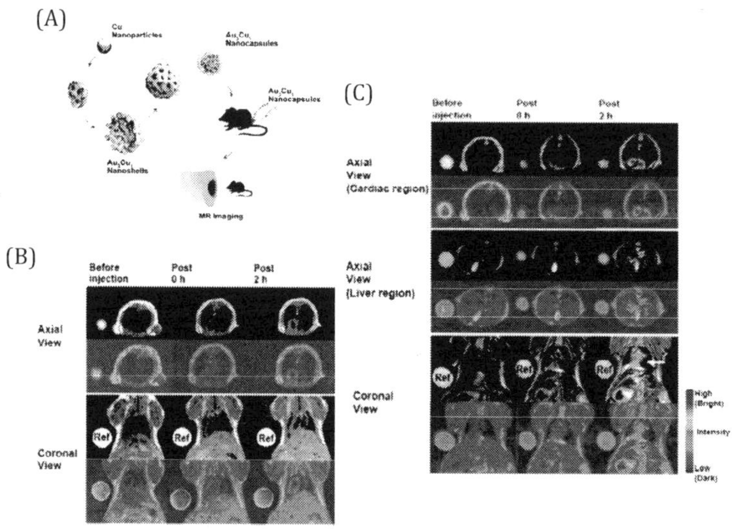

Figure 2.5

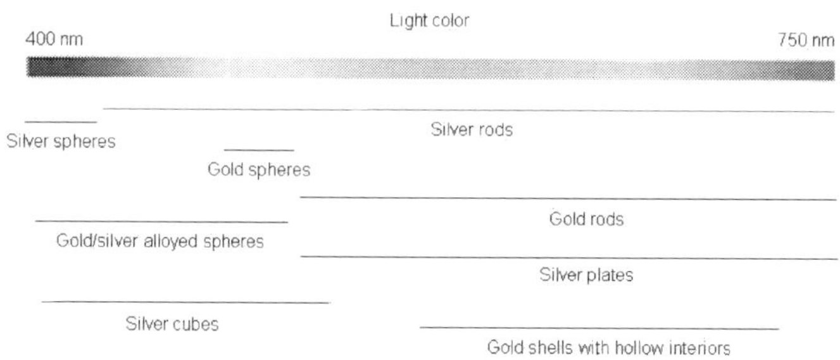

Figure 3.3

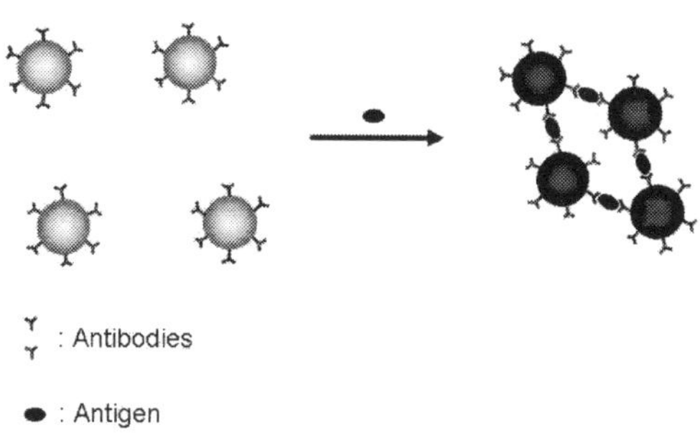

Figure 3.4

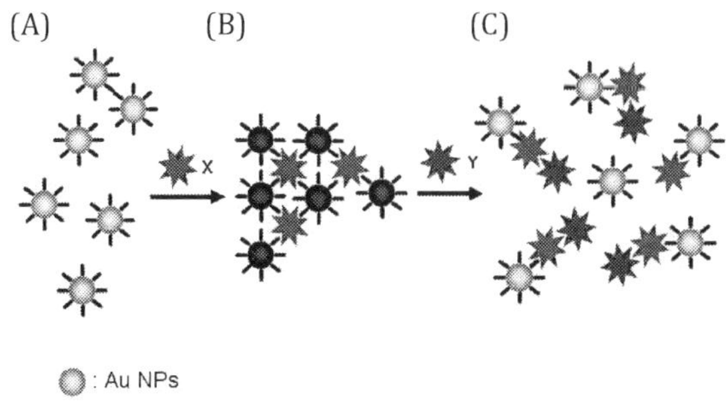

Figure 3.5

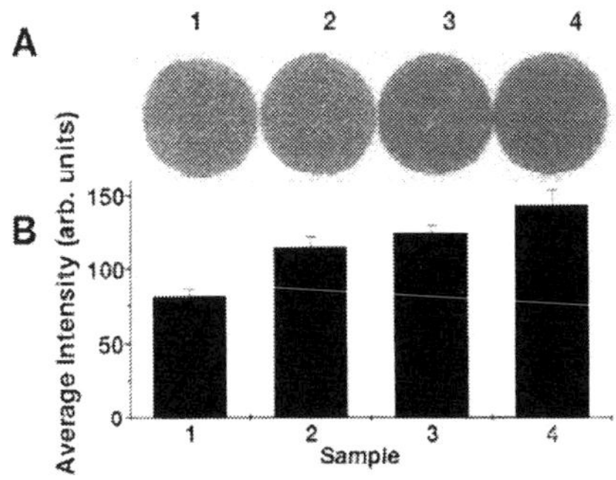

Figure 4.10

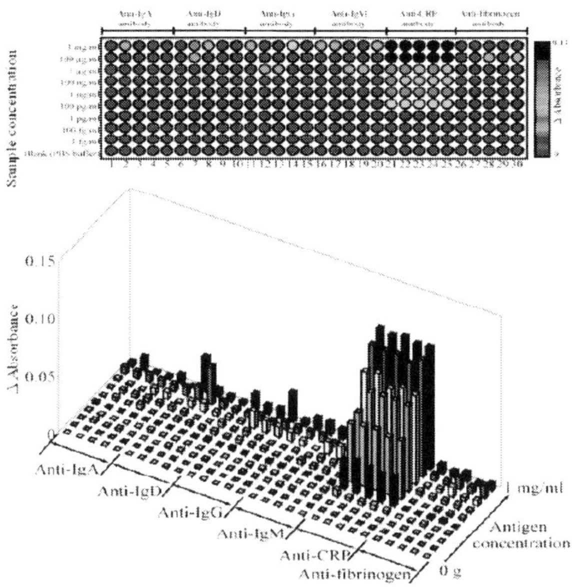

Figure 4.11

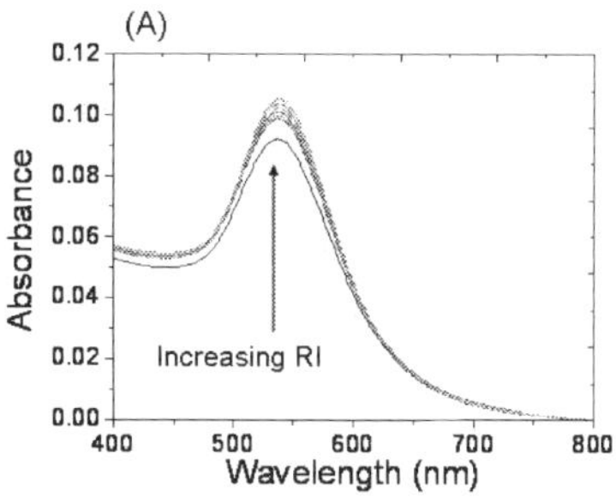

Figure 5.3

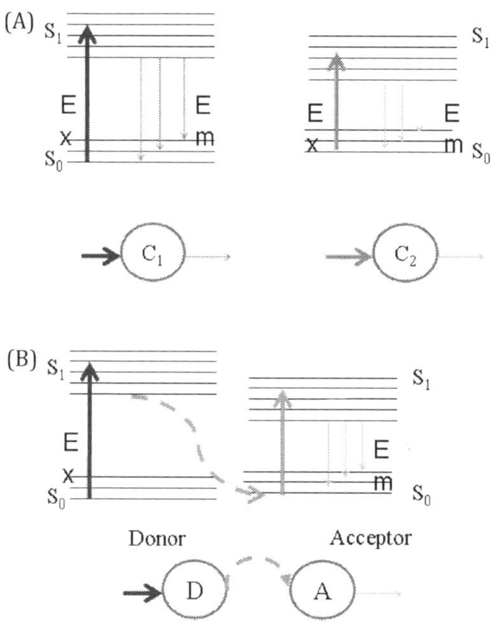

Figure 7.2

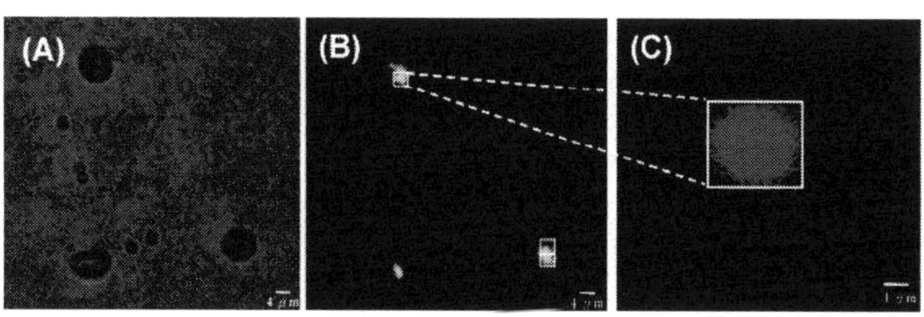

Figure 8.2

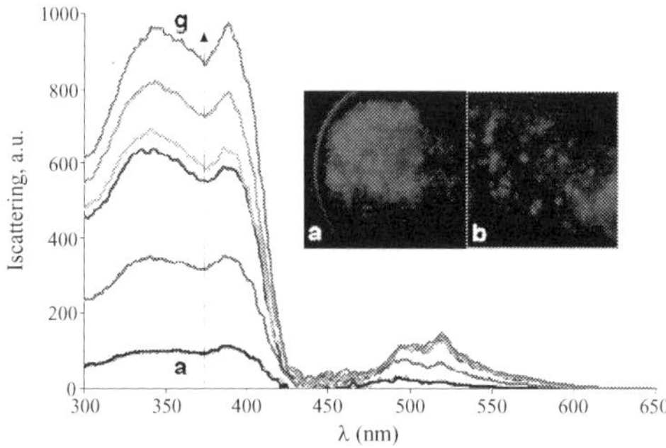

Figure 8.7

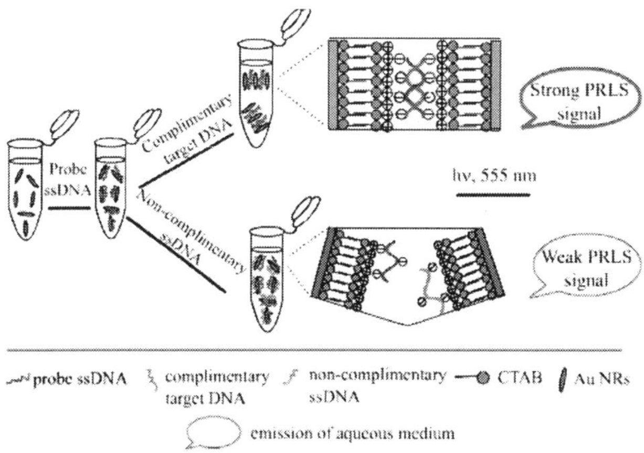

Figure 8.11

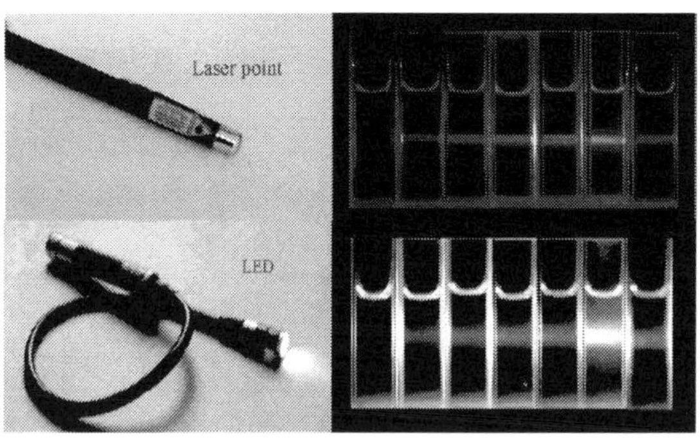

Figure 8.12

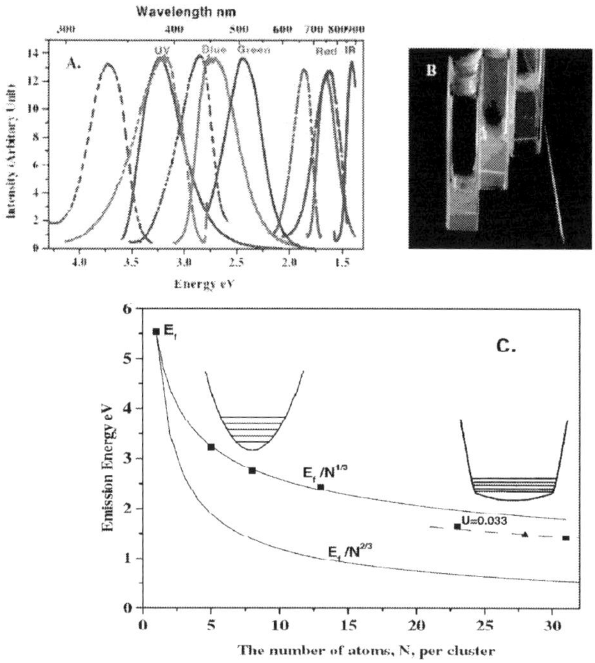

Figure 9.1

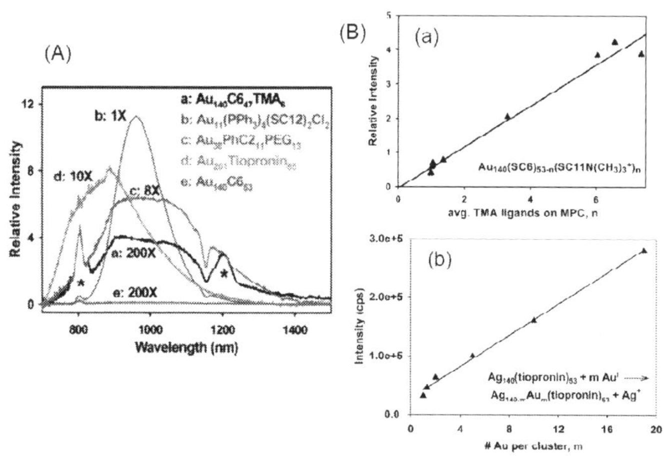

Figure 9.3

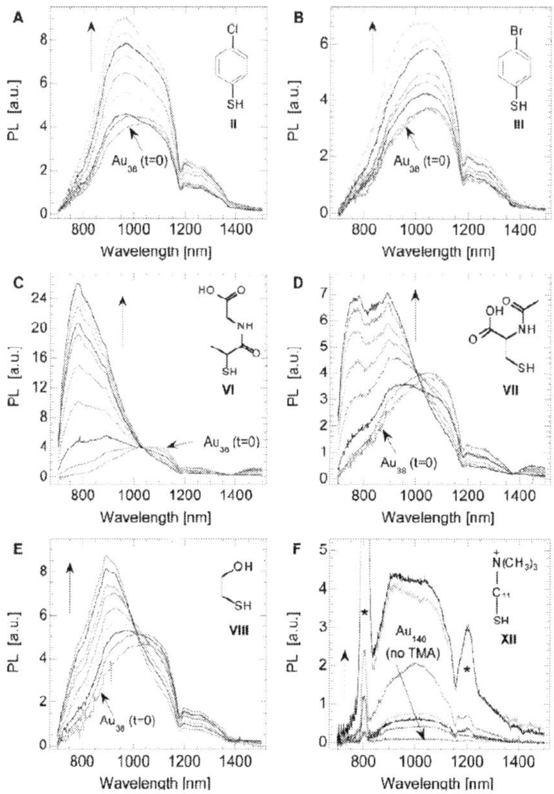

Figure 9.4

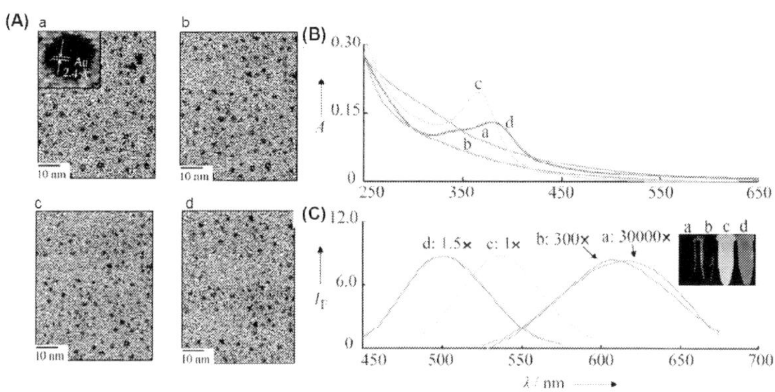

Figure 9.5

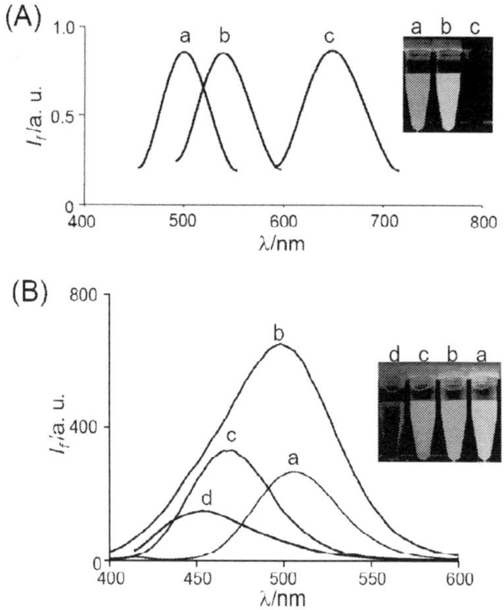

Figure 9.6

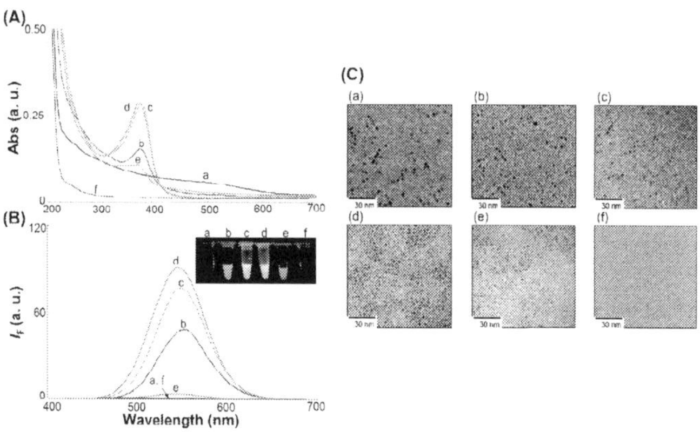

Figure 9.7

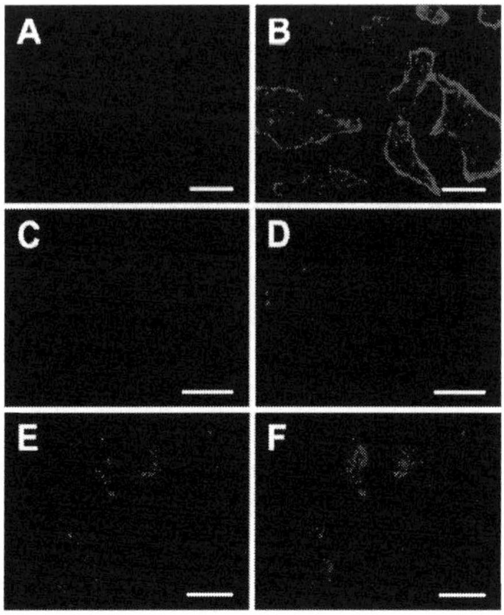

Figure 9.8

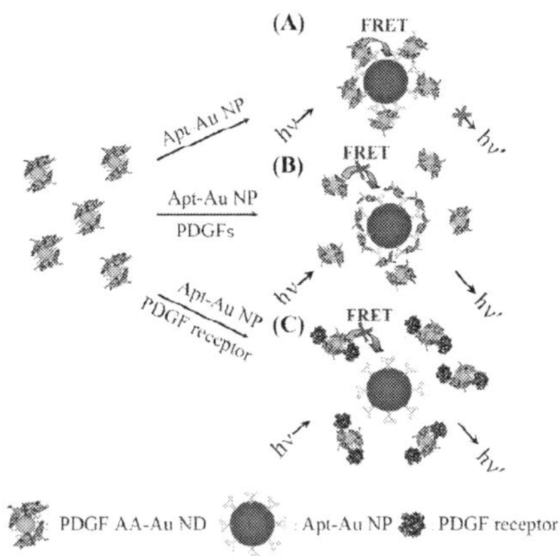

Figure 9.10

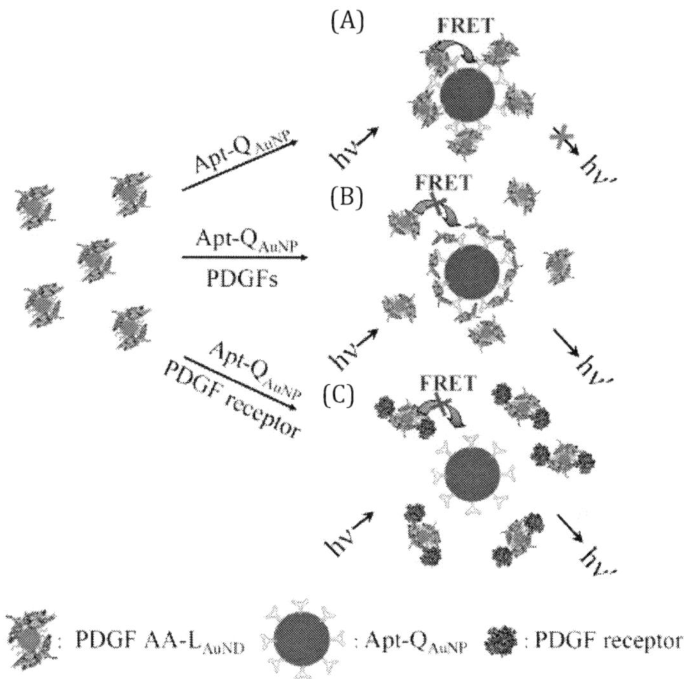

[a] h, Planck's constant; ν, frequency of light.

Figure 10.8

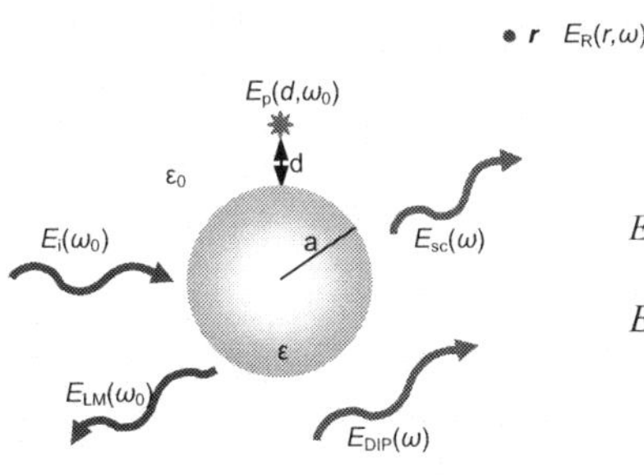

$$E_p(d,\omega_0) = E_i(d,\omega_0) + E_{LM}(d,\omega_0)$$

$$E_R(r,\omega) = E_{DIP}(r,\omega) + E_{sc}(r,\omega)$$

Figure 11.1

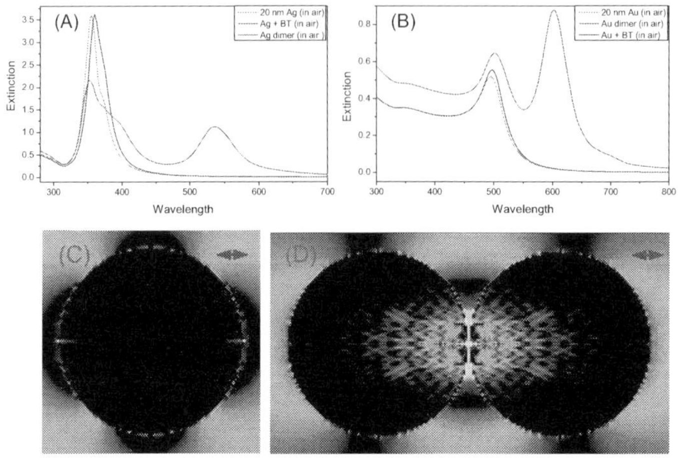

Figure 11.2

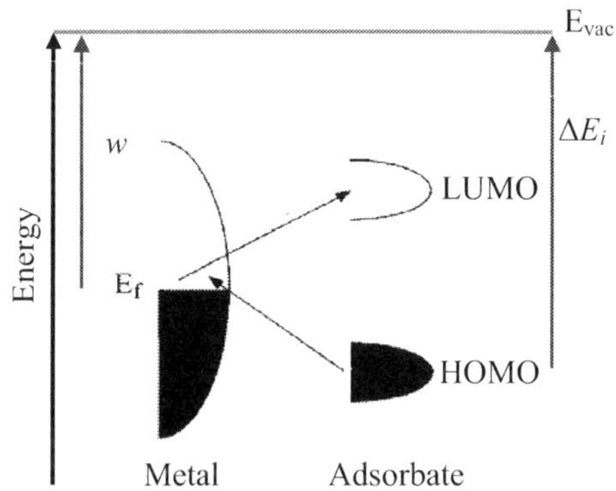

Figure 11.3

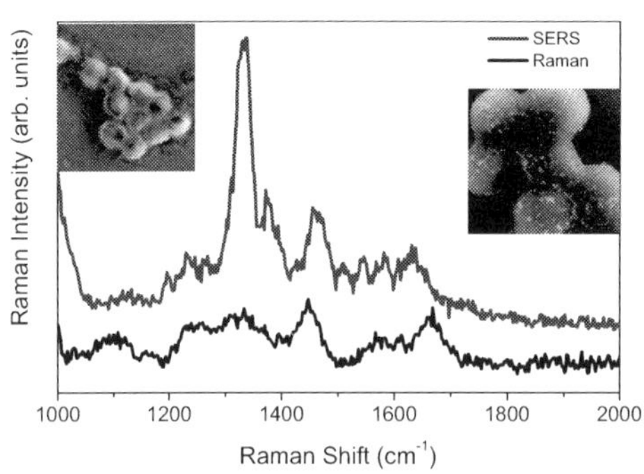

Figure 11.4

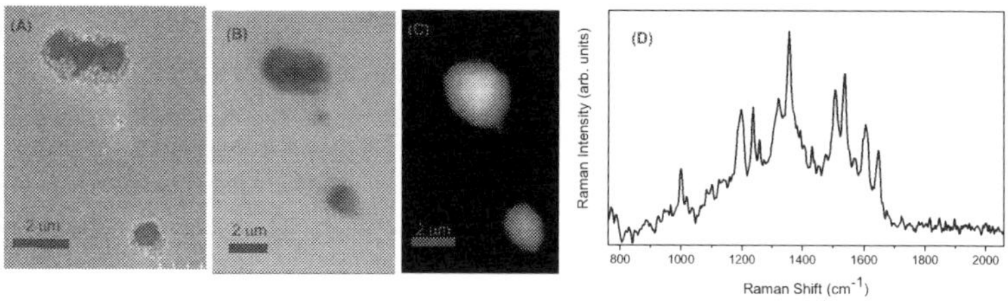

Figure 11.7

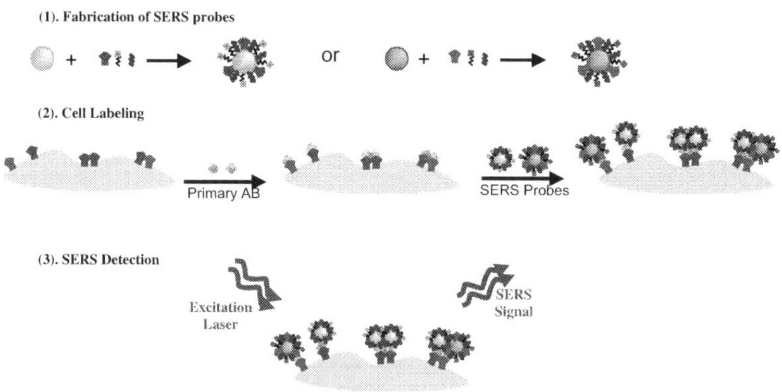

Figure 11.8

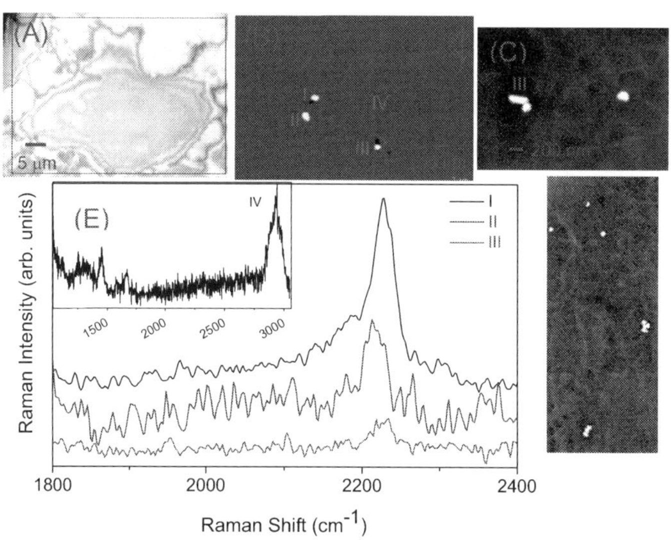

Figure 11.9

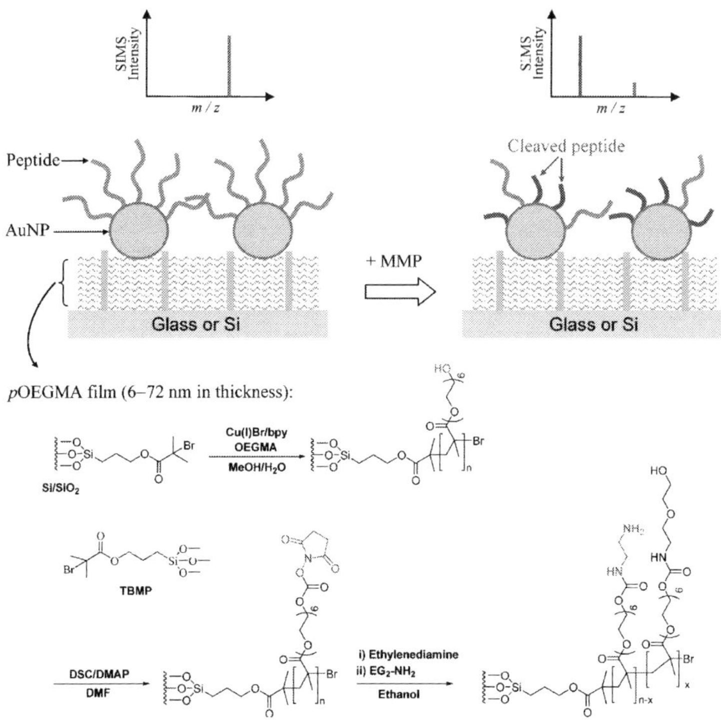
SIMS Intensity
m / z
SIMS Intensity
m / z
Peptide
AuNP
Cleaved peptide
+ MMP
Glass or Si
Glass or Si
pOEGMA film (6–72 nm in thickness):
Cu(I)Br/bpy
OEGMA
MeOH/H2O
Si/SiO2
TBMP
DSC/DMAP
DMF
i) Ethylenediamine
ii) EG2-NH2
Ethanol

Figure 12.4

Made in the USA
Las Vegas, NV
22 September 2026

b37c9d37-e5f9-4c21-bbce-471b0b83898bR02